VOIDING FUNCTION AND DYSFUNCTION
A Logical and Practical Approach

VOIDING FUNCTION AND DYSFUNCTION: A Logical and Practical Approach

Alan J. Wein, M.D.
Professor and Chairman
Division of Urology
University of Pennsylvania School of Medicine
Chief of Urology
Hospital of the University of Pennsylvania
Philadelphia, Pennsylvania

David M. Barrett, M.D.
Professor of Urology
Mayo Medical School and Mayo Foundation
Rochester, Minnesota

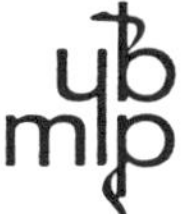

YEAR BOOK MEDICAL PUBLISHERS, INC.
CHICAGO • LONDON • BOCA RATON

1 2 3 4 5 6 7 8 9 0 CK 92 91 90 89 88

Library of Congress Cataloging-in-Publication Data

Wein, Alan J.

Voiding function and dysfunction.

Includes bibliographies and index.

1. Urination disorders. 2. Urination. I. Barrett, David M. II. Title. [DNLM:
1. Urinary Tract—physiology. 2. Urination Disorders. WJ 146 W423v]

RC901.75.W45 1988 616.6 87-24267

ISBN 0-8151-9221-5

Sponsoring Editor: David K. Marshall

Associate Managing Editor, Manuscript Services: Deborah Thorp

Production Project Manager: Max Perez

Proofroom Supervisor: Shirley E. Taylor

Preface

This work began as a textbook section only on the subject of the neurogenic bladder. Our original idea was to provide a readable, organized, and internally consistent chapter that was basic enough to facilitate an understanding of why micturition "works" (or does not) and practical enough to serve as a guide for evaluation and treatment of clinical problems. Having been privileged to be associated with a number of educational activities on the subject, and having watched some formats "bomb" and others "bloom," we borrowed liberally from the ideas of our friends and colleagues to arrive at a sequence of presentations that seem to "work." Once established, the temptation to expand this to cover most other types of voiding dysfunction was too great to resist. This book will hopefully provide easily accessible and useful information to urologists, gynecologists, neurologists, geriatricians, and other physicians and health care professionals in practice or in training who are interested in the relevant basics of voiding function and in an overall and specific evaluation and management of voiding dysfunctions. It is not meant to be an encyclopedic and lengthy compendium of contributions by respected experts, but rather an internally consistent and fairly logical and practical approach that will enable those in practice and training to understand pathophysiology, evaluation, treatment, and the basic science and clinical literature relevant to these areas. Special thanks are due to Drs. Robert Levin, Benad Goldwasser, and Jeffrey Woodside for their assistance, and to Drs. Jay Gillenwater, John Grayhack, Stuart Howards, John Duckett, and Mr. Dan Doody for their gentle reminders to finish and for their suggestion that this section of their textbook, *Adult and Pediatric Urology,* be published in a more readily available format as well.

ALAN J. WEIN, M.D.
DAVID M. BARRETT, M.D.

Contents

SECTION I

Voiding Function: Relevant Anatomy, Physiology, and Pharmacology

With the Assistance of Robert M. Levin, Ph.D.

Overview

Despite the fact that there have been an extraordinary number of good recent reviews on the subject (Tanagho, 1978; Wein and Raezer, 1979; Gosling, 1979; Andersson and Sjogren, 1982; Bradley and Sundin, 1982; Bhatia and Bradley, 1983; McGuire, 1983, 1984a; DeGroat and Booth, 1984; Mundy, 1984a), it is obvious that the anatomy, physiology, and pharmacology of the central neural and peripheral neural and muscular structures controlling micturition have not been completely elucidated. These reviews have been written from various orientations—those of anatomist, neurophysiologist, pharmacologist, and, sometimes, clinician. However, there exists in and between many of these reviews imprecise and noncomparable terminology; major conflicts regarding fundamental concepts; and very basic disagreements on fundamental facts of anatomy, physiology, and pharmacology, either by virtue of different findings and their citation, or simply by different interpretations of fundamental data. In this chapter, we hope to at least summarize many currently accepted views on the structure and function of the lower urinary tract. In many instances we will hopefully be able to present tenable hypotheses that link clinical observations to anatomic, physiologic, and pharmacologic facts.

At the outset, it might be well to briefly summarize exactly what we are trying to explain. The lower urinary tract functions as a group of interrelated structures whose joint function is to bring about efficient bladder filling and urine storage and its voluntary expulsion. During normal filling there is a very slow rise in bladder pressure, despite a large increase in volume. There is a gradual increase in proximal urethral resistance, and there is no involuntary bladder contractile activity.

Increases in intra-abdominal pressure do not cause urine leakage. At a certain intravesical pressure, the sensation of bladder distention is perceived and micturition is initiated voluntarily, proceeding to completion and involving a decrease in bladder outlet resistance and contraction of the bladder smooth musculature, with some reshaping of the proximal urethra. To explain these relatively simple-sounding phenomena, an impressive literature has been generated. It will be our goal to summarize and synthesize this literature into consistent working hypotheses. It will become readily apparent that no one prior author's viewpoint will be constantly supported. This is simply because scientists are not consistent, and no two groups of people agree about everything. We have tried to find viewpoints expressed by persons whom we respect that agree with our own particular concepts, but it will be obvious that although we may agree with and endorse one author's viewpoint in one area, this may not be the case in another area.

No matter what type of organization one uses for this subject, it is impossible to list all data in an order that seems entirely logical on first reading. We therefore suggest an initial more rapid review of this material followed by an in-depth reading. Figures are used, especially in the anatomy section, to illustrate particularly relevant points, but we have tried to avoid graphic illustration of mere laboratory data. In some cases inclusive review articles, rather than original ones, are cited; we apologize to those whose "classic" references may have been omitted.

To provide the reader with a basis for criticizing our conclusions, as well as those of others, it is well to keep in mind at the outset the following observations:

1. The bewildering array of experimental models must be carefully considered. A small change in one experimental model may make results totally noncomparable to those obtained in another.
2. Great differences may exist between species; results in certain animal models do not necessarily imply exact similarity to humans.
3. Results obtained in one type of tissue may not equal those obtained in another, even if the tissues are from the same species, seem similar, and are adjacent anatomically.
4. Significant changes in anatomy, physiology, and pharmacology may be secondary to alterations induced by or related to sex, age, hormonal status, infection, denervation or decentralization, stretch, and the effects of certain drugs, including laboratory and clinical anesthetics.

5. In vitro experimental results are not necessarily the same as in vivo experimental results, and neither of these are necessarily equivalent to "normal."
6. Anatomy (structure) does not necessarily imply function or physiology, and vice versa.
7. Receptors do not necessarily imply innervation or function.
8. The effect produced by an agonist or antagonist does not necessarily impart physiologic significance to a particular neurotransmitter, or, by inference, physiologic significance to a component of the nervous system that secretes that neurotransmitter.
9. Pressure or tension generation by a whole organ model or muscle strip is not necessarily the same as contractility, and neither of these is necessarily translatable into bladder-emptying ability. The same caveat applies to assumptions made about outlet resistance.
10. The altered physiology of an abnormal clinical state can usually be explained according to at least a part of one theory of micturition. However, this does not necessarily mean that that theory is entirely correct.
11. Authors, ourselves included, tend to be somewhat selective in their citation of references. Generally, references that support a particular viewpoint are cited more frequently, more conspicuously, and more favorably than those that do not.

Relevant Anatomy

THE BLADDER

The urinary bladder wall consists of three layers: (1) an outer adventitium composed primarily of connective tissue; (2) a smooth muscle layer; and (3) an inner mucous membrane that totally lines the interior. Although the mucosa has recently been demonstrated to contain irregularly arranged smooth muscle bundles (Dixon and Gosling, 1983), their function is uncertain, and they will not be considered further. The main smooth muscle layer of the bladder is classically divided into detrusor and trigone. Anatomically, the trigonal area is defined as that region of the posterior bladder wall between the ureteral orifices and the vesicourethral junction. This area is best divided into a superficial and a deep trigone. The deep trigone is actually continuous with, and an integral part of, the detrusor smooth muscle (El Badawi, 1982; Tanagho, 1982; Gosling and Chilton, 1984). Tanagho and Pugh (1963) seem to have been among the first to recognize the subdivision of the trigonal area, and originally described three separate layers. The superficial layer of the trigonal musculature is wholly ureteral in origin and, as such, is mesodermal in origin, while the origin of the remainder of the bladder is endodermal (Tanagho and Pugh, 1963; Woodburne, 1967). In his most recent description, Tanagho (1982) still considered the actual trigone to be divided into superficial and deep layers, both of ureteral origin (the former from the longitudinal musculature of the intravesical ureter and the latter from Waldeyer's sheath), with a separate layer of detrusor muscle below this.

The detrusor can best be described as a mesh of smooth muscle bundles that are, to a greater (Donker et al., 1982) or lesser extent (Bro-Rasmussen et al., 1965; Woodburne, 1968; Hald and Bradley, 1982; Gosling and Chilton, 1984) loosely organized in the area of the bladder base into an outer longitudinal, a middle circular, and an inner longitudinal layer. There is significant disagreement (see below) regarding the continuity of a smooth muscle layer of the bladder (including the trigone) into the urethra.

The terms "bladder body" and "bladder base" refer to a functional rather than anatomic division of the bladder smooth muscle, which is based on distinct differences in neuromorphology and neuropharmacology between the smooth muscle lying circumferentially above and below the level of the ureterovesical junction. This concept was first introduced by El Badawi and Schenk (1966), and subsequently confirmed by them and others (El Badawi and Schenk, 1968; Raezer et al., 1973; El Badawi, 1982).

THE URETHRA

Female Urethra

The adult female urethra is approximately 4 cm in length and 6 mm in diameter. It extends from the vesicourethral junction behind the symphysis pubis and is embedded in the anterior wall of the vagina. The wall of the female urethra comprises an outer muscular layer and inner epithelium, which is generally thrown into longitudinal folds and apposed to itself except during the act of voiding. The smooth muscle portion of the female urethra extends throughout its length. There is general agreement on the existence of an inner longitudinal layer (Tanagho, 1978; Gosling and Chilton, 1984), but disagreement over the extent of an outer circular or semicircular layer. Tanagho (1978) feels that the outer semicircular coat is substantial and a direct continuation of the detrusor outer longitudinal layer, but Gosling and Chilton (1984) describe only a few circularly arranged muscle fibers in the outer aspect of the smooth muscle layer. This distinction is important when considering whether or not an active urethra smooth muscle sphincteric mechanism is involved in maintaining continence. Urethral smooth muscle is embedded in a matrix of collagen, and actually collagen seems to be the major structural component of the human female urethra (Hickey et al., 1982). These collagen fibers have an orientation similar to the smooth muscle fibers.

Male Urethra

The anterior urethra (distal to the membranous portion) in the male seems to function purely as a conduit and has no role in either maintaining continence or in facilitating micturition. Gosling and Chilton (1984) described the preprostatic urethra as approximately 1–1.5 cm in length and containing smooth muscle bundles oriented as a distinct circular collar and becoming continuous distally with the prostatic capsule. These muscle bundles are separated by much connective tissue containing elastin and collagen. The prostatic urethra is approximately 3–4 cm in length. Tanagho (1986) seemed to imply that the entire male posterior urethra contains a representation of an inner longitudinal smooth muscle layer and an outer circular layer, least developed in the midline dorsally. He noted that the urethral musculature in this area is very compact and contains abundant collagen and elastic fibers. This type of arrangement also seems to be implied by Donker et al. (1982), i.e., the existence to some extent of both longitudinally and circularly oriented smooth muscle bundles in the male preprostatic and prostatic urethra. The membranous portion of the male posterior urethra extends for a distance of at least 2.5 cm distal to the prostate, to the bulb of the penis. The presence of a smooth muscular element in the wall of the membranous urethra has been described by Donker et al. (1982) and by Tanagho (1986), and it would seem from their descriptions that some such longitudinal and some circular fibers are present. Gosling (1984, 1985) describes a relatively small smooth muscle component in this area, but one which consists of outer circular and inner longitudinal components. Proximally this smooth muscle is in continuity with the fibromuscular trabeculae of the prostatic apex and distally is continuous into the bulbous part of the urethra.

Anatomic Continuity Between Bladder and Urethra

Whether bladder smooth muscle bundles are continuous into the urethra is a matter of dispute. The concept of the continuation of the inner longitudinal layer of bladder smooth muscle directly into the urethra is endorsed by Woodburne (1967, 1968), Lapides (1958, 1970), Lapides et al. (1960), Tanagho and Smith (1966, 1968), Bradley and Sundin (1982), and El Badawi (1982, 1983). Tanagho and Smith (1968) described continuation of the superficial trigonal layer into the dorsal urethral wall up to the verumontanum in the male and into the proximal two-thirds of the female urethra. Donker et al. (1982) confirm this finding relative to the superficial layer of the trigone, an idea also attributed to Hutch (1967) and to Hutch and Rambo (1967). Such an anatomical arrangement is obviously consistent with the hypothesis that opening of the bladder neck and proximal urethra during active bladder contraction is based at least in part on anatomic factors. This view, however, is disputed by McNeal (1972), Gosling (1979, 1984), Donker et al. (1982), and Gilpin and Gosling (1983). These authors regard the urethral smooth muscle system as entirely independent from that of the bladder, and developmentally unrelated to it. This would imply that the adaptive changes that occur in the bladder outlet during voiding are mediated by factors other than those related to muscular continuity and arrangement.

THE STRIATED MUSCLE COMPONENT

The classic view of the external sphincter is that of a striated muscle within the leaves of the urogenital diaphragm, which, on contraction, is capable of stopping the urinary system (Wein and Raezer, 1979). Such a structure was described by Woodburne (1967) as completely annular in the male, though decreased in bulk posteriorly, and blending with the fibers of the prostatic capsule. In the female, the muscle is classically described as tapering considerably and being deficient posteriorly.

A contemporary discussion of the striated muscle component includes both an intramural or intrinsic (to the urethra) and an extramural or extrinsic portion. The intrinsic portion, termed the "rhabdosphincter" by El Badawi (1982), denotes skeletal muscle intimately associated with the proximal (prediaphragmatic) urethra and consisting of several bundles oriented in an oblique vertical direction along the urethra, freely interdigitating with and forming an integral part of its outer muscular layer. In the male, Gosling (1979) and Gosling and Chilton (1984) described this component as being more circularly oriented and completely encircling the urethra from the verumontanum to the striated musculature of the pelvic floor. Tanagho (1986) basically endorses this description in the male, but feels that this intrinsic rhabdosphincter is deficient in the midline posteriorly. He describes some striated muscle fibers as extending over the apex of the prostate in the male and a few as being distributed up to the level of the bladder neck. In the female the intrinsic striated component is thickest in the middle third of the urethra, but was described by Gosling (1984) as being relatively deficient posteriorly in this region. Tanagho (1986), while basically agreeing with this description, simply refers to a raphe in the posterior midline.

In both sexes, the caudal end of the intramural or intrinsic striated component is classically described as adjacent to a bulky skeletal muscle structure oriented in the horizontal plane of the pelvic floor, encircling the membranous urethra, and corresponding to the so-called "external urethral sphincter" of standard anatomy textbooks. This "periurethral muscle" (Gosling, 1979, 1984; Gosling and Chilton, 1984) is related to, but structurally separate from, the urethral wall, and corresponds to Gosling's description of the medial parts of the levator ani muscles. In reviewing older literature, it is quite apparent that at least the anatomic concept of an intrinsic (intramural) vs. an extrinsic (extramural) striated component was clearly implied in the works of Woodburne (1967, 1968), Hutch (1967), Gil Vernet (1968), Tanagho and Smith (1968), and Sant (1962). Evidence presented later will show that this intrinsic striated component is also functionally different from the extrinsic component and particularly suited for the maintenance of urinary continence.

Oelrich has presented a very scholarly description of his concept of the striated muscle component in both the male (1980) and the female (1983). In the male, he described the striated urethral sphincter as being derived from a single primordium, which originally extended from the bladder to the perineal membrane. Development of the prostate occurs from the urethra and into the overlying striated muscle, thinning the overlying parts and causing a reduction or atrophy of some of the muscle in this area, while overlying it and incorporating it within the prostatic perimeter. This accounts for what appear to be isolated segments of striated sphincter muscle distributed around and in the prostate. Further, the fascia of this sphincter muscle was described as being inseparable from the prostatic sheath, oriented vertically, and passing through the urogenital hiatus to unite with the fascia of the pudendal canals at the level of the ischiopubic rami. The concept of a urogenital diaphragm comprising a transverse plane of muscle spanning between the two ischiopubic rami between a superior and inferior fascial plane, and surrounding the membranous urethra (implying the existence of an extrinsic portion of a striated urethral sphincter) was not confirmed. In the female, Oelrich described the striated component as consisting of two parts, one surrounding the urethra and the other surrounding the urethra and vagina. Both of these are infiltrated with smooth muscle, which somewhat obscures their visibility on gross dissection. The orientation of the portion that surrounds the urethra is predominantly circular, and thins out posteriorly. A separate bundle of fibers is attached to the ischiopubic rami and constitutes a compressor muscle, arching across the ventral side of the urethra. Additionally, there is a urethrovaginal sphincter surrounding the urethra and vaginal vestibule collectively. These designated muscles are in continuity with one another and are located within the pelvic cavity in the urogenital hiatus of the pelvic diaphragm.

THE SPHINCTER CONCEPT

The Smooth Sphincter

There is no anatomic sphincter at the bladder neck. Rather, there is a physiologic internal sphincter that consists of the bladder neck and proximal urethra. Both of these areas are rich in elastic fibers, and the inherent tension exerted by their walls on the lumen is dependent on these fibers and on the tone of the smooth musculature. This "smooth sphincter" tone rises during normal urine storage so that urethral pressure exceeds intravesical pressure. Normal micturition implies a number of events, one being a reduction in resistance in this "smooth sphincter" area. It is important to remember that a functional obstruction can occur at the level of the smooth sphincter either because of a failure of the usual adaptive changes that occur in this area during detrusor contraction, or because of actual simultaneous active contraction (smooth sphincter dyssynergia).

The Striated Sphincter

The striated sphincter comprises both the intramural and extrinsic striated component surrounding the urethra in the female and the posterior urethra in the male. Lapides' classical experiments involving progressive shortening of the urethra proximal to the urogenital diaphragm to within 2 cm of the bladder neck showed that the striated sphincter is not necessary for urinary continence (1957, 1958). Curarization of this striated sphincter alone does not normally result in incontinence. Incontinence may result under these circumstances, however, if the smooth sphincter apparatus has been destroyed, as with a prostatectomy. Pathologic hyperreactivity (striated sphincter dyssynergia) can produce severe functional obstruction during bladder contraction.

ANATOMIC ILLUSTRATIONS

The following figures demonstrate and will hopefully reinforce the previous discussion of relevant anatomy of the bladder and the bladder

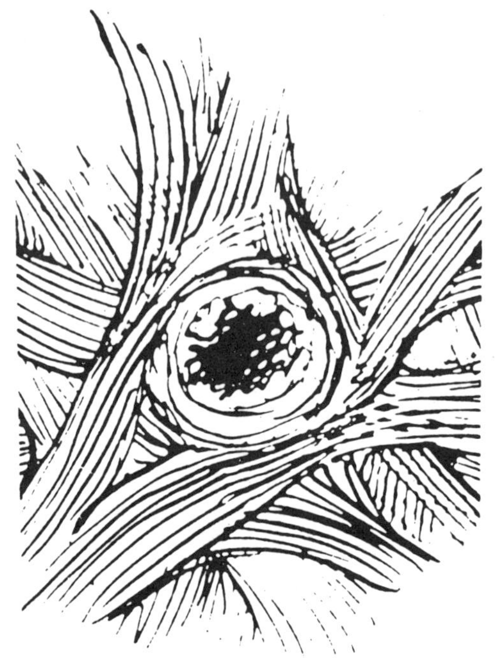

FIG 1.
Smooth muscle bundles in the area of the bladder neck. (From Woodburne RT: Anatomy of the bladder, in Boyarsky S (ed): *The Neurogenic Bladder.* Baltimore, Williams & Wilkins, 1967. Used with permission.)

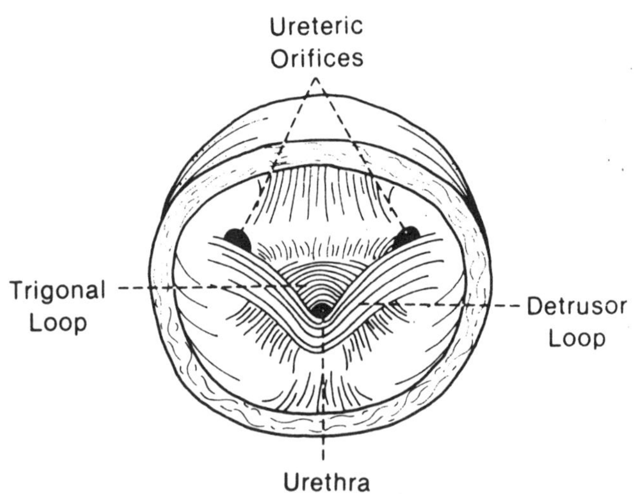

FIG 2.
Dorsal view of the bladder neck with schematic representation of the trigonal and detrusor smooth muscle loops. (From Hald T, Bradley W: *The Urinary Bladder: Neurology and Dynamics.* Baltimore, Williams & Wilkins, 1982. Used with permission.)

outlet. Figure 1 shows arching smooth muscle bundles in the area of the bladder neck. This is the only area in which there exists even a loose arrangement of the bladder smooth muscle into three vaguely distinct layers. Woodburne's concept (1967) was that the fibers at the neck are arranged in such a way that their coordinated contraction pulls the neck open rather than constricts it. This would at least seem to imply that some longitudinal component of bladder smooth muscle extends into the proximal urethra. Also, it might be inferred that bladder distention without active contraction might actually serve to constrict the vesicourethral junction. Figure 2 shows Bradley's concept of why the bladder neck opens during bladder contraction. Randomly distributed interdigitating smooth muscle fibers from the bladder dome form arcades as the bladder base is approached. The trigonal arcade intersects the detrusor arcade, which faces in an opposite direction. When normal detrusor reflex excitation occurs, there is contraction of the two smooth muscle arcades, producing separation at the bladder neck with expulsion of urine into the proximal urethra. Figure 3 diagrams Hutch's concept of the female bladder neck and proximal urethra. He pictured an "internal sphincter" as being located in the bladder base and consisting anteriorly and laterally of the fundus ring and posteriorly of the trigonal muscle. His urethral sphincter consists of the smooth muscle layers of the urethra. Both the outer circular layer and inner longitudinal layer of the urethra were described as continuous

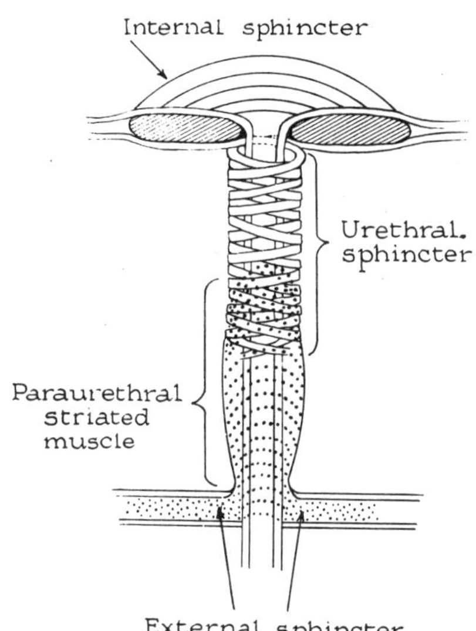

FIG 3.
The female bladder neck and proximal urethra according to Hutch. (From Hutch JA: A new theory of the anatomy of the internal urinary sphincter and the physiology of micturition: IV. The urinary sphincteric mechanism. *J Urol* 1967; 97:705. Used with permission.)

with bladder smooth muscle layers, the outer circular layer fusing caudally with the striated sphincter and the inner longitudinal layer extending down the entire urethral length. Hutch's striated sphincter consists of two parts: (1) a true "external" sphincter, consisting of striated muscle within the leaves of the urogenital diaphragm; and (2) the periurethral striated muscles, which he conceived as arising from the urogenital diaphragm, advancing upward around the lower urethra, and inserting cranially into the urethral sphincter. Figure 4 shows Hutch's concept of the male bladder neck and proximal urethra. The inner longitudinal muscle of the bladder is pictured as extending down the entire length of the posterior urethra. The outer muscular layer is similarly continuous, but only through the upper half of the posterior urethra. Figure 5 shows Woodburne's representation of the "classical" external sphincter concept in the male. Figure 6 shows Gosling's diagramatic representation of the male lower urinary tract. The lumens of the bladder and urethra are dilated and the right half of the trigone (T) in Figure 6,A, and the entire trigone in Figure 6,B are shown as surface features. The detrusor muscle (D) is in direct continuity with the deep trigone (DT), with which it is morphologically and histochemically identical. The extension of the ureteric muscle formed by the trigonal muscle is represented as a thin layer (ST) extending inferiorly as far as the verumontanum. The smooth muscle of the bladder neck forms the internal urethral sphincter (IS) and is continuous with the prostatic capsule (P). The two components of the striated sphincter are shown, ES representing the intrinsic component and PS representing the extrinsic or periurethral component. Figure 7 shows Gosling's concept of corresponding sections (to Figure 6) through the female lower urinary

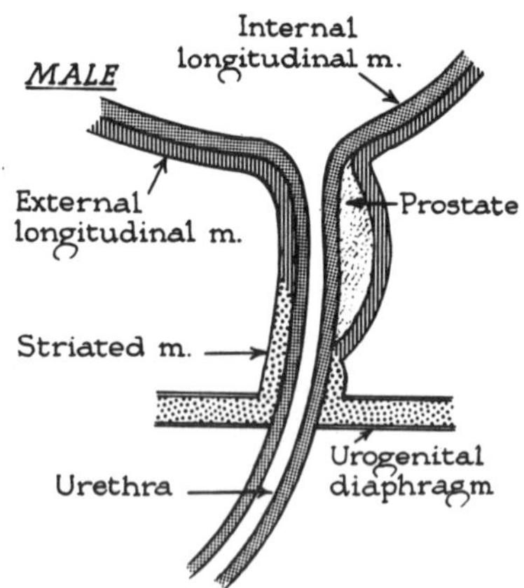

FIG 4.
Sagittal section of the male urethra according to Hutch and Rambo. (From Hutch JA, Rambo OA Jr: A new theory of the anatomy of the internal urinary sphincter and the physiology of micturition: III. Anatomy of the urethra. *J Urol* 1967; 97:696. Used with permission.)

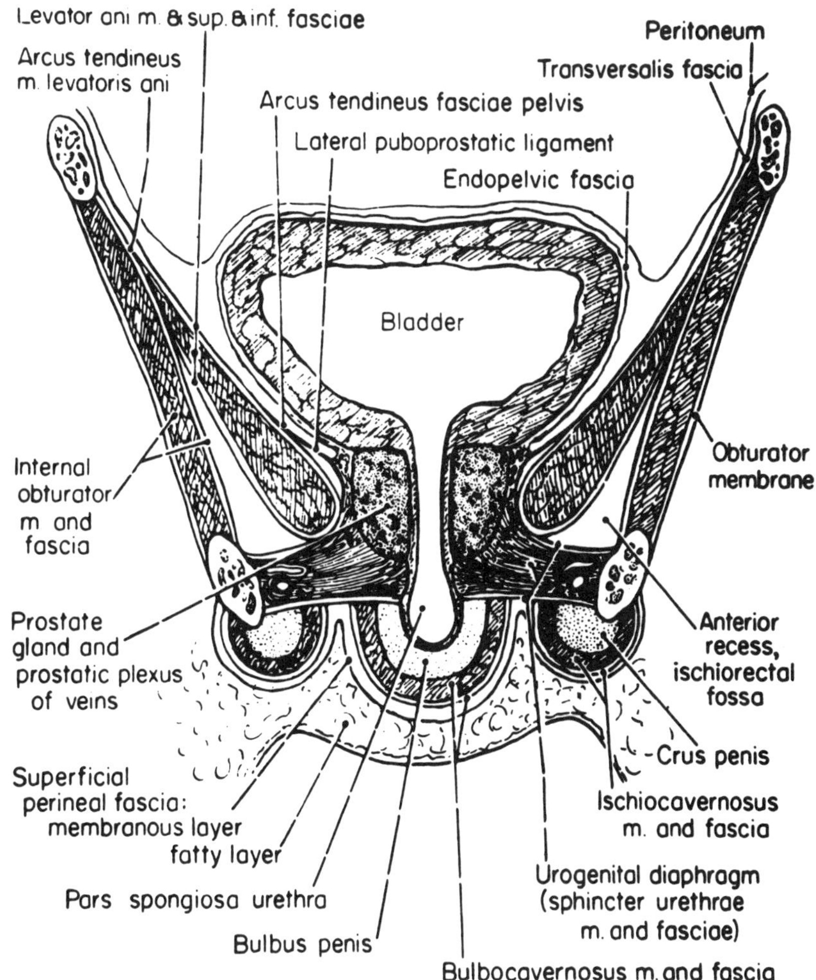

FIG 5.
The external sphincter and its relationships in the male. (From Woodburne RT: Anatomy of the bladder, in Boyarsky S (ed): *The Neurogenic Bladder*. Baltimore, Williams & Wilkins, 1967. Used with permission.)

tract. The trigone (T) is represented as a surface feature. The detrusor smooth muscle (D) continues posterior to the superficial trigone and at the bladder neck region is replaced by a thin layer of smooth muscle (SM), which extends throughout the length of the urethra. Gosling does not, however, consider the smooth muscle of the urethra actually

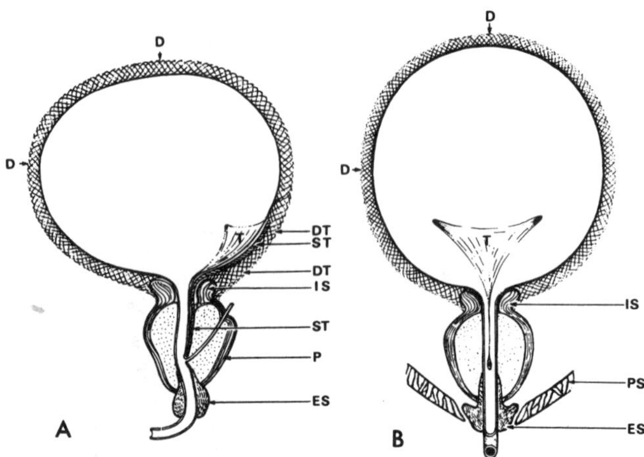

FIG 6.
A, sagittal section through the adult male lower urinary tract. **B,** corresponding coronal section. See text for more detailed descriptions. (From Gosling J: The structure of the bladder and urethra in relation to function. *Urol Clin North Am* 1979; 6(Feb):31. Used with permission.)

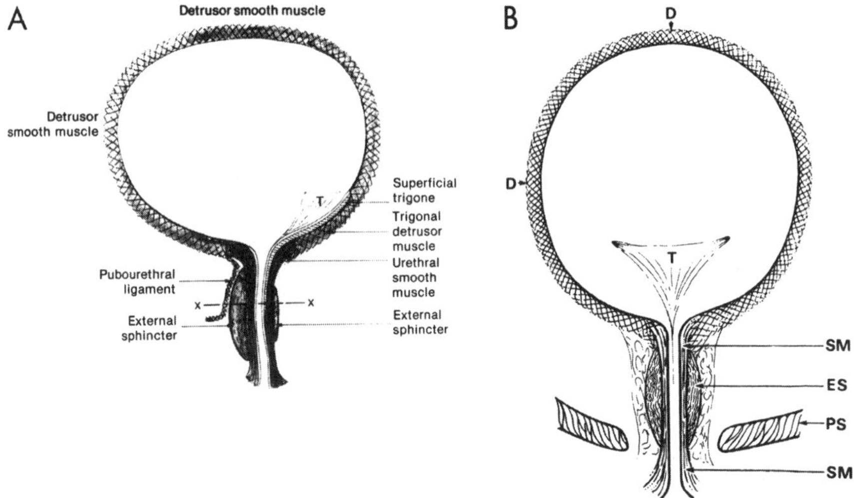

FIG 7.
A, sagittal section through the adult female lower urinary tract. **B,** corresponding coronal section. See text for more detailed description. (From Gosling J: Anatomy, in Stanton SL (ed): *Clinical Gynecologic Urology*. St Louis, CV Mosby, 1984. From Gosling J: The structure of the bladder and urethra in relation to function. *Urol Clin North Am* 1979; 6(Feb):31. Used with permission.)

continuous with the smooth muscle of the detrusor. Both components of the striated sphincter are pictured. The intramural intrinsic striated component (external sphincter [ES]) is thickest along the middle third of the urethra and relatively deficient posteriorly. This is separate from the extramural or extrinsic component, designated periurethral striated muscle (PS). The pubourethral ligament extends toward the pubis and lies anterior to the intrinsic component of the striated sphincter. Figure 8 is a cross-section of the female urethra at the plane denoted by the X in Figure 7,A. The intramural or intrinsic portion of the striated sphincter is again designated "external sphincter," an admittedly confusing term here. The smooth muscle coat consists of a relatively minor outer circular part and a thicker inner longitudinal component. Figure 9 shows El Badawi's concept of the muscular structures involved in micturition. BBD denotes the bladder body detrusor, and UT denotes the ureterotrigonal muscle unit, which extends into the proximal urethra. His "lissosphincter" consists of the periureteral sheaths, bladder base detrusor muscle, and proximal urethral smooth muscle, all of which are described as being in direct anatomic continuity. His "rhabdosphincter" corresponds to the intrinsic component of the striated sphincter and is distinct from the striated muscle of the pelvic diaphragm (PD), which encircles the urethra proximal to its pelvic subdiaphragmatic portion (SDU), comprising the extrinsic component of the striated sphincter.

The synthesis of vesicourethral structure by Khanna et al. (1981,

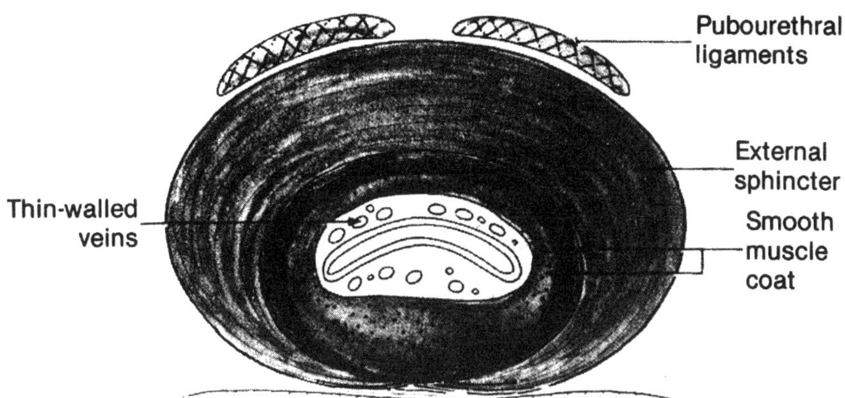

FIG 8.
Horizontal section of the female urethra in plane X—X in Fig 7,A. (From Gosling J: Anatomy, in Stanton SL (ed): *Clinical Gynecologic Urology.* St Louis, CV Mosby, 1984. Used with permission.)

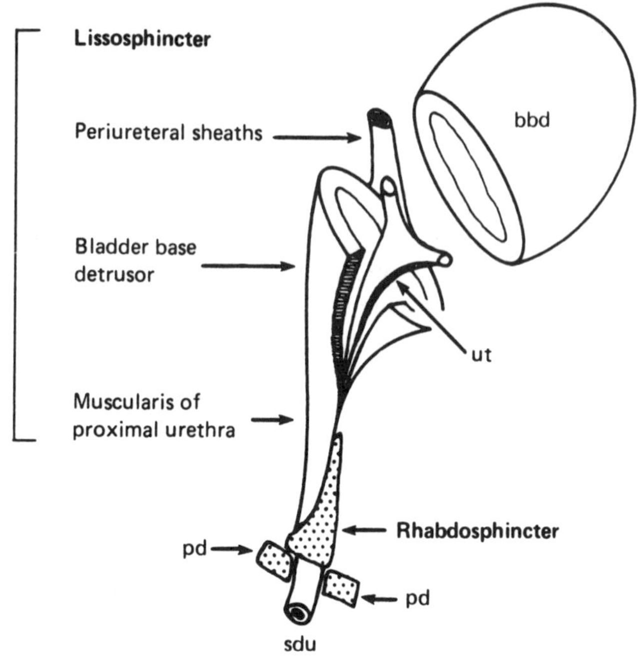

FIG 9.
Units of muscular apparatus of micturition. See text for more detailed description. (From El Badawi A: Autonomic muscular innervation of the vesical outlet and its role in micturition, in Hinman F Jr (ed): *Benign Prostatic Hypertrophy*. Berlin, Springer-Verlag, 1983. Used with permission.)

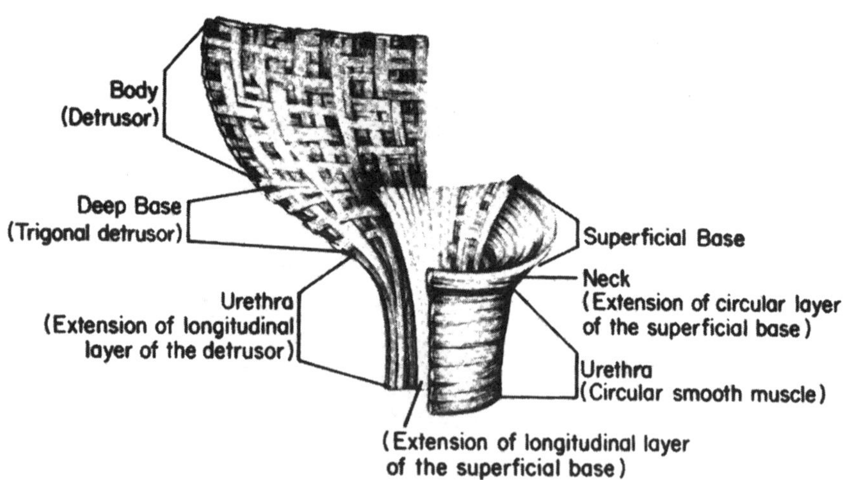

FIG 10.
Vesical neck smooth musculature. (From Khanna OP, et al: Vesicourethral smooth muscle: Function and relation to structure. *Urology* 1981; 18:211. Used with permission.)

1983) is depicted in Figure 10. They considered the predominant muscle element at the vesicourethral junction to be the superficial bladder base, the circular layer of which sweeps around to form the circular vesical neck, and the longitudinal layer of which extends to form the posterior vesical neck and urethra. They thought that this muscle element participates in active (neurally induced) closure of the outlet during bladder filling. During voiding, they thought this muscular component actively relaxed, again in response to neural stimulation. The longitudinal layer of the detrusor muscle extends to form the anterolateral and posterolateral bladder neck and urethra, providing a structural basis for adaptive funneling of the outlet and some shortening of the proximal urethra during the emptying phase of micturition. The prostatic capsule, in their schema, was felt to be simply a continuation of the smooth muscle layers of the proximal urethra in the male, constituting a single morphological unit with the bladder neck and proximal urethra.

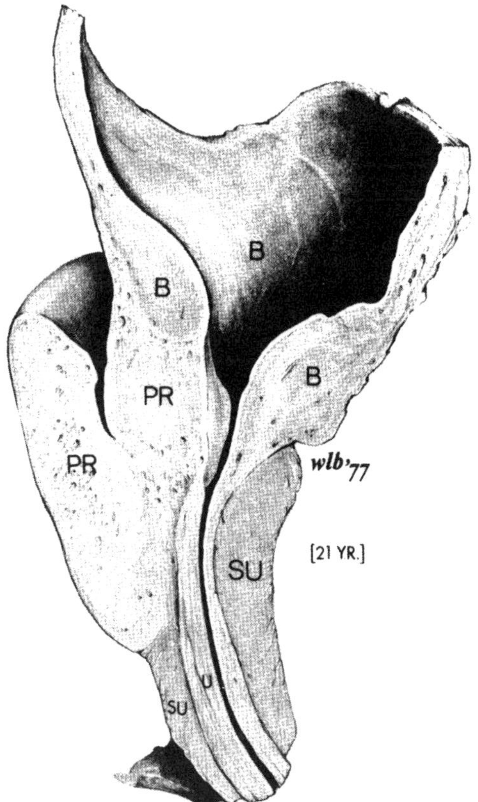

FIG 11.
Median section of bladder, urethra, prostate, and urethral sphincter in a 21-year-old man. See text for more detailed description. (From Oelrich TM: The urethral sphincter muscle in the male. *Am J Anat* 1980; 158:229. Used with permission.)

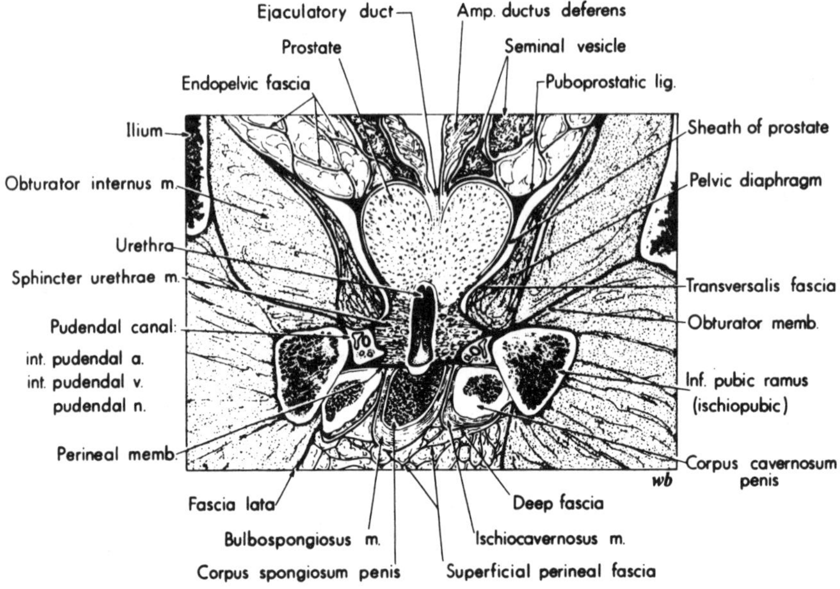

FIG 12.
Frontal section of pelvis in a 28-year-old man. (From Oelrich TM: The urethral sphincter muscle in the male. *Am J Anat* 1980; 158:229. Used with permission.)

Figure 11 shows Oelrich's illustration of a median section of the lower urinary tract of a 21-year-old man, demonstrating the extent of contact between the urethra (U) and the striated sphincter (SU, called "sphincter urethrae"). B denotes bladder and PR denotes prostate. Figure 12 shows Oelrich's diagram of a frontal section of a male pelvis taken at right angles to the perineal membrane and through the membranous urethra. The relationships of the fascial planes in the pelvis, urogenital hiatus, and perineum are demonstrated. Note the lack of a "classical" horizontally oriented urogenital diaphragm surrounded by two distinct parallel fascial layers. Figure 13 shows Oelrich's concept of an oblique view of the muscular relationships of the lower urinary tract and vagina in a 27-year-old woman. US represents the striated urethral sphincter. Distal to and directly continuous with the lower border of this is a bundle of fibers that begins as a small tendon attached to the ischiopubic ramus (IR) and extends forward toward the anterior surface of the urethra, widening to a band of approximately 6 mm, then becoming continuous with the corresponding fibers of the opposite side. This is called the "compressor urethrae muscle" (CU). The urethrovag-

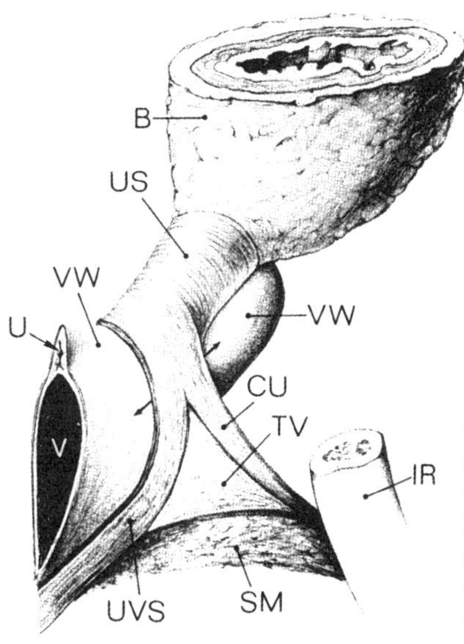

FIG 13.
Oblique view of urogenital sphincter muscles, bladder, and vagina in a 27-year-old woman. See text for more detailed description. (From Oelrich TM: The striated urogenital sphincter muscle in the female. *Anat Rec* 1983; 205:223. Used with permission.)

inal sphincter (UVS) is a thin, flat muscle that blends ventrally with the compressor urethrae. From the ventral side of the urethra its fibers extend dorsally along the lateral wall of the urethra and vagina. An additional layer of striated muscle, the transverse vaginal muscle (TV), parallels the compressor urethrae and radiates from it to attach to the anterior portion of the lateral wall of the vagina, attaching just above the urethrovaginal sphincter. SM denotes smooth muscle of the urethrovaginal compartment; VW, vaginal wall (arrow indicates continuity of this beneath the muscle); U, urethra; and B, bladder smooth muscle.

Relevant Smooth and Striated Muscle Structure and Function

SMOOTH MUSCLE

The physiology of mammalian smooth muscle has been studied far less extensively than that of skeletal or cardiac muscle, yet an extensive literature exists, including contemporary reference volumes (Bulbring et al., 1981). However, the majority of information concerning smooth muscle anatomy and physiology is derived from studies on vascular smooth muscle, with a lesser body of information available on the gut and on other smooth muscle organs. One must be careful in directly applying information and conclusions derived from one smooth muscle system to another. With this in mind, we shall briefly review only those general principles related to the structure, function, and control of the smooth muscle of the lower urinary tract.

Structure

Smooth muscle is composed of far smaller fibers than skeletal muscle—usually 2–5 μ in diameter and 50–200 μ in length, although ranging up to nearly 1 mm in some organs (Gabella, 1981; Guyton, 1986). Cell length is an uncertain parameter, as cells can shorten and elongate over a wide range. The cell membrane is similar to that of other cell types, but presents numerous in-pocketings known as "caveolae," whose significance remains obscure, but which seem to be closely associated with portions of the abundant sarcoplasmic reticulum. Smooth muscle contains both actin and myosin filaments, which have chemical characteristics similar to but not exactly like those of the filaments in skeletal muscle. Smooth muscle also contains tropomyosin, but probably not troponin or a troponin-like substance. However, as in skeletal muscle, a chemical interaction between actin and myosin forms the basis for the contractile process and, as in skeletal muscle, although the details differ, this contractile process is activated by calcium ions, with ATP ultimately providing the energy source for this process. The actin and myosin filaments lack the periodic spatial arrangement found in striated muscle, and thus no cross-striations are visible microscopically—hence the term "smooth" muscle. However, smooth muscle does contain large numbers of thin actin filaments attached to so-called dense bodies (Fig 14). Some of these dense bodies are attached to the cell membrane, whereas others seem held in place by a scaffold of structural protein forming attachments from one dense body to an-

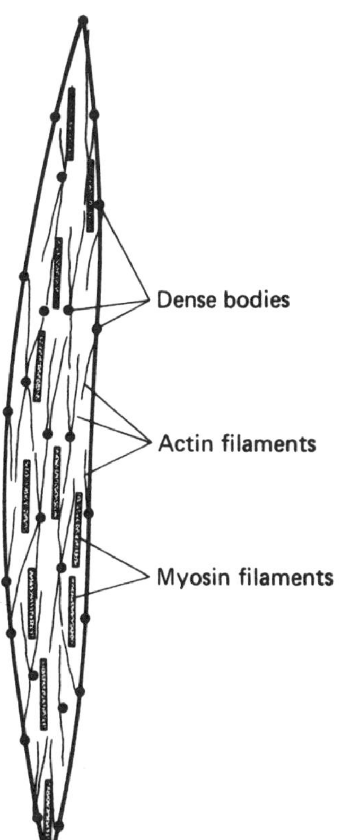

FIG 14.
Arrangement of actin and myosin filaments in smooth muscle cell, showing dense bodies. (From Guyton AC: *Textbook of Medical Physiology*. Philadelphia, WB Saunders, 1986. Used with permission.)

other. Thick filaments about 2.5 times the diameter of the thin actin filaments, and assumed to be myosin, are interspersed throughout. Despite the fact that these are only 1⁄12–1⁄15 as numerous as the actin filaments, it is presumed that there are sufficient cross-bridges to interact with the actin filaments and cause contraction by a sliding filament mechanism similar to that of skeletal muscle. Although the contractile process seems relatively similar, contraction in smooth muscle develops much less rapidly.

Fiber Arrangement and Spread of the Contractile Impulse

Bozler (1941) originally proposed two categories of smooth muscle—multiunit and unitary—on the basis of general physiologic properties. Multiunit smooth muscle receives an extensive innervation, often having a 1:1 ratio between nerve endings and muscle fibers. Motor coordination is effected primarily through the nervous system, and fibers appear to be organized in some sort of a motor plan. Spontaneous activity generally does not occur. The outer surfaces of these fibers are covered by a thin layer of glycoprotein that seems to help insulate the separate fibers from each other (Guyton, 1986). Typical examples of multiunit smooth muscle include the fibers of the ciliary muscle and iris of the eye, piloerector muscles, and the muscle of many larger blood vessels. Unitary smooth muscle, often called visceral smooth muscle, receives a much less extensive innervation, and the muscle fibers are usually arranged in sheets or bundles such that the cell membranes contact each other at multiple points to form "gap junctions" through which ions can flow from one cell to the next. These fibers usually form a functional syncytium whose motor coordination is primarily dependent on myogenic conduction from muscle fiber to fiber. Classical unitary smooth muscle is found in the wall of the gut, bile duct, ureter, and uterus.

The smooth muscle of the bladder seems to share characteristics of both multiunit and unitary type. Most authors agree on an abundant cholinergic innervation of the bladder smooth muscle, but there was originally some disagreement as to the degree of innervation, some authors arguing for a nearly 1:1 nerve-muscle cell basis (El Badawi and Schenk, 1966, 1968; Schulman et al., 1972; Taira, 1972), while others argued for a nerve-muscle cell ratio of considerably less than 1:1 (Raezer et al., 1973). El Badawi's ultrastructural studies, however, clearly indicate that no part of the vesicourethral smooth muscle is supplied by nerves on a one-to-one basis (El Badawi, 1982). Daniel et al. (1983), studying adult human female detrusor muscle, found many nerve profiles (about one for each eight cells cut in cross-section) and felt that the muscle cells did not possess any large gap junctions such as would provide typical low-resistance contacts between cells. There were observed, however, some regions of contact that might represent small gap junctions, and there were close apposition contacts and intermediate contacts between cells. Fletcher and Bradley (1978) also summarized morphologic evidence of close contact between adjacent bladder smooth muscle cells. However, they felt that neurotransmitter was delivered to a "domain" within a bladder muscle fascicle. From the site of each varicosity, they hypothesized neurotransmitter molecules diffusing in all directions, exciting whichever smooth muscle cells the transmitter reached in sufficient quantity. This theory necessitates bladder smooth muscle having an extensive coating with receptor sites.

Thus, the bladder does not seem to fit exclusively in either category of smooth muscle, but seems to possess properties more of a multiunit than a unitary smooth muscle, with some morphologic substrates compatible with cell coupling and the capability of impulse propagation from cell to cell. Few data are available regarding the path of spread of the contractile sequence during an emptying bladder contraction. Experimentally, it has been shown by Conway and Bradley (1969) that bladder contraction during reflex micturition begins in the dorsal urethrovesical junction area and spreads to the fundus, probably ventrally.

Innervation

Burnstock and Bell (1974) and Burnstock (1977, 1985, 1986) has extensively reviewed and updated current concepts of the structural relationships of peripheral autonomic nerves and smooth muscle. The neuroeffector junction differs significantly from the synapses of skeletal muscle and those of ganglia, both of which are elaborate, with separation of specialized presynaptic and postsynaptic membranes by about 20–50 nm. Transmitters are released from presynaptic sites, diffuse across a narrow cleft, and occupy receptors located on the postsynaptic or postjunctional membrane. Peripheral autonomic nerve fibers have extensive terminal varicose regions, which are free of Schwann cell envelopments. In these areas vesicle-filled varicosities, 1–2 μ in diameter, release transmitter *en passage*. Prejunctional varicosity membranes sometimes show thickenings, but there are rarely postjunctional specializations, and there is a variable and often wide (20–120 nm) cleft, allowing the potential for significant modulation (Fig 15). Vesicles are the most characteristic component of peripheral autonomic nerve end-

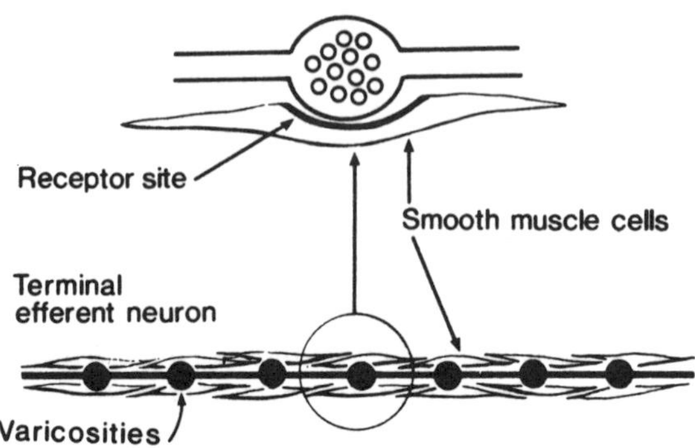

FIG 15.
Peripheral autonomic neuroeffector junction. (From Mundy AR: Clinical physiology of the bladder, urethra and pelvic floor, in Mundy AR, Stephenson TP, Wein AJ (eds): *Urodynamics: Principles, Practice, and Application.* New York, Churchill Livingstone, 1984. Used with permission.)

ings. Since these contain neurotransmitters and are believed to be involved in their release, attempts to classify nerve endings rest mainly on the identification of the neurotransmitters at the EM level. Endings containing a large majority of small agranular (clear) vesicles are considered to be cholinergic, those containing numerous small granular vesicles are considered to be adrenergic (Gabella, 1981). Varicosities are also seen that contain large granular vesicles, and these have been considered to be purinergic (containing ATP).

Excitation, Excitation-Contraction Coupling, and Contraction

Excitation of smooth muscle cells can occur in a number of different ways (Guyton, 1986). The intracellular calcium concentration in smooth muscle is maintained at less than 10^{-7}M via active extrusion against an electrochemical gradient across an essentially impermeable plasma membrane. With excitation, whether by direct membrane depolarization or receptor activation, calcium acts as the predominant messenger linking stimuli from extracellular origin to the intracellular environment (Kuriyama, 1981; Movsesian, 1982; Droogmans et al., 1985). The threshold for mechanical activation of the contractile process occurs at a calcium concentration of about 10^{-7}M and full activation occurs at a free calcium concentration in the cytosol of about 10^{-5}M.

The increase in intracellular calcium occurs as a result of an increased permeability of the membrane to extracellular calcium with resultant influx, and from a secondary release of calcium from intracellular stores. The importance of this latter pathway varies from tissue to tissue, but the location of these stores seems to be the sarcoplasmic reticulum and storage sites on the inner surface of the plasma membrane. In general, smooth muscle is considerably more dependent on extracellular calcium translocation than is skeletal muscle. Excitation, with increase in cytosol calcium concentration, can occur by a number of different mechanisms, which can be briefly summarized as follows (Kuriyama, 1981; Movsesian, 1982; Droogmans et al., 1985; Guyton, 1986): (1) action potentials can produce associated calcium influx through potential dependent channels (voltage-regulated channels); (2) agonist-induced receptor activation can induce calcium influx by causing depolarization, but such excitation may also occur with no depolarization at all, through so-called receptor-dependent channels.

Membrane potential varies from one type of smooth muscle to another, but is generally of the order of −50 to −60 mV, about 30 mV less negative than in skeletal muscle. Action potentials in visceral (unitary) smooth muscles are qualitatively similar to those in skeletal muscle. However, it is said that action potentials probably do not occur in pure multiunit smooth muscle (Guyton, 1986). Some types of visceral smooth muscle generate a slow-wave rhythmic fluctuation of the membrane potential that is similar to that seen in true pacemaker cells. These waves cannot cause muscle contraction, but when they rise above the approximately −35 mV threshold potential, an action potential develops and spreads over the visceral muscle mass with resultant contraction. When visceral smooth muscle is stretched, spontaneous action potentials are usually generated, and these are thought to result from a combination of a decrease in the membrane potential caused by the stretch itself plus the normal slow-wave potentials. The question of whether bladder smooth muscle exhibits "spontaneous activity" has not been settled. The presence of "slow-wave fluctuations" is not the same as spontaneous activity. Although spontaneous activity is a property of some smooth muscle, it is not a property of all. The function of most smooth muscle organs is to slowly move contents through their length via peristalsis (such as the gastrointestinal tract and the renal collecting system and ureter). Thus, spontaneous activity would be a mechanism for initiation and control of peristalsis. Unlike most other smooth muscle organs, the urinary bladder functions to passively store its contents at low pressure until micturition occurs, at which time the bladder undergoes a coordinated contraction of sufficient magnitude to fully empty its contents. The presence of spontaneous activity in this system would be counterproductive. This topic will be discussed in greater detail later.

The actual contractile process in smooth muscle fibers is different from that in skeletal and cardiac muscle (Perry and Grand, 1979; Movsesian, 1982; Guyton, 1985). Smooth muscle probably does not have an effective tropinin complex, which regulates arrangement of the contractile proteins of skeletal muscle. The sequence of excitation-contraction coupling is as follows: (1) excitation of the muscle leads to the depolarization of the cell membrane and translocation of extracellular calcium into the cell; (2) this extracellular calcium can trigger the release of intracellular calcium, which increases the cytosol calcium concentration above 10^{-7}M; (3) the intracellular calcium binds to calmodulin (a calcium-binding protein) and the combination activates myosin kinase; (4) the activated myosin kinase phosphorylates myosin via adenosine triphosphate (ATP) hydrolysis and results in actin-myosin interaction; (5) the actin and myosin filaments slide past each other, resulting in contraction; (6) relaxation occurs following repolarization of the cell membrane and the resultant decrease in intracellular free calcium (mediated by both sequestration within intracellular storage sites and active calcium translocation back across the cell membrane). In the absence of sufficient free cytosol calcium, myosin kinase inactivates, myosin dephosphorylates, and the muscle relaxes.

What actually causes the signal transduction between excitation and the intracellular processes that cause contraction or relaxation is a field that is of great interest at this time, and a few relevant facts bear mentioning. The signaling system using cyclic adenosine monophosphate (cAMP) as a second messenger may be best known. There is a reasonable rationale for the hypothesis that cAMP can induce smooth muscle relaxation by stimulating calcium uptake into the sarcoplasmic reticulum or perhaps by stimulating calcium extrusion from the cytosol (Hardman, 1981). Cyclic guanosine monophosphate (GMP) may mediate smooth muscle relaxation, at least in vascular smooth muscle, by likewise somehow antagonizing the accumulation of free cytosolic calcium (Ignarro and Kadowitz, 1985). Most recently, inositol triphosphate has been proposed as a link between the plasma membrane and the increase in cytosol calcium (which occurs with smooth muscle contraction), especially in pharmacomechanical coupling, the type that occurs with the various physiological neurotransmitters (Berridge and Irvine, 1984; Somlyo, 1985).

Tonus

Tonus can be considered as a state of continuous stress in muscle maintained by activity of the contractile elements. Such activity may be contributed to by the intrinsic characteristics of smooth muscle, which are responsible for its response to stretch and for its spontaneous activity (where this exists), by prolonged direct smooth muscle excitation via local tissue factors or circulating hormones, and by tonic activity initiated extrinsically in the autonomic nervous system (Wein and Raezer, 1979; Guyton, 1986). The status of the intravesical pressure during bladder filling—which, up to a certain point, normally rises very little as a function of volume—is thought to be a result of this inherent tonus, the presence or absence of phasic excitatory or inhibitory neuronal impulses acting at the cell membrane or ganglia, and those important characteristics of smooth muscle that describe its ability to change length greatly without marked changes in tension, its elastic properties.

The urinary bladder appears to have intrinsic tone (in the absence of neuronal influences). Using an isolated whole bladder model, Levin et al. (1984) demonstrated that, in the absence of any extrinsic influences, the cystometric curve could be shifted to the right (more compliant) by diltiazem (calcium-channel blocker), EGTA (calcium chelator), or isoproterenol (β-adrenergic agonist).

Elasticity and Viscoelasticity

The bladder wall is composed of passive elements and active elements. The passive elements consist of collagen, elastic, and those elements of smooth muscle that do not require energy utilization for their function. The passive properties attributable to these elements account for much of the reason why a very gradual increase in bladder volume, with consequent stretch on the bladder wall elements, results in only a very low increase in pressure or wall tension, whereas a rapid stretch results in a large increase in pressure or tension, but one that begins to disappear immediately and that gradually returns almost to the prestretch level, even though the muscle is still lengthened. Similarly, if a segment of smooth muscle is rapidly shortened, all tension will be immediately lost, but over a period of time much of the tension again returns (Guyton, 1986). These properties collectively describe the elastic and viscoelastic properties of the bladder wall. They constitute the so-called passive characteristics that are extremely important in determining the bladder response to filling, and may be important as well in determining contractility characteristics during the emptying phase of micturition. These properties, and their measurements, have been described by a number of authors. Note, however, that the spherical bladder and its pressure volume relationships during storage and active contraction may not be directly related to those of a longitudinal length-tension muscle system. Further, unfortunately, terminology is not consistent, and makes comparison of one author's viewpoint to that of another quite difficult (Kondo et al., 1972; Van Mastrigt et al., 1978; Zinner et al., 1983; Coolsaet, 1984; Griffiths, 1984; Van Duyl, 1985).

STRIATED MUSCLE

Skeletal muscle is generally divided into slow-type fibers and twitch-type fibers. Slow-type fibers, not to be confused with slow-twitch-type fibers, are widely distributed in animals, but in mammals are found only in the extrinsic muscles of the ear and in the extraocular muscles, and will not be considered further (Kirchberger and Schwartz, 1985).

Twitch-type fibers have been further classified into subtypes on the basis of their metabolic and functional characteristics. Such classification was initiated about 15 years ago, and now eight such classification systems are listed by Kirchberger and Schwartz (1985). Speed of contraction seems to correlate with histochemical reaction for adenosine triphosphatase (ATPase) at an alkaline pH. Fibers strongly reactive are fast-twitch, whereas those that are weakly reactive are slow-twitch. Resistance to fatigue is directly related to the intensity of oxidative enzyme staining in the same fibers. Slow-twitch fibers are high in oxidative enzyme activity and are relatively fatigue-resistant. Fast-twitch fibers may be fatigable or relatively fatigue-resistant. Gosling et al. (1981) stated that the entire intramural (intrinsic) striated sphincter is composed of slow-twitch type fibers, whereas the periurethral levator ani (the extramural or extrinsic component) consist of both slow-twitch and fast-twitch fibers. Teleologically, this would be convenient because the intramural striated component would then consist of specialized fibers functionally capable of maintaining tension over prolonged time periods without fatigue. Their data indicated that the extramural component of the striated sphincter is also composed of a majority of slow-twitch type fibers rather than fast-twitch. They postulated this might be related to a role played by this muscle in actively supporting the pelvic viscera, and that the slow-twitch fibers are responsible for "background activity" during electromyographic (EMG) recordings. The fast-twitch population of the extramural component of the striated sphincter is functionally associated with rapid, forceful muscle contraction. It is these fibers, then, that are recruited to increase the force and speed of contraction of the levator ani during those events that might otherwise cause stress incontinence by raising intra-abdominal pressure.

Bazeed et al. (1982), studying the dog, reported a different fiber distribution in the intramural component of the striated sphincter. They found that only 35% of the intramural striated sphincter consisted of slow-twitch fatigue-resistant fibers. Like Gosling, they felt that it was these fibers that were responsible for the contribution of the striated sphincter to continence at rest. Of the fast-twitch fibers, they reported that fatigue-resistant ones constituted 20%, with fatigable fibers constituting the remainder. The intramural striated sphincter in the rabbit was found by Tokunaka et al. (1984) to consist solely of fast-twitch fatigue-resistant striated muscle. Bowen et al. (1976) stated that the intramural striated sphincter of the cat was fast-twitch fatigable muscle, but El Badawi and Atta (1985) showed ultrastructural evidence that it consists of both fast- and slow-twitch fibers.

It is tempting to look upon the physiology of the striated sphincter as changeable (Schmidt, 1983), change potentially occurring in response to a change in the type of stimuli or innervation. Such a change causing an increase in the proportion of slow-twitch fibers or nonfatigable fast-twitch fibers might augment sustained outlet resistance during urine storage.

Neural Control of Muscle Function

AUTONOMIC VS. SOMATIC NERVOUS SYSTEM

The physiology of smooth muscle cannot be separated from that of the autonomic nervous system, which includes all efferent pathways having ganglionic synapses outside the central nervous system, and therefore includes the efferent innervation of all smooth muscle cells, cardiac muscle cells, and several types of secretory cells (see references cited by Wein and Raezer, 1979; Appenzeller, 1982; Guyton, 1986). There are no efferent somatic nerve cell body synapses outside of the central nervous system. Other differences between autonomic and somatic nerves include the following: (1) autonomic nerves may form extensive peripheral plexuses, while somatic nerves generally do not; (2) the most distal autonomic motor neurons are generally nonmyelinated, while somatic neurons are myelinated; (3) neurotrophic atrophy occurs when the somatic nerve supply to a skeletal muscle is sectioned, whereas such changes do not generally occur in a smooth muscle structure whose autonomic nerve supply has been destroyed.

CLASSICAL ANATOMY AND FUNCTION OF THE AUTONOMIC NERVOUS SYSTEM

The terms sympathetic and parasympathetic refer only to anatomic divisions of the autonomic nervous system (Wein and Raezer, 1979; Appenzeller, 1982; Guyton, 1986). The sympathetic division consists of fibers originating in the thoracic and lumbar regions of the spinal cord, while the parasympathetic division consists of fibers originating in the cranial and sacral spinal nerves. The classical view of the peripheral autonomic nervous system, necessary for a full understanding of contemporary modifications, was described by us in a previous chapter (Wein and Raezer, 1979), based on the schema outlined by Jacobowitz (1974) (Fig 16). Each division was thought to generally involve a two-neuron system: "preganglionic" neurons emanating from the central nervous system and making synaptic contact with cells within ganglia, from which "postganglionic" neurons emerge to innervate peripheral organs. Three classes of ganglia were described in the sympathetic division: (1) those located adjacent to the spinal cord (paraganglia); (2) those located between the paravertebral ganglia and the end organ (preganglia); and (3) those located adjacent to or within the end organ (peripheral ganglia). In the parasympathetic system, ganglia were described as generally located in or near the innervated organs. Peripheral sympathetic ganglia were described that were close to peripheral parasympathetic cell bodies, providing an anatomic substrate for sympathetic influences on parasympathetic ganglion cell transmission. Afferent or sensory fibers from any autonomically innervated organ pass uninterruptedly through peripheral (infraspinal) autonomic ganglia to end in a neurosynapse only in the spinal cord. According to the clas-

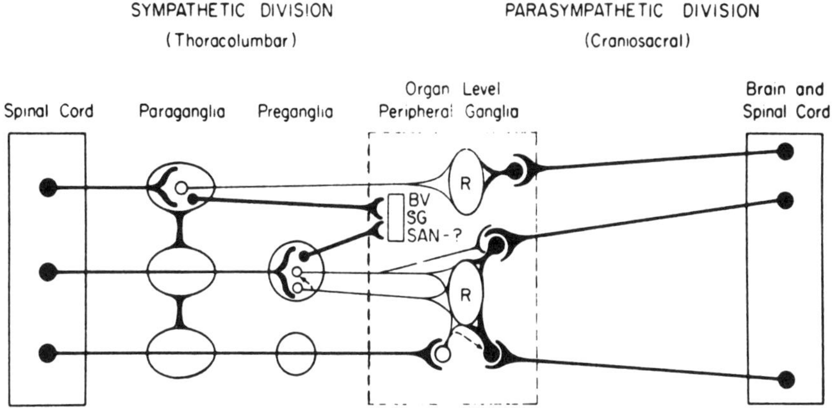

FIG 16.

Classical view of the autonomic nervous system. Black circles represent cholinergic cell bodies; white circles, adrenergic cell bodies; R, receptor organ; BV, blood vessel; SG, sweat gland; and SAN, sinoatrial node. *Small dotted arrow* indicates intraganglionic adrenergic system of fibers. (From Jacobowitz DM: The peripheral autonomic system, in Hubbard JI (ed): *The Peripheral Nervous System.* New York, Plenum Press, 1974. Used with permission.)

sical scheme then, spinal neural control of an autonomically innervated organ is achieved by a "reflex arc" type of arrangement involving three or perhaps four neurons establishing an organ–spinal cord–peripheral autonomic ganglion–organ neural circuit.

CONTEMPORARY MODIFICATION OF CLASSICAL AUTONOMIC NERVOUS SYSTEM SCHEME

Some of these traditional concepts of the autonomic nervous system require modification to be able to understand the extensive literature that exists about innervation and neural control of the lower urinary tract. El Badawi (1982, 1983, 1984, 1985) has very nicely summarized the anatomic aspect of these modifications and the following represents what seems to us to be a synthesis of his conclusions (Fig 17). The muscular innervation of the lower urinary tract is derived exclusively from postganglionic neurons of what is termed "the urogenital short neuron system." Although paraganglia and preganglia exist, actual innervation predominantly (or exclusively) emanates from peripheral ganglia that are at a short distance from, adjacent to, or within the organs they innervate, thus the name "short" (as opposed

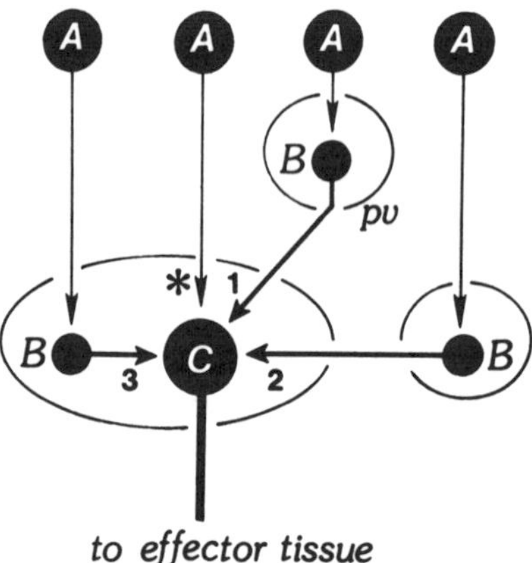

FIG 17.
Basic and simplified scheme of neural control of vesicourethral smooth muscle. **A,** preganglionic spinal cord–derived neurons; **B,** postganglionic modulator neurons; **C,** postganglionic effector neurons innervating vesicourethral muscularis and other effector tissues. Whether cholinergic or adrenergic, effector neuron **C** can be influenced by multiple neurosynapses established by its corresponding preganglionic neuron *(asterisk)*, a modulator sympathetic adrenergic neuron derived from paravertebral ganglia (pv; terminal 1), a modulator sympathetic adrenergic or parasympathetic cholinergic or SIF cell catecholaminergic neuron that is located in the same ganglion of the urogenital short neuron system (terminal 2), or in a more proximal ganglion of the same system (terminal 3). (From El Badawi A: Autonomic muscular innervation of the vesical outlet and its role in micturition, in Hinman F Jr (ed): *Benign Prostatic Hypertrophy*. Berlin, Springer-Verlag, 1983. Used with permission.)

to the "long" postganglionic fibers from cell bodies that lie away from the target organ in paraganglia or preganglia). The ganglia themselves are composed of three cell types: cholinergic principal neurons, adrenergic principal neurons, and small intensely fluorescent (SIF) cells (see also Jacobowitz, 1974). The latter cells are thought to play an important role in the modulation of interganglionic vasomotor function and ganglionic transmission and are identifiable both histochemically and ultrastructurally. Urogenital ganglia also include a complex intraganglionic network of cholinergic and adrenergic fibers that either pass uninterruptedly through the ganglion or terminate in it as neuron synapses with one or more of its cell populations. Thus, the efferent autonomic pathways of the lower urinary tract do not necessarily conform to the classical autonomic bineuronal efferent model, as they may be interrupted by more than one synaptic relay. Postganglionic neurons innervate effector tissues, but also may terminate within ganglia of the same system, or in relation to its individually distributed neurons, similar to the depiction in the "classical" scheme of postganglionic sympathetic terminations on parasympathetic ganglion cells. Finally, some urogenital nerve fibers may establish infraspinal sensory synapses in the urogenital short neuron system or central ganglia to form organ-to-ganglion-to-organ neural circuits that bypass and function independently of the spinal cord.

Another relatively contemporary concept requires mention for subsequent understanding of studies involving autonomic stiumulation and blockade. For many years the only autonomic neurotransmitters recognized were acetylcholine and norepinephrine. However, it has become obvious that other transmitters might indeed be present in components of the autonomic nervous system. Burnstock (summarized in Burnstock, 1985, 1986) has repeatedly emphasized this concept and the concept of modulatory transmitter mechanisms, including prejunctional inhibition or enhancement of transmitter release, postjunctional modulation of transmitter action, and the secondary involvement of locally synthesized hormones and prostaglandins. Cotransmitters may be released along with a classical neurotransmitter in response to nervous activation and may interact at the level of the receptor and/or second messenger before evoking a functional response. The cotransmitter may have a direct action on postjunctional cells, or may facilitate the action of the classical neurotransmitter or/and act as an inhibitor of its release. Cotransmitter and classical transmitter may be stored in the same vesicle, and therefore be released in a parallel fashion at all impulse frequencies, or be stored in separate vesicle types, in which case differential release at different impulse frequencies might be possible.

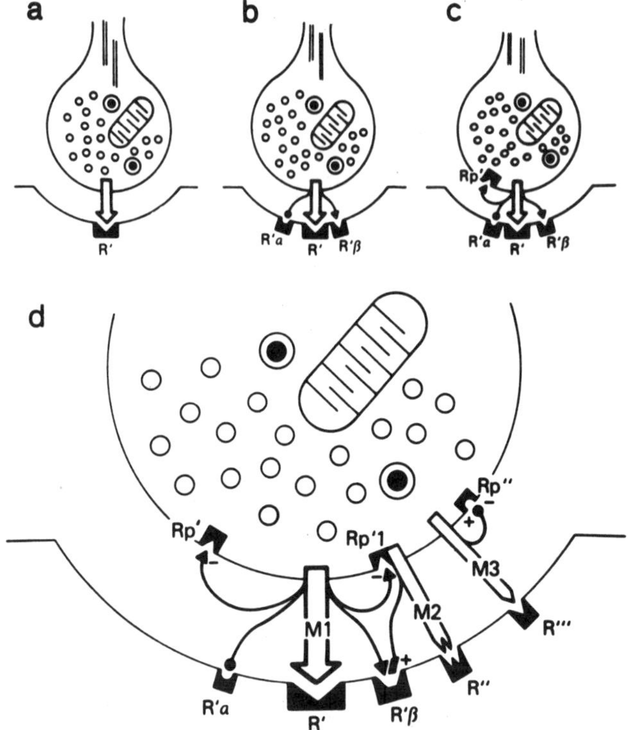

FIG 18.
Development of the concept of chemical neurotransmission. Schematic illustration of the development of the concept of chemical transmission. One transmitter *(a)* acts on one postsynaptic receptor (R′). One transmitter *(b)* acts on multiple types of postsynaptic receptors (R′α,R′β). The transmitter *(c)* acts in addition on a presynaptic receptor (Rp′). Multiple compounds (M1–3), possibly differentially stored in small vesicles (classical transmitter) and in large dense-core vesicles (classical transmitter plus peptide), are released from the same nerve ending *(d)*. The main possible interactions indicated are: (1) inhibition of release of the second messenger (peptide M2) by the classical transmitter (M1) via presynaptic action (Rp′1); (2) interaction at the postsynaptic receptor (R′β) level between M1 and M2; (3) facilitation or inhibition of release of the classical transmitter by the peptide (M3) via action on a presynaptic receptor (Rp″); and (4) activation by the peptide (M3) of electrical activity in the presynaptic neuron via action on a presynaptic receptor (Rp″). (From Lundberg JM, Hokfelt T: Coexistence of peptides and classical neurotransmitters. *Trends Neurol Sci* 1983; 6:325. Used with permission.)

This concept may explain why pharmacologic blockade of classical receptors may only partially abolish the effects of neural stimulation. These somewhat complicated concepts and possibilities are nicely summarized in a diagram by Lundberg and Hökfelt (1983) (Fig 18).

NEUROTRANSMISSION AND RECEPTORS

Although smooth muscle cell contraction can occur via excitation in a variety of different ways (see previous discussion), the classical model involves synaptic release of a neurotransmitter in response to neural stimulation, with subsequent conbination of the transmitter agent with a recognition site, or receptor, on the postsynaptic smooth muscle cell membrane. The transmitter receptor combination then initiates changes in the postsynaptic effector cell, which ultimately result in what we consider to be the "characteristic" effect of that particular neurotransmitter. Although other mechanisms exist, classical synaptic neurotransmission involves a vesicular-exocytotic mechanism (see Cooper and Meyer, [1984] for review). According to this theory, an action potential initiates an influx of calcium ions into the presynaptic nerve terminal, resulting in a process of exocytosis of the neurotransmitter in the presynaptic nerve terminal. The molecular mechanism for this remains obscure.

Clinicians are often confused because they assume that the terms "sympathetic" and "parasympathetic" necessarily imply particular neurotransmitters. As previously stated, these terms imply strictly anatomic origin, whereas in both subsystems of the autonomic nervous system other adjectives are used to describe the nature of the neurotransmitter involved in the chemical transmission of impulses from nerve to smooth muscle.

Cholinergic Receptor Sites

The term "cholinergic" refers to those receptor sites at which acetylcholine is the neurotransmitter. Peripheral cholinergic fibers are thought to include somatic motor fibers, all preganglionic autonomic fibers, and all postganglionic parasympathetic fibers. Classically, cholinergic receptor sites have been subdivided into two major classes: muscarinic and nicotinic receptors. These divisions are based on the original observations that the alkaloid muscarine mimics the effects of acetylcholine at some cholinergic sites, while low doses of nicotine mimic the effects of acetylcholine at other sites. Muscarinic sites include all autonomic effector cells (postsynaptic autonomic cholinergic receptors), whereas nicotinic sites are located on autonomic ganglia and motor end plates of skeletal muscle. These nicotinic sites are not identical. Atropine competitively inhibits muscarinic receptors, whereas high doses of nicotine inhibit nicotinic sites. Large concentrations of atropine may, in addition to blocking muscarinic receptors, exert some inhibitory effect on nicotinic receptors as well.

During the last ten years there have been major technical advances in receptor physiology and pharmacology, including the development of highly specific agonists and antagonists, along with specific radioligands to label and quantitate these, and more exact characterization of the intracellular changes that occur as a result of receptor-effector coupling. Although the identification of receptor subtypes may be confusing at times, the concept does provide a basis to explain the differing actions sometimes exhibited by a neurotransmitter at different effector junctions, and also offers the opportunity for the development of more selective pharmacologic tools for the therapy of effector dysfunctions. The distinction between nicotinic and muscarinic cholinergic receptors has already been mentioned. There are at least two subtypes of muscarinic receptors: M_1 and M_2 (Hammer and Giachetti, 1982; Eglen and Whiting, 1985). The M_1 class was originally defined as exhibiting a high affinity toward the antagonist pirenzepine, and was thought to be located primarily in the central nervous system, while M_2 receptors were described as exhibiting a low affinity toward this antagonist and thought to be located mainly on peripheral effector organs. Further subclassification (an M_3 receptor has already been proposed) will doubtless occur (Nilvebrant, 1986).

Events at the cholinergic neuromuscular junction were described by Burnstock (1974) and Burnstock and Bell (1977) and summarized by Benson (1983) (Fig 19). Acetylcholine is synthesized from acetyl coenzyme A and choline by the enzyme choline acetyltransferase (*a* in Fig 19). It is then stored in agranular vesicles (*b*) and is released from the nerve terminal into the synaptic cleft with nerve stimulation (*c*). It then diffuses to receptor sites on the smooth muscle membrane (*d*). Inactivation is due primarily to local hydrolysis by postjunctional acetylcholinesterase (*e*). A small fraction may diffuse away to be hydrolyzed elsewhere in the effector or in the general circulation. Active reuptake of choline by the nerve terminal does occur (*f*) but active reuptake of acetylcholine does not.

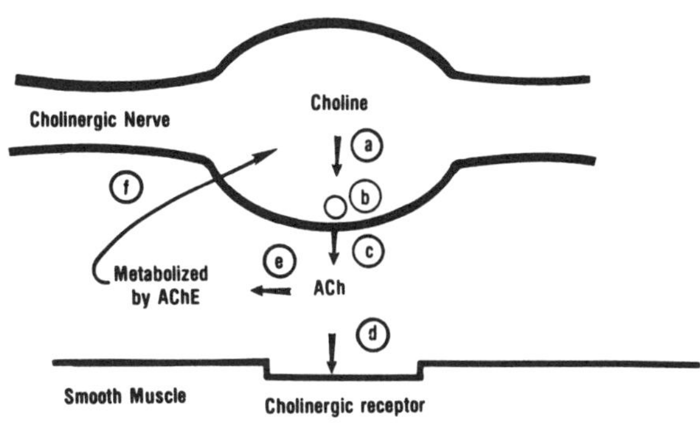

FIG 19.
Events at the peripheral cholinergic nerve terminal. See text for more detailed description. (From Benson GS: Mechanisms of autonomic drug action on the bladder outlet, in Hinman F Jr (ed): *Benign Prostatic Hypertrophy*. Berlin, Springer-Verlag, 1983. Used with permission.)

Adrenergic Receptor Sites

Receptor sites at which a catecholamine is the neurotransmitter are termed adrenergic and include most postganglionic sympathetic fibers (including those to the lower urinary tract smooth muscle), where the catecholamine responsible for neurotransmission is norepinephrine. Adrenergic receptor sites are further classified as α or β on the basis of the differential effects elicited by a series of catecholamines (see Wein and Raezer, [1979] for references). Classically, α-adrenergic effects consist of vasoconstriction and contraction of the smooth musculature. These effects are stimulated most potently by norepinephrine and methoxamine and cannot be elicited by isoproterenol. α-Adrenergic effects were described originally as being inhibited by phentolamine and phenoxybenzamine, though a number of other selective inhibitors now exist. β-Adrenergic effects are classically considered to include cardiac stimulation, vasodilation, bronchodilatation, and other types of smooth muscle relaxation. These effects are stimulated most potently by isoproterenol, less so by epinephrine, and least by norepinephrine.

Events at the peripheral adrenergic neuromuscular junction have been described by Burnstock (1974) and Burnstock and Bell (1977) and summarized by Benson (1983) (Fig 20). Norepinephrine is synthesized from tyrosine through steps involving the synthesis of dopa and do-

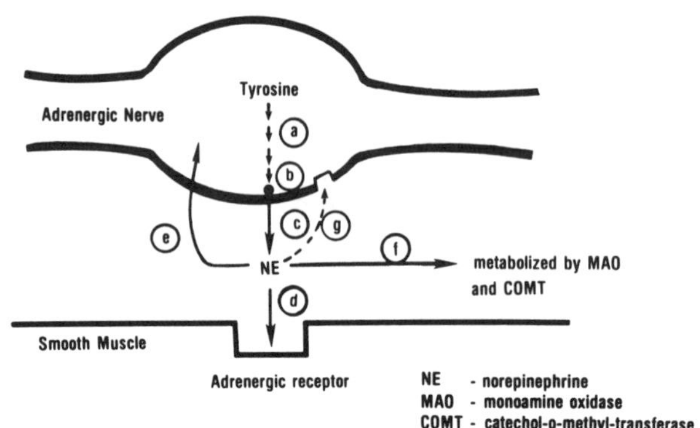

FIG 20.
Events at the peripheral adrenergic nerve terminal. See text for more detailed description. (From Benson GS: Mechanisms of autonomic drug action on the bladder outlet, in Hinman F Jr (ed): *Benign Prostatic Hypertrophy*. Berlin, Springer-Verlag, 1983. Used with permission.)

pamine. The rate-limiting step is the tyrosine hydroxylase–induced transformation of tyrosine to dopa (*a* in Fig 20). The norepinephrine is then stored in granular vesicles (*b*), and in response to a nerve stimulus, the transmitter is released from the nerve terminal (*c*) and diffuses to a receptor site on the smooth muscle membrane (*d*). Inactivation occurs largely through active reuptake into peripheral nerve terminals (*e*), where granular reincorporation and/or degradation by monamine oxidase and catechol-O-methyltransferase occurs. Inactivation also occurs to a lesser extent by uptake into smooth muscle cells, where enzymatic inactivation occurs, and by similar enzymatic inactivation in other tissues, primarily the liver and kidneys. Site *g* in Figure 20 depicts the ability of norepinephrine to interact with presynaptic receptors and thereby regulate its own rate of release from the nerve terminal (see below). In the adrenal medulla, an additional synthetic change occurs—the synthesis of epinephrine from norepinephrine by the enzyme phenylethanolamine-*N*-methyltransferase.

Much attention has been paid to the identification and subclassification of adrenergic receptor subtypes. α-Adrenergic receptors were originally classified into two subtypes, defined by their anatomic location on presynaptic and postsynaptic sites (Berthelson and Pettinger, 1977; Lavin et al., 1981; Kalsner, 1984; Ruffolo, 1984; Wein, 1986 [and references contained therein]). Presynaptic α-receptors were thought to mediate feedback inhibition of the release of norepinephrine from nerve terminals (site *g* in Fig 20), whereas postsynaptic receptors were thought to mediate the typical responses exhibited by effector organs, such as smooth muscle contraction. Originally, postsynaptic receptors were termed α_1, and presynaptic autoreceptors termed α_2. Phentolamine and phenoxybenzamine are both nonspecific α-adrenergic antagonists and, like dihydroergocryptine, bind to both α_1 and α_2 sites. Prazosin is a relatively selective antagonist of α_1 receptor sites, whereas rauwolscine and yohimbine are relatively selective antagonists of α_2 sites. The agonist clonidine appears to selectively bind to α_2 receptor sites. Although the anatomic subclassification of presynaptic as equivalent to α_2 and postsynaptic as equivalent to α_1 subtype is generally true, recent studies have indicated that not all α_1-adrenergic receptors are located postsynaptically, and not all α_2 adrenergic receptors are located presynaptically.

β-Adrenergic receptors are generally likewise agreed to exist in two forms (see references in Minneman and Molinoff, 1980; Lefkowitz et al., 1984). β_1-Adrenergic receptors are postsynaptic, produce an increase in the rate and force of cardiac contraction, and stimulate lipolysis and amylase secretion by salivary glands. Norepinephrine is considered to have a selectivity for β_1 receptors, and epinephrine for β_2, whereas isoproterenol has no distinct selectivity but is a more potent stimulator (effective at lower concentrations) of both subtypes. Propranolol and alprenolol antagonize both β_1 and β_2 effects, but β_1 effects are preferentially inhibited by metoprolol and betaxolol. β_2-Adrenergic receptors are present both presynaptically and postsynaptically. They mediate smooth muscle relaxation in bronchi, blood vessels, and the genitourinary and gastrointestinal tracts; facilitate norepinephrine release from presynaptic nerve terminals; increase glycogenolysis in liver and muscle; increase gluconeogenesis in liver; increase insulin and glucagon secretion by pancreatic cells; and stimulate renin release by juxtaglomerular cells in the kidney. β_2-Adrenergic receptors are also selectively stimulated by salbutamol and soterenol.

Signal transduction from receptor to effector mechanism is thought to depend on adenyl cyclase stimulation in the case of β receptors, on inhibition of adenyl cyclase or an increased calcium influx through the cell membrane in the case of α_2 effects, and on alteration of cellular calcium ion fluxes for α_1 (perhaps an increased release of intracellular calcium) (Andersson, 1985) and muscarinic cholinergic receptors. In dog bladder body muscle strips Rohner and Hannigan (1980) have shown that β-adrenergic–induced relaxation (and that induced by theophylline) increases cAMP content. Contractions in response to cholinergic and α-adrenergic stimulation were not associated with changes in cAMP.

Other Receptors

Excitatory and inhibitory effects are produced by various endogenous compounds in the central and peripheral nervous system in addition to acetylcholine and norepinephrine. Some of these substances may serve as modulators of transmission rather than as actual excitatory or inhibitory neurotransmitters. It should be noted, however, that when a proposed transmitter substance causes a tissue to respond, this does not necessarily imply that the tissue is innervated under normal circumstances by nerves releasing that substance. Specific criteria must be satisfied before a substance can be established as a neurotransmitter in a particular tissue (Burnstock, 1977, 1985, 1986; Wein and Raezer, 1979). This mistake is often made in the urologic literature, i.e., ascribing neurotransmitter status to a substance that is simply active in an in vitro or in vivo preparation. Substances besides acetylcholine and norepinephrine that have been proposed as neurotransmitters are listed in Table 1. Those that are particularly relevant to lower urinary tract function are discussed in subsequent sections.

TABLE 1.
Proposed Neurotransmitters and Neuromodulators in Addition to Acetylcholine and Norepinephrine*

	Central	Peripheral
Adenosine triphosphate (ATP)		X
Prostaglandins (F_2, E, E_2)		X
Peptides		
Opioids	X	X
Vasoactive intestinal polypeptide (VIP)	X	X
Substance P	X	X
Neuropeptide Y		X
Somatostatin		X
Bradykinin		X
Amines and amino acids		
Dopamine	X	X
Serotonin	X	X
Histamine	X	X
γ-Amino butyric acid (GABA)	X	X
Glycine	X	X
Glutamate	X	X
Taurine	X	
Proline		X
Carnosine		X
Octopamine		X

*Data from Wein and Raezer, 1979; Anderson and Sjogren, 1982; Hald and Bradley, 1982; Burnstock, 1985.

DENERVATION

When smooth muscle is denervated its sensitivity to neurohumoral transmitters increases, and the increase is greater when postganglionic rather than preganglionic fibers are destroyed (Wein and Raezer, 1979). The resultant supersensitivity of smooth muscle so produced has been elegantly reviewed by Westfall (1981), and has direct potential application to the lower urinary tract. Supersensitivity may be experimentally manifested by one of three states: (1) the maximal response of a tissue may increase with no change in the dose required to produce a response that is 50% of maximum (ED_{50}); (2) there may be a decrease in the ED_{50} with no change in the maximum response; and (3) there may be both an increase in the maximum response and a decrease in the ED_{50}. Westfall divides supersensitivity into two broad categories. Deviation supersensitivity implies an increased percentage of the administered drug or neurotransmitter reaching the receptors. It does not involve a change in the actual responsiveness of target cells. This type of change is termed "prejunctional" in some of the older (and current) literature. This type of change usually develops relatively rapidly, and is specific for a given agonist or neurotransmitter. The mechanisms involved are either a loss of neuronal uptake or inactivation mechanisms or loss of extraneuronal uptake or inactivation mechanisms. Nondeviation supersensitivity, sometimes called postjunctional or postsynaptic, involves an actual change in the responsiveness of the effector (smooth muscle) cells. This type of response generally requires time to develop, several days up to weeks. It is a nonspecific type response in that drugs besides the specific neurotransmitter originally involved may likewise produce a supersensitive response. The mechanism seems to be related to a chronic interruption, pharmacologic or surgical, of the normal pattern of neurotransmission to effector cells. In other words, it is a consequence of a chronic decrease in the normal contact between an excitatory neurotransmitter and its effector cells. It is intriguing to speculate that some receptor alteration may be involved, but studies have shown no change in receptor affinity, and thus far no increase in receptor density in smooth muscle, though such an increase does occur in skeletal muscle. There appears to be some electrophysiologic alteration that, in some smooth muscles, involves a change in the state of depolarization—the resting potential is decreased but the threshold potential is not changed so that the magnitude of depolarization necessary to move the membrane potential from resting to threshold is decreased. Sensitivity of the effector would then be expected to increase to any agonist that induces contraction by cell membrane depolarization. If this is so, the ED_{50} should decrease. Another possibility is that the threshold potential itself may increase (become less negative and require less depolarization to achieve). An increase in maximum response may also occur because of what is termed an improvement in the electrical coupling between cells, leading to enhanced synchronization of agonist-induced contractions. Alterations in calcium homeostasis may also play a part in the development of non-deviation supersensitivity at the molecular level.

It should be remembered that when we speak of "denervation" regarding the lower urinary tract, that we are more often talking about "decentralization." Denervation implies a loss of the postsynaptic neuron that innervates the muscle, whereas decentralization refers to the loss of intermediate neuron(s) between the central nervous system and the final postsynaptic neuron. Because of the nature of the short neuron system innervating the smooth muscle of the bladder and urethra, surgical "denervation" distal to the spinal cord generally affects only nerves that are proximal to the ganglia from which originate the final postganglionic efferent neurons.

Peripheral Innervation of the Lower Urinary Tract

GROSS NEUROANATOMY

The pelvic and hypogastric nerves supply the bladder and urethra with efferent parasympathetic and sympathetic neurons, and both convey afferent (sensory) neurons from these organs to the spinal cord (Fig 21) (Bors and Comarr, 1971; Bradley et al., 1974; Fletcher and Bradley, 1978; Bradley and Sundin, 1982; El Badawi, 1982, 1983). The parasympathetic efferent supply is classically described as originating in the intermediolateral region of the gray matter of sacral spinal cord segments S2–4, and emerges as preganglionic fibers in the ventral nerve roots. This parasympathetic preganglionic supply is ultimately conveyed by the pelvic nerve, which courses deep in the pelvis on each side of the rectum as three or four trunks in man. Efferent sympathetic nerves to the bladder and urethra are thought to originate in the intermediolateral nuclei of spinal cord segments T11–L2 (Norlen, 1982), although El Badawi (1982) mentions only an upper and midlumbar origin. These nerves traverse lumbar sympathetic (paravertebral) ganglia and branches of these ganglia join the presacral nerve (superior hypogastric plexus), which is a plexiform nerve arrangement in the lumbosacral area anterior to the aorta. This divides into the right and left hypogastric nerves, each of these actually being an elongated plexus. Bilaterally, at a variable distance from the bladder and urethra the hy-

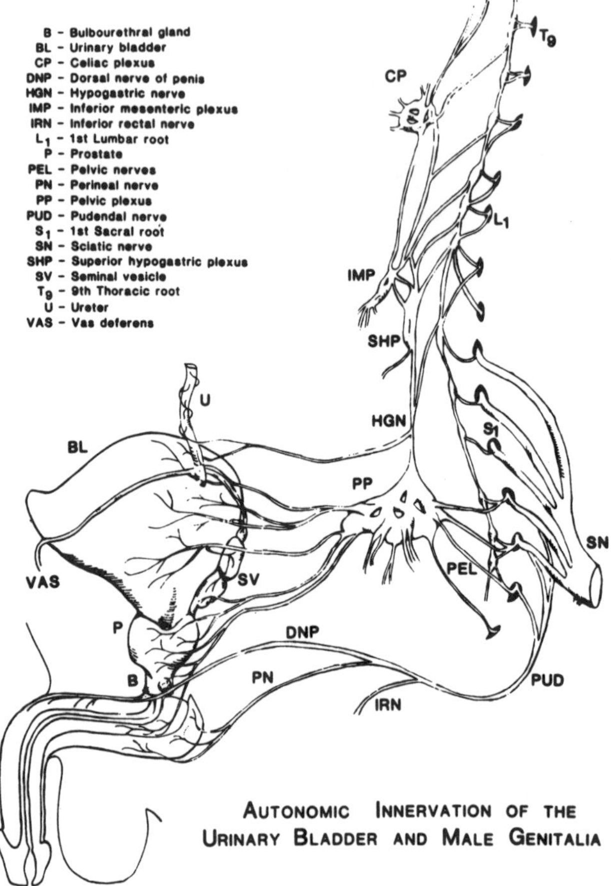

FIG 21.
Autonomic innervation of the lower urinary tract (in the male). (From DeGroat WC, Booth AM: Autonomic systems to the urinary bladder and sexual organs, in Dyck PJ, Thomas PK, Lambert EH (eds): *Peripheral Neuropathy.* Philadelphia, WB Saunders, 1984. Used with permission.)

pogastric and pelvic nerves meet and branch to form the pelvic plexus, sometimes known as the inferior hypogastric plexus or plexus of Frankenhauser. This is a plexus of freely interconnected nerves in the pelvic fascia that is lateral to the rectum, internal genitalia, and lower urinary organs. Divergent branches of this plexus innervate these pelvic organs. Afferent neurons are conveyed by both the hypogastric and pelvic nerves to the dorsal columns of the lumbosacral spinal cord. Most of the afferent fibers reach the spinal cord through dorsal nerve roots, but some through ventral roots (El Badawi, 1982, 1983). As would be expected, the main trunks of both nerves contain nonmyelinated (preganglionic efferent) and myelinated (sensory) nerve fibers.

As has been previously mentioned, the actual neuronal innervation of bladder and urethral smooth muscle emanates from ganglia, which theoretically may be located anywhere between the spinal cord and organ of innervation. Ganglia that innervate the bladder and urethral smooth musculature generally lie close to or within these structures, and give rise to "short neurons," which comprise the bulk of the nerves that actually innervate these structures. All peripheral ganglia are composed of cholinergic, adrenergic, and small intensely fluorescent cells, and represent one morphological substrate in which modulation of one neural component by another can occur. Dixon et al. (1983) feel that the intramural autonomic ganglion cells of the bladder (at least those in the dome and lateral walls) possess only cholinergic neurons, and distinguish these from those in the pelvic plexus. Other authors have not made this distinction.

Efferent innervation of the striated sphincter is likewise classically thought to emanate from the sacral spinal cord, via the pudendal nerve (Fletcher and Bradley, 1978; El Badawi, 1982, 1983). However, some think that the striated sphincter is innervated primarily by the autonomic nervous system through the hypogastric plexus (Donker et al., 1982), while Gosling thinks that the slow-twitch fibers in both the intramural and extramural component of the striated sphincter are innervated by somatic fibers within the pelvic nerve (1979). In the cat at least, El Badawi and others (El Badawi and Schenk, 1974; El Badawi, 1982, 1983; El Badawi and Atta, 1985) think that the intramural component of the striated sphincter possesses somatic and autonomic (both cholinergic and adrenergic) innervation. It is interesting to note that using studies employing retrograde axonal transport of horseradish peroxidase, Tanagho et al. (1982) and Morita et al. (1984) came to different conclusions regarding the innervation of the striated sphincter in the dog. Tanagho thought that the pudendal nucleus was the only motor center, whereas Morita et al. thought that the pelvic nerve might contain some somatic fibers innervating the striated sphincter. Electrophysiologic studies in the human by Vodusek and Light (1983) seemed to show that the intramural component of the striated sphincter is innervated by the pudendal nerve, but the authors did not exclude the possibility that the autonomic nervous system also innervates this muscle. These somewhat contradictory (and therefore confusing) views of the neural supply of the striated sphincter are summarized in Table 2.

TABLE 2.
Nerve Supply of the Striated Sphincter (Intramural and Extramural)

View	Selected References
Pudendal nerve only (both components, somatic fibers only)	Traditional (see text) Fletcher and Bradley (1978) Kluck (1980) Tanagho et al. (1982)
Pelvic plexus only (both components)	Gil Vernet (1968) Donker et al. (1982)
Pudendal nerve—fast-twitch fibers (extramural only)	Gosling (1979)
Pelvic nerve—slow-twitch fibers (both components, somatic fibers only)	
Somatic via pudendal nerve	El Badawi (1982, 1983) El Badawi and Atta (1985)
Autonomic cholinergic via pelvic nerve Autonomic adrenergic via hypogastric, perhaps pelvic and pudendal nerve	

BLADDER AND URETHRAL SMOOTH MUSCLE

Abundant cholinergic innervation of the bladder has been demonstrated by histochemical and ultrastructural technology in a variety of experimental animals (El Badawi and Schenk, 1968, 1974; Raezer et al., 1973; Alm and Elmer, 1975; Fletcher and Bradley, 1978; El Badawi, 1982). There is some disagreement as to regional variation of the degree of innervation. At this time there does not seem to be any clear consensus regarding this (El Badawi, 1982), and functionally these subtleties would seem unimportant, because of the overall relative abundance of the cholinergic innervation. These observations regarding cholinergic innervation in animals seem to be applicable to and to extend at least into the proximal urethra (El Badawi, 1982; Ekstrom and Malmberg, 1984). Adrenergic innervation of the bladder and urethral smooth musculature has been likewise extensively studied in animals using similar techniques (El Badawi and Schenk, 1966 and 1968; Oman et al., 1971; Raezer et al., 1973; Wein et al., 1974; Alm and Elmer, 1975; Benson et al., 1976; Fletcher and Bradley, 1978; El Badawi, 1982). These animal studies show that the smooth musculature of the bladder base and proximal urethra has a rich adrenergic innervation, while the bladder body has sparse but definite such innervation. The density of innervation seems in all areas to be less than that of the cholinergic system.

Studies of cholinergic and adrenergic nerve endings in the smooth muscle of the human bladder and urethra have produced inconsistent conclusions. Ek et al. (1977) described an abundance of cholinergic nerves in all parts of the bladder musculature of both sexes, and a similar less extensive cholinergic innervation of the urethra. Kluck (1980), Daniel et al. (1983) and Gosling (1984) supported this view of an extensive cholinergic innervation of the human bladder body smooth musculature. Gosling stated that this type of cholinergic innervation extended throughout the human bladder base, except for what he termed the "superficial trigonal muscle," an area that he considers to be of little functional significance. Gosling made a distinction between the bladder neck and what others term the "bladder base," and he noted that bladder neck smooth muscle is histologically, histochemically, and pharmacologically distinct from the remainder of the bladder. He described the male bladder neck as having a very sparse cholinergic innervation, but the female bladder neck as being supplied with cholinergic fibers (1979, 1985). Kluck (1980) described the trigonal musculature (of at least the male) as having a relatively sparse distribution of cholinergic nerves, but described cholinergic innervation of the remainder of the bladder base and of at least the ventral part of the urethra, with no differences between male and female.

Mobley et al. (1966) described adrenergic fibers in the anterior wall of the human bladder; Sundin et al. (1977) and Benson et al. (1979) showed clear evidence of sparse but definite innervation of the human bladder body. Kluck (1980), however, did not find adrenergic innervation in the human female bladder body, while Daniel et al. (1983) found that small granular vesicles (presumably adrenergic) were the predominant vesicle type in approximately 15% of the nerve profile seen before 5-hydroxydopamine treatment (which generally makes adrenergic fibers more prominent), and 23% afterward. Both Ek et al. (1977) and Sundin et al. (1977) described a dense adrenergic innervation of the human trigone. Nordling (1983) stated that superficial trigonal musculature possesses a moderately dense adrenergic innervation (though ascribes little anatomic mass or significant function to this area), and that an otherwise sparse supply of adrenergic nerves exists in the bladder base. Norlen (1982) agreed with this. The male bladder neck was described by Gosling (1985) and Kaneko et al. (1980) as possessing a rich adrenergic innervation, but Kluck (1980), in specimens that he described as being from the dorsal part of the male bladder neck, failed to find adrenergic nerve fibers. Gosling (1985) found human female bladder neck to contain relatively few adrenergic nerves; no other authors have made definite statements about the morphology of this area in the female. Kluck (1980) reported no adrenergic innervation of the ventral part of the female urethra, but evidence of a sparse adrenergic innervation of his only biopsy sample of anterior female urethra. Gosling stated that the smooth muscle of the female urethra is associated with relatively few adrenergic nerves, but that the preprostatic urethra in the male possesses a rich adrenergic innervation (1984).

El Badawi (1985) wisely commented on the extreme heterogeneity of findings related to cholinergic and adrenergic innervation of the human lower urinary tract. He stated that all human material thus far studied morphologically cannot be considered as representative of the adult norm in either sex for a variety of reasons, and cautioned likewise against the unqualified acceptance of the existence of sex differences in vesicourethral innervation, without further confirmation of standardly processed truly "normal" specimens. The functional aspects of adrenergic and cholinergic stimulation will be discussed subsequently, but an obvious question to ask is, how much of a particular type of innervation is actually necessary to subserve a physiologic function, and the answer, of course, is unknown.

Other neuroactive substances have been identified in the autonomic nerves supplying the lower urinary tract. Leucine enkephalin was found present in preganglionic terminals in cat bladder ganglia (deGroat et al., 1983). ATP and a number of peptides have been shown to exist in bladder nerves in a variety of animals and in man (El Badawi, 1982; Gu et al., 1984; Mundy, 1984b). These other peptides include vasoactive intestinal polypeptide (VIP), substance P, and neuropeptide Y and somatostatin. An independent purinergic (Burnstock et al., 1972) and peptidergic (Alm et al., 1977) population of efferent autonomic nerves has been postulated, but El Badawi (1982) stated that no unequivocal morphologic evidence exists that such nerves exist as a separate and independent population in the bladder or urethra smooth musculature. He pointed out that although these substances may function as neurotransmitters or neuromodulators, the vesicles containing them may simply be stored in an otherwise classical cholinergic or adrenergic nerve (1982).

STRIATED SPHINCTER

Most authors agree that the striated sphincter, including both components—the intramural (intrinsic) and extramural (extrinsic)—is innervated only through motor end plates, implying purely somatic innervation, though there may be differences in opinion regarding the actual nerve trunks carrying these fibers (Fletcher and Bradley, 1978; Gosling, 1979, 1984). El Badawi reviewed his evidence for triple innervation (somatic plus cholinergic and adrenergic autonomic) of the intramural striated sphincter of the male cat (1982) and updated this with ultrastructural evidence of such innervation in the same species (El Badawi and Atta, 1985). Additionally, his laboratory (Atta and El Badawi, 1985) studied the effects of bilateral ventral sacral rhizotomy and found that autonomic cholinergic and adrenergic innervation was preserved (and exhibited sprouting), whereas somatic axons totally degenerated. Morphologic evidence of autonomic innervation of the striated sphincter has not yet been demonstrated in other species or in man (Fletcher and Bradley, 1978; Gosling, 1979, 1984; Wein et al., 1979; Kluck, 1980). El Badawi (1982) pointed out that his conclusions are applicable only to the intramural portion of the striated sphincter, and that other authors' conclusions regarding the intramural component may have been erroneously drawn from specimens from the adjacent extramural component. Further studies will obviously be necessary to settle this question.

SENSORY INNERVATION

Afferent nerve fibers have been demonstrated in the pelvic, pudendal, and hypogastric nerves (Kuru, 1965). Fletcher and Bradley (1978) concluded that most vesical afferent axons terminate as free nerve endings, and that no specialized receptors are identifiable, except for sparse pacinian corpuscles. Afferent terminals are found in the submucosa and muscularis; Fletcher and Bradley stated that, in the cat at least, a greater terminal density of afferent fibers to the pelvic nerve exists in the muscularis, while a greater density of afferents to the hypogastric nerve exists in the submucosa (1978). deGroat and Booth (1984) and deGroat and Kawatani (1985) state that afferent fibers subserving the sensation of bladder distention originate in tension receptors in the bladder wall and travel in the pelvic nerves, while mechanoreceptor afferents are present in the hypogastric nerve. Further, according to them, both pelvic and hypogastric afferent pathways carry nociceptive afferents, while afferent pathways from the striated sphincter and from the urethra transmit sensations of temperature, pain, wall distention (urethra), and urine passage, and travel in the pudendal nerve. Fletcher and Bradley (1978) summarized studies in the cat that they interpreted as consistent with the fact that afferents subserving the sensation of distention (and active therefore in evoking micturition), are more prominent in the muscle layer than in the submucosa and are distributed evenly to all regions of the bladder, whereas afferents traveling in the hypogastric nerve are most dense in the trigone and anterior bladder neck region, and subserve the sensations of pain, conscious touch, and distention.

Peripheral, Neural, and Humoral Influences on Lower Urinary Tract Function

CHOLINERGIC RECEPTOR DISTRIBUTION, STIMULATION, AND BLOCKADE

Cholinergic contractile receptor sites that can be blocked by atropine (muscarinic) have been demonstrated in the bladder body and bladder base in the rat (Elmer, 1974), cat (Nergardh and Boreus, 1973; Nergardh, 1975), dog (Leoni et al., 1973; Raezer et al., 1973), rabbit (Levin et al., 1980), and man (Todd and Mack, 1969; Benson et al., 1976; Levin et al., 1983a). Khanna et al. (1981) studied the differential effects of cholinergic stimulation on the different layers of the rabbit bladder body and base. They found that acetylcholine had a marked stimulatory effect on both longitudinal and circular bladder body smooth musculature, a moderate contractile effect on the longitudinal and circular (less so) layers of the bladder base, a weak contractile response from the longitudinal layer of the urethra, and none from the urethral circular layer. In vitro studies of human urethral strips by Ek et al. (1977b) demonstrated a very low contractile response to acetylcholine, and the responses that did occur could be blocked with atropine. Similar data were presented by Persson and Andersson (1976) for the cat and guinea pig. Abdel-Rahman et al. (1983) showed a very minor contractile effect of cholinergic stimulation on the longitudinal and circular smooth muscle of the cat proximal urethra, contrasted with a moderate contractile effect in the bladder. Ekstrom and Malmberg (1984), however, recorded rapid and marked contractile responses of the rat urethra to cholinergic stimulation and felt that these effects were exerted by a direct action on muscarinic receptors.

Levin et al. (1980) found that the response to cholinergic stimulation in the rabbit bladder was not uniform, and was substantially greater in the bladder body than in the bladder base. They were the first to use radioligand-binding technology to quantitate the muscarinic cholinergic receptor density in animal and man (Levin et al., 1980, 1982, 1983a), and found, using tritiated (^{3}H-QNB) as a binding agent, that the distribution of receptor sites was qualitatively similar. Nilvebrant et al. (1983, 1985) confirmed, in the bladder body of the rabbit and human, the presence of a single population of noninteracting binding sites with pharmacologic specificity characteristic of muscarinic receptors. Lepro and Kuhar reported similar findings in the rabbit bladder (1984). Anderson and Marks (1982) reported considerable "spare" cholinergic receptors in the bladder, implying that one could inhibit a significant proportion of muscarinic receptors without affecting cholinergically induced contractile function. Levin et al. (1983c) found no such evidence of spare muscarinic receptors in the rabbit, a finding supported by Nilvebrant et al. (1985) in human bladder. Adami et al. (1985) demonstrated the muscarinic receptors in rat bladder are of the M_2 variety, a finding recently confirmed in our laboratory in both rabbit and human bladder body (Ruggieri et al., 1986).

PARASYMPATHETIC NERVOUS SYSTEM FUNCTION

Stimulation and Blockade

A sustained bladder contraction is produced by stimulation of the pelvic nerves (Ursillo and Clark, 1956; Ingersoll et al., 1957; Gyermek, 1961; Kuru, 1965). It is generally agreed that reflex activation of this pelvic nerve excitatory outflow tract is responsible for the emptying bladder contraction of normal micturition. Whether acetylcholine is the sole neurotransmitter released during such stimulation is highly controversial. Muscarinic blockade only partially antagonized the bladder response to pelvic nerve stimulation (Ambache, 1955; Ursillo and Clark, 1956; Ambache and Zar, 1970; Burnstock et al., 1972; Elmer, 1975). Some urethral responses to pelvic nerve stimulation and cholinergic stimulation have also shown atropine resistance (Tanagho et al., 1969a, 1969b; Nergardh and Boreus, 1973; Khanna et al., 1975). These authors found increased urethral resistance to flow in response to cholinergic stimulation, attributed by Khanna et al. and Nergardh and Boreus to be mediated by intramural ganglion cells belonging to the short adrenergic system. McGuire (1978) and McGuire and Herlihy (1978) presented compelling evidence, however, that urethral smooth muscle relaxation occurs during detrusor activity, and they attributed those apparent increases in urethral "resistance" previously described in response to pelvic nerve stimulation to simple transmission of an intravesical pressure head to an open urethral chamber. They explained that this occurred normally after an initial prevoiding urethral relaxation, following which the bladder and urethra become essentially isobaric. McGuire (McGuire, 1977, 1978; McGuire and Herlihy, 1978, 1979) obviated this experimental problem of pressure transmission by diverting the urinary stream. He then reported urethral smooth muscle relaxation in response to pelvic nerve stimulation, which was blocked after propranolol administration, implying that this is a β-adrenergic response to pelvic nerve and presumably short adrenergic stimulation. This is an important observation, as it forms the basis for one theory of the mechanism of relaxation of the bladder neck and proximal urethra at the onset of voiding.

Field stimulation of isolated bladder strips has been used to reproduce the effects of nerve-mediated activity. Hindmarsh et al. (1977) showed that such electrical stimulation produced contractions in human bladder strips that were only partially blocked by atropine. The variable blockade achieved by atropine of pelvic nerve–induced and field stimulation–induced bladder contractile activity has given rise to an exceptionally large literature having to do with "atropine resistance" of the urinary bladder. In many ways, atropine resistance is a clinically convenient concept, as it can be invoked to explain our clinical difficulty in abolishing involuntary bladder contractions with anticholinergic agents, and it can be invoked also to support the rationale of the treatment of such types of bladder activity with more than one pharmacologic agent with different mechanisms of action (Wein, 1986). Typical examples of such atropine resistance in field-stimulated specimens include data reported by Krell et al. (1981), showing a maximum inhibitory ability of 55%–60% for guinea pig bladder strips, by Nergardh (1981) showing less than 20% inhibition in the cat, by Adami et al. (1985) showing 50% inhibition in the rat, and by Cowan and Daniel (1983) showing 50% inhibition in human female bladder body smooth muscle. Atropine resistance in human bladder muscle, however, is by no means agreed upon, and there is some evidence that it may not in fact occur in normal bladder. Sibley (1984) studied bladder strips from rabbit, pig, and man in the same experimental model. In the rabbit, he found that atropine was at most 56%–64% effective in blocking the response to field stimulation (at higher frequencies only—the response at low frequency was only 14%), and that this atropine-resistant response was completely abolished by the addition of tetrodotoxin, indicating that it was nerve-mediated. In the pig, he found that up to 83% of the contractile response was abolished at higher frequencies of stimulation. In the human, atropine produced an effective blockade at all frequencies of stimulation, with only 1%–7% of the response persisting, and this persistent response was not significantly reduced by tetrodotoxin, indicating that the nerve-mediated contractile responses were purely cholinergic. These human strips were obtained from patients undergoing surgery for lower urinary tract disorders or from patients undergoing donor nephrectomy; no difference was found between specimens from the two sources. Kinder and Mundy (1985a) demonstrated an almost total inhibition by atropine of the response of human bladder body strips to field stimulation. In those strips in which there was some resistance to inhibition by atropine, the residual contractile response to stimulation was only minimally affected by tetradotoxin. The 13 patients from whom the samples were taken all had normal bladder function on urodynamic study. Sjogren et al. (1982) demonstrated marked atropine inhibition (more than 95% at higher concentrations) of field stimulation responses in bladder preparations from young patients and from those undergoing cystectomy for cancer. However, in bladder strips from patients who either had a diagnosis of bladder instability or who exhibited bladder hypertrophy, atropine was markedly less effective, a maximum inhibitory effect of approximately 50% being obtained. The reasons for this were not obvious, but it is tempting to speculate that noncholinergic nonadrenergic activation of the contractile apparatus may be more prominent in patients with bladder dysfunction than in those with normal bladder function.

Atropine Resistance and the Role of Adenosine Triphosphate

Many theories have been proposed to explain those instances of the relative insensitivity of bladder contractility, elicited by pelvic nerve or field strip stimulation, to atropine. Historically these hypotheses have included the following: (1) that at least some of the cholinergic receptors in the bladder are nicotinic rather than muscarinic (Gyermek, 1961); (2) that the nerve impinges so closely on the muscarinic receptor complex that atropine cannot penetrate this sufficiently to produce complete inhibition (Ursillo and Clark, 1956; Elmer, 1975; Carpenter, 1977); and (3) that a major portion of the parasympathetic transmission is noncholinergic (and nonadrenergic) (Ambache and Zar, 1970; Burnstock, 1972; Johns and Paton, 1976). Most contemporary literature points to hypothesis no. 3 as the most probable explanation of this phenomenon. In this regard, ATP (Burnstock et al., 1972; Burnstock, 1985, 1986) and prostaglandins (Kuru, 1965; Johns and Paton, 1976) have been the substances most frequently proposed as noncholinergic nonadrenergic parasympathetic neurotransmitters. Burnstock (1972, 1977, 1985, 1986) has provided evidence that ATP is an excitatory neurotransmitter involved in the bladder response to pelvic nerve stimulation. Further, he has proposed that this concept explains atropine resistance in those species where it in fact does occur. In 1978 he and co-workers presented evidence (quinacrine fluorescence histochemistry) of what were presumed to be purinergic nerves in the guinea pig urinary bladder and evidence that field stimulation produced a bladder contraction that was predominantly noncholinergic, associated with ATP release, and, further, that the release could be blocked by tetrodotoxin but not by adrenergic nerve destruction (Burnstock et al., 1978a, 1978b). Downie and Dean (1977) and Dean and Downie (1978) showed that a noncholinergic excitatory substance was involved in motor neurotransmission in rabbit bladder and concluded that this probably was ATP. Further work from Burnstock's laboratory (Kasakov and Burnstock, 1983) showed that mechanical responses to ATP and field stimulation in guinea pig bladder strips were simultaneously abolished after desensitization of these strips by a slowly degradable analogue of ATP, α, β-methylene ATP. Recent studies have shown that desensitization with this compound blocks not only the atropine-resistant contractile response to field stimulation but the atropine-resistant excitatory junction potential as well (Hoyle and Burnstock, 1985). Arylazido aminopropionyl ATP ($ANAPP_3$) is a photoaffinity analogue of ATP that antagonizes contractile responses to it. Theobald (1983) reported that this compound blocks ATP-induced contractions in the cat urinary bladder. Most recently, he has shown this antagonism is restricted to one purinergic receptor subtype (P_2 as opposed to P_1; see Theobald [1986] and Burnstock [1986] for discussion). Theobald has looked quite carefully at the bladder response in this animal to parasympathetic nerve–induced contraction. Two distinct components could be observed. The initial or first response was a sharp transient spiked rise in pressure (phase 1), as opposed to a second phase that consisted of a tonic maintenance of contraction during stimulation. This second phase was maintained at a certain level or fell slowly to a lower pressure level as long as the pelvic nerves were stimulated. He showed that $ANAPP_3$ partially blocked the first phase of the response to parasympathetic nerve–induced contraction. Atropine had no effect on phase 1 response or on ATP-induced contraction, but blocked the second phase of the pelvic nerve contraction, changing the character of this response so that it resembled that of an ATP-induced contraction. These data indicate that the second phase of the pelvic nerve–induced contraction is atropine-sensitive and produced by the release of acetylcholine. These data also suggest that acetylcholine is not solely responsible for the first phase of the nerve–induced contraction, but that ATP, released by pelvic nerve stimulation, is at least partially responsible for this event. The fact that the first phase of pelvic nerve–induced contraction is only partially antagonized by $ANAPP_3$ while ATP-induced contractions are completely antagonized suggests further that there may be another transmitter involved in the first phase of these contractions. This other transmitter may be acetylcholine or another neurotransmitter released on pelvic nerve stimulation (Theobald, 1983). Maggi et al. (1985c) came to similar conclusions regarding two components of the twitch response to field stimulation of rat bladder strips. They found that the inhibition of atropine of the second or tonic component was much greater (over 60%) than of the early or phasic component (less than 10%). Both were almost completely inhibited by tetrodotoxin.

Levin et al. (1986) likewise found that the response of their whole bladder model responded to field stimulation with a biphasic response: an initial rapid rise in tension followed by a plateau period of increased intravesical pressure. Functionally, virtually all bladder emptying occurred during the plateau period. Although purinergic stimulation accounted for approximately 50% of the initial phase of bladder contraction, because of the phasic nature of the purinergic response, it mediated virtually no bladder emptying. These authors concluded that whereas purinergic stimulation may play a role in initiating micturition, bladder emptying appears to be primarily a cholinergic phenomenon. Further, work from this laboratory has shown that β,γ-methylene ATP is approximately 100 times more potent than ATP itself in stimulating this initial phasic contractile activity. Studies on ATPase activity have demonstrated that this activity is too slow to account for this difference in potency, and studies on enzyme kinetics have demonstrated that this analogue of ATP does not bind to ATPase, indicating that purinergic response is not mediated by activation of a surface membrane ATPase (Levin et al., 1983b, 1986). Although high-affinity binding of ^{3}H-ATP to membrane fractions of rabbit bladder has been demonstrated, distribution of these binding sites is not consistent with those of neurotransmitter receptor sites, and probably represents other specific binding sites for ATP.

Nicotine induces an increase in intravesical pressure in cats that is atropine resistant and not mediated either through adrenergic or cholinergic mechanisms. However, Koley et al. (1984) felt that a purinergic mechanism was involved, and in fact quinidine (which is felt under some circumstances to block ATP-induced contractions) and ATP desensitization (which also inhibits the response to subsequent exogenous ATP) abolish the response to nicotine.

PROSTAGLANDINS

In the lower urinary tract, prostaglandins have been prominently mentioned as perhaps having a potential role in excitatory neurotransmission, contractile activity, and, perhaps, an involvement in the response to ATP. Pharmacologic evidence for the role of prostaglandins in bladder contractility has been succinctly and well summarized by Andersson and Sjogren (1982). Evidence that various prostaglandins of the E and F types produce contraction of bladder muscle strips is summarized, and the point made that the contractions were slower in development and with a longer duration than those produced by acetylcholine. These contractions likewise were reported as not influenced by tetrodotoxin, atropine, or phenoxybenzamine (Bultitude et al., 1976; Abrams and Feneley, 1976; Andersson et al., 1977). Khanna et al. (1978) suggested the existence of a specific prostaglandin receptor in the bladder.

Khalaf et al. (1981) showed that distention of the dog bladder and pelvic nerve stimulation both caused a release of prostaglandins. Bultitude et al. (1976) summarized evidence that prostaglandin synthetase inhibitors decreased spontaneous activity and basal tone of the rabbit bladder, effects that were antagonized by prostaglandin $F_{2\alpha}$, suggesting a connection between contractile effects mediated by acetylcholine and by prostaglandins. Johns and Paton (1976) suggested that prostaglandins are liberated during neural excitation of bladder contraction and contribute to the atropine-resistant portion of this response. Andersson and Sjogren (1982) summarized evidence that indicates that it is unlikely that these agents are directly involved in bladder emptying, but more probable that they contribute to tone or spontaneous activity in the bladder muscle, or that they may be modulators of transmission, increasing the release of or the effectiveness of excitatory neurotransmitters.

There is some evidence that prostaglandins may be involved in the contractile response of bladder smooth muscle to ATP. Andersson et al. (1980) showed that the response to ATP in rabbit bladder strips consisted of an initial sharp phasic component, then a tonic maintained component, whereas in the guinea pig, there was only the phasic component. Prostaglandin synthetase inhibitors abolished only the tonic portion in the rabbit and had no effect in the guinea pig. Downie and Larson (1981) found a similar response to ATP in the rabbit, and found further that prostaglandin synthetase inhibition decreased the second tonic portion of the response to 30% of control but did not affect the initial phasic response. Husted et al. (1983) found that indomethacin abolished the second tonic phase of the response of rabbit and human bladder muscle strips to ATP and reduced the first phasic response by about 30%. They pointed out, however, that the ATP response was heavily dependent on extracellular calcium, and therefore that the inhibitory action of indomethacin might be attributable to a calcium antagonist effect rather than to an exclusive effect on prostaglandin synthesis. They also noted parenthetically that hypertrophic detrusor seemed to be more sensitive to the action of ATP than normal detrusor.

Downie and Karmazyn (1984) have presented interesting findings that suggest a different type of contractile influence of prostaglandins on detrusor muscle. They found that mechanical irritation of the epithelium of rabbit bladder increased basal tension and spontaneous activity in response to electrical stimulation of bladder muscle, and that these responses were related to the intensity of the irritative trauma. The effects were mimicked by prostaglandins of the E, F, and I series, and the transfer effect was significantly reduced by pretreatment of the epithelium, but not the muscle, with prostaglandin synthetase inhibitors. Certainly this suggests a potential role of prostaglandins in the pathophysiology of hyperactivity secondary to traumatic changes of the bladder urothelium. These prostaglandin products would be capable of causing muscle contraction per se and enhancing neurotransmission in the muscle layer of the bladder. In a similar vein, Maggi et al. (1984a) found that the ability of various prostaglandin synthetase inhibitors to block rhythmic contractions induced by distention in the rat bladder was proportional to their anti-inflammatory effectiveness. Although prostaglandin release during bladder distention has been classically described as mediated from the muscle layer, it may be that this occurs from the epithelial layer.

It is interesting that at least some prostaglandins have been shown to cause relaxation of urethral preparations as well as increased contractility of bladder. Andersson et al. (1977) showed that prostaglandin E_1 (PGE_1) and PGE_2 relaxed urethral preparations that had been contracted by norepinephrine, epinephrine, or PGF_2. Khalaf et al. (1981)

similarly found that PGE_2 produced a decrease in resting urethral pressure in the dog, and Finkbeiner and Bissada (1981) found that a similar effect was produced in guinea pig by PGE_2, PGE_1, PGF_1, and PGF_2. It should be noted that Finkbeiner and Bissada are the only authors who note relaxation of urethral smooth muscle with PGF_2; all others have noted contraction.

Prostaglandins, then, have been potentially implicated in bladder contractility or tension development that occurs during bladder filling and also in the emptying contractile response of bladder smooth muscle to neural stimulation. It has also been suggested that they are involved in the maintenance of urethral tone during the storage phase of micturition, and also in the release of this tone during bladder contraction. As has been implied, the mechanisms surrounding the maintenance of continence during the filling phase of micturition have not been established, and, also, there is no agreement regarding what causes opening of the bladder outlet with reflex-induced bladder contraction during the emptying phase of micturition. Ito and Kimoto (1985) have suggested the involvement of prostaglandins in maintenance of tension in the rabbit proximal urethra and in its reduction during micturition. They found that indomethacin and a specific prostaglandin antagonist markedly reduced the resting tension of urethral muscle strips and that activation of intrinsic inhibitory nerve fibers failed to evoke muscle relaxation at this reduced muscle tone (after treatment with indomethacin or the specific inhibitor). In other words, the amplitude of muscle relaxation invoked by field stimulation was dependent on the pre-existent level of muscle tone of the urethral strips, and the data indicate that endogenous prostaglandins play a role in maintaining this muscle tone. Electrical field stimulation evoked a phasic contraction followed by relaxation, and guanethidine, phentolamine, and atropine each reduced the amplitude of the electrical changes so produced during the phasic contraction portion of the response as well as of the mechanical responses. The combined application of guanethidine and atropine further reduced the amplitude of these changes. The muscle relaxation phase was not affected by propranolol, phentolamine, guanethidine, or atropine. These results taken together indicate that proximal urethral smooth muscle cells in the rabbit are innervated by adrenergic and cholinergic excitatory fibers, and by noncholinergic, nonadrenergic inhibitory fibers. Thus, the muscle tone of the proximal urethra may be maintained by endogenous prostaglandins and by adrenergic and cholinergic excitatory neural stimuli, and reduction in the muscle tone may occur by the activation of noncholinergic, nonadrenergic inhibitory fibers.

It is interesting that a similar concept of the role of nonadrenergic, noncholinergic inhibitory fibers in the opening of the bladder outlet during micturition was expressed by Andersson et al. (1983) and Klarskov et al. (1983) in closely related articles that appeared within a few months of one another. Andersson et al. showed that field stimulation caused a contraction of isolated rabbit and human urethral smooth muscle when the resting tension was low, and that this response was abolished by tetrodotoxin. The contractions were markedly but not completely reduced by α-adrenergic blockade. When the preparations were contracted by norepinephrine, however, which might mimic the state of the proximal urethra during bladder filling, electrical stimulation produced relaxation, and this response was inhibited by tetrodotoxin, suggesting the involvement of nerves and the release of a relaxation-producing transmitter. The electrically induced relaxation was not blocked by indomethacin, propranolol, acetylcholine, atropine, or metoclopramide. The authors speculated that, during transmural electrical stimulation of the urethra, both excitatory and inhibitory transmitters may be released, and the ultimate effect might depend on initial baseline tension. When the tension is low, the excitatory effect predominates, probably through α-adrenergic neurotransmission and effect. When the tension is increased, which may mimic the physiologic situation during bladder filling, the inhibitory effect of the neurotransmitter is demonstrable. Klarskov et al. (1983) exposed human and pig urethral, bladder neck, and trigonal smooth muscle to field stimulation. Responses were composed of different combinations of relaxation and contraction, but there were no significant consistent differences in the responses from various areas. The configuration of the response was slightly shifted in favor of contraction by β-adrenergic blockade and prostaglandin synthetase inhibition. The reverse effect was seen, with augmentation of the relaxation phase after α-adrenergic blockade and muscarinic cholinergic blockade. Cholinergic blockade had the most pronounced effect and, in some strips, changed a pure contraction into a relaxation. α-Adrenergic blockade diminished the contraction and β-adrenergic blockade inhibited it. Relaxation was slightly diminished, and contractions slightly enhanced, by prostaglandin synthetase inhibition. However, after blockade of all transmitter systems, the major part of the relaxation was still present during electrical field stimulation, and this relaxation phase was totally abolished by tetrodotoxin. It was concluded then that this relaxation phase was nerve mediated through noncholinergic, nonadrenergic, nonprostaglandin transmitter or modulator systems.

ADRENERGIC RECEPTOR DISTRIBUTION, STIMULATION, AND BLOCKADE

Regardless of controversies surrounding the presence or absence of adrenergic innervation, there is general agreement that the smooth muscle of the bladder body, bladder base, and proximal urethra in a variety of animals and in man contains both α-adrenergic receptors and β-adrenergic receptors. Originally, functional studies done on isolated bladder strips showed that responses to β-adrenergic stimulation were greatest in the bladder body, whereas α-adrenergic responses predominated in the bladder base and proximal urethra (Edvardsen, 1968a, 1968b, 1968c, 1968d; Edvardsen and Setekleiv, 1968; Todd and Mack, 1969; Anderson et al., 1971; Rohner et al., 1971; Donker et al., 1972; Leoni et al., 1973; Raezer et al., 1973; Awad et al., 1974; Elmer, 1974; Benson et al., 1976). Some investigators found no smooth muscle response in the bladder body to α-adrenergic stimulation (Nergardh and Boreus, 1972; Sundin et al., 1977). In all other studies, the β-adrenergic effect in this area simply predominated over the α-adrenergic effect. At the bladder neck area, β-adrenergic responses have been found to be weak and inconsistent (Nergardh and Boreus, 1972; Raezer et al., 1973; Caine et al., 1975; Benson et al., 1976). Urethral strips in both humans and animals show a predominance of α-adrenergic responses over β-adrenergic responses with no gradation from the bladder neck, at least through the proximal urethra (Raz et al., 1972a; Ek et al., 1977). Studies have demonstrated that the distribution of α- and β-receptors parallels the functional responses to adrenergic stimulation. β-Adrenergic receptors predominate in the bladder body and α-adrenergic receptors predominate in the bladder base of man, dog, and rabbit (Wein and Levin, 1979; Levin and Wein, 1979a, 1979b; Levin et al., 1980). Attempts to subcategorize the β-adrenergic receptors in bladder body have not produced a great degree of consistency. Nergardh et al. (1977) found the cat bladder body to contain β_1 receptors, whereas they found a third type of β-adrenergic receptor in human bladder, corresponding neither to β_1 nor β_2. Larsen (1979) found β_2-adrenergic receptors in the detrusor muscle of the pig, but also found β-adrenergic receptors in the human bladder with neither β_1 nor β_2 characteristics. Maggi and Meli (1982) found that the rat bladder contains β_2-adrenergic receptors, while Anderson and Marks (1984) found the rabbit bladder body to contain primarily β_2-adrenergic receptors but with a minor population (13%–23%) of classical β_1-adrenergic receptors.

Andersson et al. (1984) used radioligand-binding techniques to evaluate the proportion of α_1- and α_2-adrenergic receptors in female rabbit bladder base and urethra. In membrane preparations, they found 25% α_1- and 75% α_2-adrenergic receptors. Functional experiments of the urethral smooth muscle determined that both α_1 and α_2 subtypes were present postjunctionally, since norepinephrine, phenylephrine, and clonidine all caused contraction; prazosin inhibited norepinephrine-induced contraction by 84%, and rauwolscine by 52%. Larsson et al. (1986) reported that the number of α-adrenergic receptors in the female bladder base and urethra increased toward the urethral meatus, but that this increase was due primarily to a selective increase in the number of α_2-adrenergic receptors. The distal urethra was more responsive to clonidine than the proximal portion (contractile response—indicating postjunctional α_2-adrenergic receptors), while no such difference in responses to norepinephrine occurred. If, as some have suggested (Langer and Shepperson, 1982), the α_2 postsynaptic receptor responds to humoral stimulation, while the α_1 postsynaptic receptor responds to neural stimulation, the two subtypes in the urethra may serve different functions, i.e., a greater tonic-type response in the distal urethra (Larsson et al., 1986). Yablonsky et al. (1986) reported a sex-related difference in regional α subtypes in the rabbit urethra. They found the relative proportion of α_1- and α_2-adrenergic receptors corresponded to 20% and 80% of the total α-adrenergic receptor number in the female (about the same as reported by Andersson et al., 1984), whereas it was 65% and 35% in the male. Additionally, they reported that α_2-adrenergic receptor-binding capacity and affinity were 6.6 times higher and 2 times lower, respectively, in the female than in the male. Mattiasson (1984) found that in the human, however, the urethral contractile response was mediated by postjunctional α_1-adrenergic receptors. He found α_2-adrenergic receptors as well, but these were of the presynaptic autoregulatory type. Similarly, Kunisawa et al. (1985), Honda et al. (1985), and Tsujimoto et al. (1986) reported that postjunctional α_1-adrenergic receptors mediate contractile responses in the human and rabbit bladder base.

SYMPATHETIC NERVOUS SYSTEM FUNCTION

The role of the sympathetic nervous system in lower urinary tract function has been a fertile issue for research, discussion, and debate since the early 1900s. Those who advocate a major role for the sympathetic nervous system in lower urinary tract function generally do so

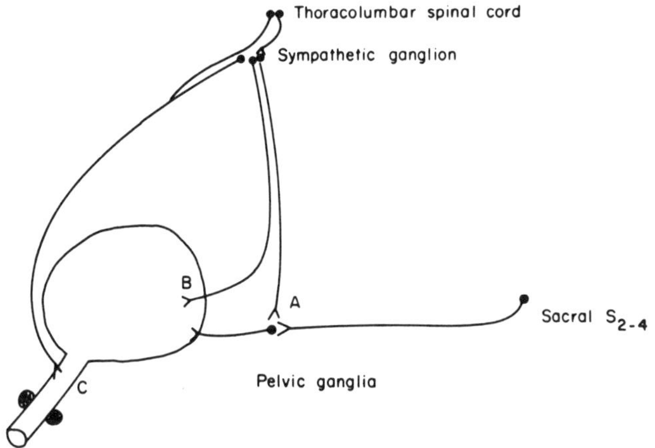

FIG 22.
Summary of potential effects of the sympathetic nervous system on the lower urinary tract. **A,** inhibition of parasympathetic ganglionic transmission. **B,** increased accommodation during filling/storage by stimulation of the predominantly β-adrenergic receptors of the bladder body. **C,** increased outlet resistance by stimulation of the predominantly α-adrenergic receptors of the bladder base and proximal urethra. All tend to facilitate the filling/storage phase of micturition. (From McGuire EJ: Clinical evaluation and treatment of neurogenic vesical dysfunction, in Libertino J (ed): *International Perspectives in Urology*. Baltimore, Williams & Wilkins, 1984. Used by permission.)

along the lines of McGuire's figure (Fig 22), the implications of which have been recently summarized by multiple authors (Wein and Raezer, 1979; Norlen, 1982; El Badawi, 1982; McGuire, 1984a; deGroat and Booth, 1984). According to evidence cited by these authors (which will be summarized below), the sympathetic nervous system acts primarily to facilitate the filling/storage phase of micturition, and does so by three mechanisms: (1) increasing accommodation, by stimulation of the β-adrenergic receptors in the bladder body; (2) increasing outlet resistance, by stimulation of the predominantly α-adrenergic receptors in the bladder base and proximal urethra; and (3) inhibiting bladder contractility via a blocking effect on parasympathetic ganglionic transmission. Evidence to support this view comes mainly from animal experimentation. Inferences are made about human physiology primarily on the basis of (1) similar effects of adrenergic stimulation and blockade on isolated bladder muscle strips; (2) urodynamic studies of bladder and outlet function during filling/storage and emptying in normal individuals, and in individuals with various voiding dysfunctions; and (3) the pathology produced by various lesions of the neural axis thought to result in relatively pure sympathetic neural deficits. There is considerable disagreement, however, regarding the role of the sympathetic nervous system in human lower urinary tract function. Many are of the opinion that it plays a very minor role, and this side of the controversy is well summarized by Tanagho (1978), Gosling (1979), Nordling (1983), and Mundy (1984a).

The results of hypogastric nerve stimulation in different experimental animals are sometimes contradictory, probably because of (1) species differences in the relative densities of α- and β-adrenergic receptors in different areas of the bladders; (2) stimulation of different populations of α- and β-adrenergic receptors according to different stimulus characteristics used by different investigators; (3) varying effects, through ganglionic interactions, on postganglionic cholinergic and nonadrenergic noncholinergic neurons; and (4) the presence of nonadrenergic postganglionic fibers in the hypogastric nerves of some animals. Kuru (1965) summarized experiments in the cat that show that hypogastric stimulation produces an initial transient rise of intravesical pressure, thought to be primarily due to trigonal contraction, followed by inhibition of spontaneous or evoked bladder contractions. deGroat and Saum (1971, 1972, 1976) showed that this inhibition is mediated by two distinct mechanisms: (1) a direct depression of bladder smooth muscle brought about by activation of primarily β-adrenergic receptors and (2) a depression of transmission in parasympathetic ganglionic cells mediated by α-adrenergic receptors. deGroat and Theobald (1976) showed that this inhibitory, sympathetic efferent pathway is activated only by afferent impulses in the pelvic nerves, thought to occur as a response to bladder filling. This is thus a spinal reflex whose efferents were originally thought to emanate from the lower thoracic and upper lumbar spinal cord segments (deGroat, 1975). Recent anatomic and physiologic studies by deGroat's group (Kuo et al., 1984) have shown that the sympathetic pathways to the lower urinary tract of the cat originate in the sacral sympathetic chain as well as in the upper lumbar and inferior mesenteric ganglia. Edvardson (1968a, 1968b) likewise postulated a spinal reflex in the cat—with afferents in the pelvic nerves and efferents in the hypogastric nerves—causing bladder relaxation during filling and, therefore, an increased volume threshold for micturition. Consistent with this hypothesis is the fact that, in the cat, β-adrenergic blockade or surgical sympathectomy has been reported to increase bladder activity, decrease bladder capacity, and produce a shift to the left of the accommodation limb of the cystometric curve (Gjone, 1965; Edvardson, 1968a, 1968b, 1968c, 1968d; deGroat and Saum, 1972; deGroat and Theobald, 1976). Chemical and surgical sympathectomy have been found to produce similar results in the dog (Wein et al., 1974; Nishizawa et al., 1985). Fall et al. (1977) showed that intravaginal electrical stimulation at a low intravesical pressure induced detrusor inhibition in cats via the hypogastric nerve and that this inhibition was eliminated by β-adrenergic blockade. Pudendal nerve afferent stimulation was noted by Sundin et al. (1974) to similarly produce detrusor inhibition in the cat. Creed (1979) showed that hypogastric nerve stimulation in the dog increased urethral pressure, but she also found that this increased bladder pressure as well. The urethral response was attributed to direct adrenergic innervation. The bladder response was attributed to an indirect action via ganglia in the pelvic plexus but also a probable direct action as well. Ohtsuka et al. (1980) stimulated the hypogastric nerve of dogs and observed a rapid transient increase in bladder pressure but an inhibition of bladder contraction induced by stimulation of the pelvic nerve proximal to the pelvic plexus. Two mechanisms of inhibition were thought to exist, one at the level of the ganglia in the pelvic plexus, mediated by α-adrenergic receptors, and one peripherally at or in the bladder wall, mediated by β-adrenergic receptors.

Elliot (1907) reported that the bladder neck of the monkey contracted in response to sympathetic stimulation. Kleeman (1970) reported that electrical stimulation of the presacral nerves and the administration of α-adrenergic agonists caused bladder neck closure in dogs. He also made what seems to be the first observation that sympatholytic drugs were capable of facilitating bladder emptying in certain patients. Krane and Olsson (1973a, 1973b) described the concept of a physiologic internal sphincter, controlled partially via tonic stimulation from the sympathetic nervous system of contractile α-adrenergic receptors in the smooth muscle of the bladder neck and proximal urethra. Awad and Downie (1976a, 1976b, 1977) likewise endorsed the concept of sympathetic nervous system involvement in the continence mechanism at the level of the bladder outlet. McGuire (1984a, 1984b) not only supported the concept of a sympathetically induced β-adrenergically mediated moderating effect on bladder tone during filling, but also endorsed the concept of a major influence of the sympathetic nervous system on proximal urethral activity. His observations were a synthesis of data from the literature plus experimental observations on urethral closure pressure and pressure profiles made in his laboratory on the cat (McGuire, 1977; McGuire and Herlihy, 1978, 1979), and from clinical observations made by him and his associates in patients with nonfunctional bladder outlets (Woodside and McGuire, 1979; McGuire, 1984a, 1984b). He postulated that during bladder filling there was an excitatory influence on urethral closing pressure mediated by the sympathetic nervous system through α-adrenergic receptors. Urethral smooth muscle closure function was felt to be totally independent of preganglionic parasympathetic influences and totally lost when the thoracolumbar sympathetic outflow was destroyed in man. He argued strongly that bladder filling clearly results in a sympathetic motor response, normally resulting in vasomotor changes that are best seen when profoundly augmented in spinal cord injury patients with autonomic hyperreflexia. Further, he stated that smooth sphincter activity increases with bladder filling as a result of this sympathetic efferent activity, and that this rise can be blocked with α-adrenergic blocking agents. Additionally, he hypothesized an involvement of the adrenergic component in the opening of the bladder outlet that occurs at the initiation of the emptying phase of micturition. This was felt to be a result of β-adrenergic stimulation of the outlet smooth musculature, but through parasympathetic stimulation. In other words, this theory involves preganglionic parasympathetic stimulation not only as the prime factor in bladder contraction (through postganglionic primarily cholinergic fibers), but also as a major contributing factor to the decrease in outlet resistance seen during the empyting phase of micturition (through postganglionic adrenergic fibers—the "short adrenergic system"). This short adrenergic component activates β-adrenergic receptors (not α-adrenergic) in the outlet.

El Badawi (1982), on reviewing the available physiologic and pharmacologic data, totally endorsed the view that "the storage phase of micturition is controlled primarily by sympathetic, and the voiding phase by parasympathetic vesicourethral innervation." Further, he endorsed the concept of β-adrenergic–induced relaxation of the smooth sphincter at the outset of voiding, and synthesized this with his own view that unitary contraction of the body detrusor and smooth sphincter occurred during micturition and was essential for the maintenance of the voiding phase. As he put it, "This proposal does not contradict McGuire-Herlihy's thesis of lissosphincter relaxation at the outset of voiding, which the present author endorses unreservedly, believing that relaxation of a continent lissosphincter, maintained under sympathetic α-adrenergic excitation during the storage phase, must be replaced by parasympathogenic contraction, to sustain a rigidly open vesicourethral outlet in the face of the pressure force of the urine stream." Our interpretation is that this proposal involves a sympathetic α-adrenergic contribution to smooth sphincter tone during storage, replaced by a parasympathetic short adrenergic β-receptor–induced relaxation at the onset of emptying. During emptying, parasympathetic cholinergic stimulation of this also keeps it rigid (in the "open" position) to prevent ballooning and loss of the pressure force.

An equally impressive body of evidence and opinions by equally impressive investigators, however, argues against a significant role of the sympathetic nervous system during either the filling/storage or the emptying phase of micturition. Klevmark (1977) failed to demonstrate a significant bladder pressure rise in anesthetized cats with an intact neural axis at physiological (very low) filling rates (one hourly diuresis [HD] equilvalent to 1.1 ml/kg/hr). At rates of 3–4 HD the intravesical pressure gradually increased. No change occurred after sympathectomy, whether at high or low volume, leading Klevmark to conclude that no significant influence on bladder activity during filling was exerted by the sympathetic nervous system. Clinically significant alteration of bladder capacity with β-adrenergic antagonists does not occur in normal individuals, though there is some suggestion that some change might occur in selected individuals with a decreased bladder capacity (Wein, 1986). Tanagho (1978) has very nicely summarized some of the impressive array of his work on the dog, which has led him to raise significant questions regarding the reality of a sympathetic effect on the intrinsic smooth musculature of the urethra. His group (Tanagho and Myers, 1969; Tanagho et al., 1969a, 1969b; Tanagho and Miller, 1970) did not find a consistent and lasting response of the urethra in response to sympathetic stimulation, but did find that this smooth musculature responded uniformly to parasympathetic and cholinergic stimulation, and that its activity was obliterated by muscarinic antagonists. The effects of adrenergic stimulation and blockade were attributed to receptors in the vasculature of the urethra rather than on the smooth muscle itself. A definite adrenergic influence was postulated for a genital sphincter in the male that prevents retrograde ejaculation. This genital sphincter consists of smooth muscle in the supramontanal male urethra, a view that is similar to that of Gosling, who postulated a similar role for adrenergic innervation in the lower urinary tract of the male, but restricted this area more precisely to the area of the bladder neck (Bruschini et al., 1978; Gosling, 1979; Gosling and Chilton, 1984).

Finally, Nordling (1983) summarized an impressive amount of data relative to the role of the sympathetic nervous system in lower urinary tract function and concluded that, at least in the normal individual, the role is indeed a minor one. He pointed out that "sympathectomy" and operations that affect sympathetic ganglia, such as retroperitoneal lymphadenectomy, rarely if ever cause a lasting effect on the micturition of a normal individual. Studying urethral pressure changes in response to α-adrenergic blocking agents in a group of patients with localized neurologic lesions of the spinal cord, cauda equina, or peripheral nerves, he concluded that only lesions of the peripheral sympathetic nervous system caused a decreased effect of α-adrenergic blockade on maximum urethral pressure. He felt that this did confirm the existence of urethral α-adrenergic innervation-induced tonus at rest, but found no evidence for a significant influence of the sympathetic system on bladder function at rest or during voiding. Additionally, he questioned the classic localization of the origin of the sympathetic nervous supply to the lower urinary tract by pointing out that in the patients whom he studied, no specific level of the spinal cord could be demonstrated to act as a center for sympathetic innervation of the lower urinary tract. He added that this might be due to an extension of the sympathetic origin over so many spinal segments that damage to only a few would not significantly alter sympathetic influence on the urethra. Attempts to correlate the appearance of an open bladder neck with the bladder at rest and the level of spinal cord or peripheral neurologic lesion produced the conclusion that an intact parasympathetic rather than sympathetic innervation was the prerequisite for keeping the bladder neck closed at rest. Severe stress on the bladder neck produced by strong detrusor contractions in the presence of sphincter dyssynergia was also noted as a possible cause of the "open bladder neck." On the basis of experiments done in normal females, Nordling suggests that urethral pressure is partly maintained through peripheral α-adrenergic receptors in the urethral vessels rather than the smooth muscle itself, and by α-adrenergic receptors in the central nervous system that are more involved in the regulation of striated sphincter tone than smooth sphincter tone.

α-Adrenergic Effects on the Striated Sphincter

Much of the confusion relative to whether or not the sympathetic nervous system has an effect on the striated sphincter relates to the interpretation of clinical observations and experimental data referable to the effect of α-adrenergic blocking agents on urethral pressure in the region of the urogenital diaphragm and on electromyographic (EMG) activity in the periurethral striated muscle of this area. Nanninga et al. (1977) found that the EMG activity recorded in the "external sphincter" decreased after phentolamine administration in three paraplegic patients. They attributed the effect to a peripheral blockade of a direct sympathetic action on the striated sphincter (through sympathetic innervation). Nordling et al. (1981) demonstrated that clonidine and phenoxybenzamine (both of which pass the blood-brain barrier) decreased urethral pressure and EMG activity from the area of the striated sphincter in five normal women, but that phentolamine (which does not pass the blood-brain barrier) also decreased urethral pressure in this area, while it had no effect on the EMG activity. The authors concluded that phentolamine's effect was due purely to smooth muscle relaxation, while the effect of clonidine (and, possibly, phenoxybenzamine) was elicited mostly through centrally induced changes in striated urethral sphincter tonus, but that these agents also had an effect on the smooth muscle component of urethral pressure. These pressure effects were measured as effects on the maximum urethral pressure during urethral profilometry. It should be noted, however, that none of the drugs affected the reflex rise in urethral pressure or the reflex increase in EMG activity seen during bladder filling. Likewise, there was no drug-induced decrease in the urethral pressure or EMG activity response to voluntary contraction of the pelvic floor striated musculature. Pedersen et al. (1980) studied the effects of thymoxamine on the urethral pressure profile in ten patients with spastic paraplegia and on striated sphincter EMG activity in five. This drug is an α-adrenergic blocking agent that passes the blood-brain barrier. Peak urethral pressure was reduced in all patients studied, and EMG activity was likewise decreased, leading the authors to speculate that the drug had its action on the striated sphincter on a central basis.

Gajewski et al. (1984) conducted an elegant series of experiments on cats to explore the effect of α-adrenergic blocking agents on the striated sphincter. They found that hypogastric and pudendal nerve stimulation produced rises in urethral perfusion pressure, and that prazosin and phentolamine decreased the response only to hypogastric nerve stimulation. However, when the striated sphincter response was evoked indirectly, by stimulating the central cut end of the contralateral pudendal nerve, the urethral pressure response was significantly decreased by α-adrenergic blockade, more by prazosin than by phentolamine. The EMG potentials elicited by the indirect stimulation were completely abolished by prazosin, while the potentials elicited by direct stimulation remained unchanged, but did disappear after gallamine, a striated muscle blocker, was administered. Hypogastric nerve stimulation produced no EMG activity. The calculated reflex characteristics that were elicited by the contralateral pudendal cut-end stimulation were determined to be characteristic of a multisynaptic pathway in a spinal reflex. The authors concluded that α-adrenergic blocking agents do not influence the pudendal nerve–dependent urethral response through a peripheral action, but that at least prazosin can significantly inhibit this response at a central level.

PERIPHERAL PEPTIDES

The word "peptide" loosely refers to any member of a class of compounds of low molecular weight that yields two or more amino acids on hydrolysis. Those mentioned as putative neurotransmitters affecting the lower urinary tract are listed in Table 1. Of these, one large family is composed of the opioids. This term refers to any directly acting compound with effects that are stereospecifically antagonized by naloxone. This definition does not exclude the possibility that an opioid or part of it may have additional actions not antagonized by naloxone and therefore not mediated by opioid receptors. The term "opioid peptide" is usually applied to a naturally occurring peptide with opiate-like biological properties, i.e., at least some of the characteristic properties of morphine, which effects should be reversible by naloxone (Hughes and Kosterlitz, 1983; Morley, 1983; Mundy, 1984b). The terminology in this field is just becoming established and is still somewhat confusing. There are three distinct families of endogenous opioid peptides—enkephalins, endorphins, and dymorphins. These families are distinguished by genetically distinct precursor polypeptides and by characteristic anatomical distributions. To further complicate matters, there is reasonably firm evidence for at least four major categories of opioid receptors, designated μ, κ, δ, and σ. There may in fact be as many as eight different types of opioid receptors. A full discussion of the general pharmacology of this area, still developing, is beyond the scope of this chapter, and the interested reader is referred to the symposium edited by Hughes (see Hughes and Kosterlitz, 1983) and to Jaffee and Martin (1985), though both these reference sources will probably be out of date at the time of, or shortly after, the publication of this text.

Substance P

Substance P is an undecapeptide originally detected in extracts of gut and brain, and prepared as a powder, hence the designation "P." The pharmacologic effects of substance P include vasodilation; stimulation of intestinal, bronchial, and other smooth muscles; stimulation of salivary secretion; diuresis and natriuresis; and a variety of effects on peripheral and central neurons apparently attributable to depolarization (Douglas, 1985). It is found in small amounts in the human bladder, mainly in a suburothelial position, and in the dorsal root ganglia and dorsal horn of the spinal cord, particularly in the lumbosacral cord (Alm et al., 1978; Mundy, 1984b). In vitro, substance P produces a contractile effect on the canine bladder (Norlen et al., 1983), which is atropine-resistant (Mundy, 1984b). Lack of effect of the substance P antagonist on contractile responses to electrical field stimulation in rabbit and guinea pig muscle strips, and an increase in response in rat bladder strips, suggests that substance P is not, however, a mediator of excitatory noncholinergic activation (Husted et al., 1981), though a role as a local neuromodulator cannot be excluded. deGroat and Kawatani (1985) have identified substance P in 22% of bladder afferents identified in feline sacral dorsal root ganglia. They speculated that substance P may be a sensory neurotransmitter, and this is consistent with experiments that indicate that the systemic administration of capsaicin, an agent that depletes substance P and other peptides in small-diameter afferents, depressed the micturition reflex in rats and caused urinary retention (Maggi et al., 1984b).

Vasoactive Intestinal Polypeptide

Vasoactive intestinal polypeptide (VIP) is a peptide that contains 28 amino acid residues and was first isolated from the small intestine, hence its name. Its range of effects is very broad and includes potent vasodilation, stimulation of cardiac contractility, stimulation of glycogenolysis, and relaxation of many smooth muscles. It also stimulates secretion of several pituitary and hypothalamic hormones and of pancreatic, salivary, intestinal, and other exocrine secretions (Douglas, 1985). Of the peptide-containing nerves in the bladder, those containing VIP are the most abundant. VIP is found in all bladder layers, but especially beneath the transitional epithelium, around blood vessels, and in the muscle layers (Polak and Bloom, 1984; Mundy, 1984b). Although Finkbeiner (1983) found no significant effect of VIP on the spontaneous activity of guinea pig bladder muscle or that induced by acetylcholine or electrical stimulation, others (Levin and Wein, 1981; Larsen et al., 1981; Klarskov and Gerstenberg, 1984; Kinder and Mundy, 1984b) have shown an inhibitory effect on muscle strip spontaneous contractility and on that evoked by electrical field stimulation or stimulation with various pharmacologic agonists. This effect, also seen in urethral smooth muscle, was not affected by tetrodotoxin (Klarskov and Gerstenberg, 1984), β-adrenergic blockade (Levin and Wein, 1981; Klarskov and Gerstenberg, 1984), or prostaglandin synthesis blockade (Klarskov and Gerstenberg, 1984). Sjogren et al. (1985) reported similar inhibition effects on rabbit bladder strip preparations but not on human specimens. They also noted an inhibitory effect of VIP on the contractile response of the rabbit urethra to electrical stimulation and norepinephrine, but a less marked effect on human urethral response to norepinephrine and no consistent effect on the response of this tissue to field stimulation.

Gu et al. (1983) have reported a markedly reduced concentration of

VIP in the "unstable bladder" as compared with the normal. This observation, with the results of some of the experiments just cited, has led to speculation regarding a possible role of VIP as a modifier of bladder activity during filling. There is by no means agreement on this hypothesis (Sjogren et al., 1985). In the pharmacologic literature the emerging view of VIP seems to be that of a neuroeffector agent involved in the control of flow in local vascular beds and in the modulation of cholinergic transmission (Haynes, 1985). deGroat and Kawatani (1985) showed that 24% of bladder afferents in sacral dorsal root ganglia contained VIP. Sixty-two percent of the VIP bladder afferent neurons also contained substance P. This raises speculation as to a potential afferent neurotransmitter role for this substance as well, especially since VIP-positive nerves have also been found in the spinal cord (Mundy, 1984b).

Neuropeptide Y

Neuropeptide Y is a 36 amino acid peptide found to occur in various peripheral locations, including the bladder (Lundberg et al., 1984). Mundy (1984b) describes its bladder distribution as similar to that of VIP, and describes it as a potent contractor of smooth muscle. Varied potential functions in the mammalian nervous system have been hypothesized. Although it does cause generalized vasoconstriction, it also inhibits contractile responses to electrical stimulation in vas deferens and cervix smooth muscle (Gray and Morley, 1986). Lundberg et al. (1984) found NP-Y to induce a reversible reduction of the noncholinergic, nonadrenergic contractile response to field stimulation of the guinea pig urinary bladder. Gu et al. (1984) report numerous neuropeptide Y–containing nerves in the human bladder, primarily in the muscle layer, and particularly in the trigonal region.

Peripheral Opioids

Most discussions on the potential role of the opioids as a major influence on lower urinary tract function concern a central inhibitory role, but there is some suggestion that enkephalins may function as an inhibitory neuromodulator at the peripheral level as well (deGroat and Kawatani, 1985), at the ganglionic level. A full discussion of the potential role of opioid mechanisms influencing lower urinary tract activity will be presented in the section on central mechanisms.

OTHER SUBSTANCES

The effects of histamine are mediated through specific H_1 and H_2 receptors, so classified by their susceptibility to blockade by pyrilamine and burimamide (Khanna, 1983; Caine, 1984). Contractile H_1 receptors have been demonstrated in rabbit (Fredericks, 1975), guinea pig (Khanna et al., 1977), and dogs and humans (Van Buren and Anderson, 1979; Khanna, 1983). No H_2 receptors have been identified in bladder smooth muscle. Atropine partially blocks the response to histamine, and so muscarinic receptors may be involved in this response (Fredericks, 1975).

Serotonin (5-hydroxytryptamine [5-HT]) produces a contractile response in guinea pig, dog, and cat urinary bladder (Gyermek, 1962; Erspamer et al., 1973; Saum and deGroat, 1973). The bladder effect is biphasic, consisting of an initial transient contraction due to stimulation of the autonomic ganglia, followed by a more prolonged contraction due to a direct effect on the smooth muscle itself (Caine, 1984). There is an additional inhibitory effect on parasympathetic ganglia produced by serotonin as well (Saum and deGroat, 1973). Two types of excitatory serotonin receptors have been identified in the cat urinary bladder, the so-called M and 5-HT_2 type (Saxena et al., 1985). The physiologic significance of the action of serotonin on urinary bladder is open to speculation. Vaidyanathan et al. (1981a) have shown that administration of clomipramine, an inhibitor of serotonin uptake, decreased bladder capacity, and cite other work reporting the occurrence of urinary frequency with this drug, suggesting that serotonin might have a potentiating effect on excitatory bladder reflex activity.

γ-Aminobutyric acid (GABA) is thought to be primarily a central inhibitory neurotransmitter. However, GABA receptors have been shown to be present in guinea pig bladder dome strips. Maggi et al. (1985a, 1985b) have shown that GABA may transiently enhance excitatory neurotransmission early in the phase of neurogenic activation, and then exhibit a more sustained inhibition of contractility, mediated by both $GABA_A$ and $GABA_B$ receptors. In the mouse bladder, Santicioli et al. (1986) postulated that prejunctional $GABA_B$ receptors are present in the postganglionic excitatory innervation and act to reduce neurotransmitter release when stimulated.

Involvement of a nonadrenergic, noncholinergic neurotransmitter in the urethral relaxation that occurs during bladder emptying has already been somewhat considered in the section on prostaglandins. Additionally, Mattiasson et al. (1985) have reported that the electrically induced contraction of urethral smooth muscle from rabbit and man consists of two main components, one adrenergically mediated and one nonadrenergic and atropine-resistant. This suggests an unknown contractile neurotransmitter released by stimulation of known nerves or by stimulation of another type of nerve yet to be established.

Central Nervous System Influences on the Lower Urinary Tract

Micturition is basically a function of the peripheral autonomic nervous system. However, the ultimate control of lower urinary tract function, including that of the periurethral striated musculature, obviously resides at higher neurologic levels. At any of these levels, and within the pathways that connect them, facilitation and inhibition of various aspects of bladder and outlet activity during the filling/storage and emptying phases of micturition can occur. There is considerable disagreement regarding details of the location and relative importance of central nervous system structures regulating micturition, and as well about ascending and descending pathways connecting these structures to each other and to the thoracic, lumbar, and sacral spinal cord. In this section we shall attempt to summarize the most widely quoted views that are consistent with our present working knowledge of micturition and its disorders.

NEURAL PATHWAYS

Spinal Cord

The micturition center in the spinal cord is primarily localized to three spinal nerve segments, S2–4, with its major part focused at S3 (Bradley et al., 1974; Fletcher and Bradley, 1978; deGroat and Booth, 1980; Hald and Bradley, 1982; Bradley and Sundin, 1982; Bhatia and Bradley, 1983; Schmidt, 1983). This is anatomically located at vertebral levels T12–L1. Rockswold et al. (1980a) reported that the origin of vesical pelvic nerve fibers in the rhesus monkey was S1–2 and in the chimpanzee S1–4. They also noted that the spinal origin of the pudendal nerve was one segment rostral (Rockswold et al., 1980b). Schmidt (1983) nicely summarized the neuroanatomy of the conus medullaris in the dog as follows. The gray matter is divided into a series of zones, and the parasympathetic preganglionic motor neurons lie within an intermediolateral gray column. The cells extend in a vertical plane along the border between the white and gray matters, and in a horizontal plane at the base of the dorsal horn at lamina 7 and lamina 5, the former serving as the center for bladder control, and the latter more medial group of parasympathetic cells serving as the center for rectal control. Between the rectal center and the bladder center lies a zone of interneurons believed to be a site of convergence for afferent input to these two visceral centers. Somatic nerve fibers originate from the nucleus of Onuf, in the midventral spinal gray matter at the level of S1 (in animals), drifting laterally to the edge of the spinal white and gray matters at S2. This area corresponds to human levels S2–3. The innervation to most striated muscles of the pelvic floor, including those of the periurethral and anal sphincters, originates within the nucleus of Onuf. Figure 23 conceptualizes Schmidt's description. Hald and Bradley's cross-sectional diagrams at the level of the sacral cord (Fig 24) and

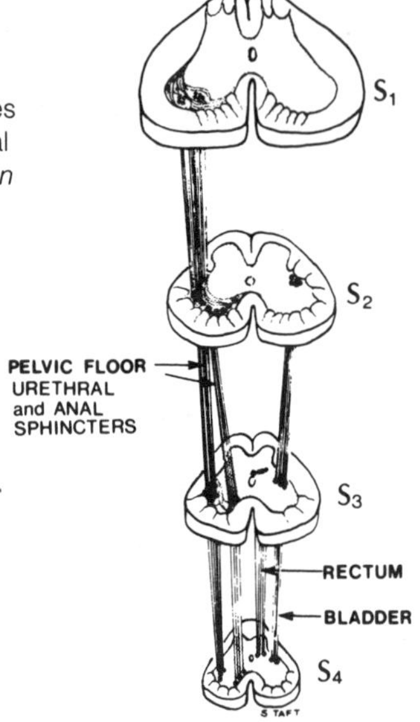

FIG 23.
Micturition center (sacral spinal cord) in the human. Based on horseradish peroxidase transport studies in animals and the results of sacral root stimulation studies in humans (see text). (From Schmidt RA: Urethrovesical reflexes and their inhibition, in Hinman F Jr (ed): *Benign Prostatic Hypertrophy*. Berlin, Springer-Verlag, 1983. Used with permission.)

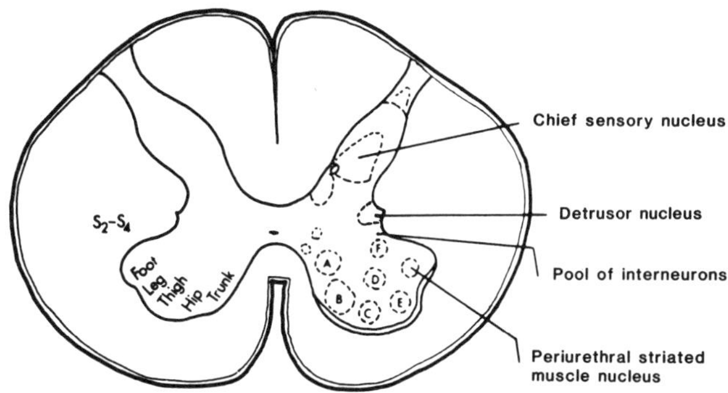

FIG 24.
Spinal cord at level S2–4. Location of detrusor and pudendal motor nuclei. Bilateral representation, though not pictured, exists. (From Hald T, Bradley W: *The Urinary Bladder: Neurology and Dynamics*. Baltimore, Williams & Wilkins, 1982. Used with permission.)

above (Fig 25) are likewise helpful in understanding the efferent innervation of the lower urinary tract at the spinal cord level.

Ascending sensory stimuli from the lower urinary tract include exteroceptive (pain, temperature and touch—generated in the urothelium) and proprioceptive sensory impulses (initiated in the bladder muscle and periurethral striated muscle). Exteroceptive impulses ascend in the spinothalamic tract, while proprioceptive impulses travel in the posterior columns (Hald and Bradley, 1982; Bradley and Sundin, 1982; Bhatia and Bradley, 1983) (Figs 26 and 27). Proprioceptive axons

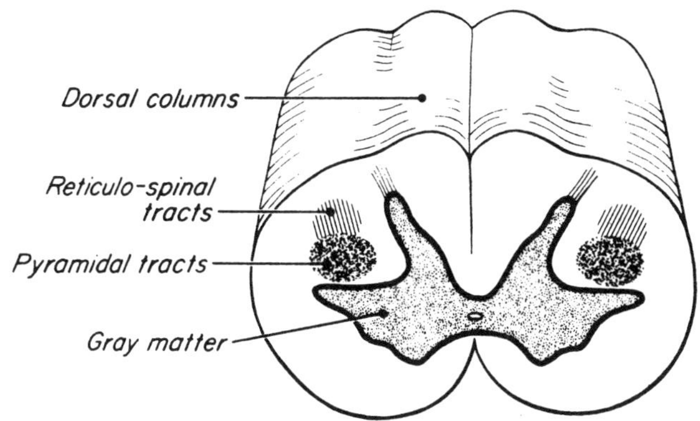

FIG 25.
Spinal tracts innervating the bladder (reticulospinal tracts) and striated periurethral musculature (pyramidal or corticospinal tracts.) (From Hald T, Bradley W: *The Urinary Bladder: Neurology and Dynamics*. Baltimore, Williams & Wilkins, 1982. Used with permission.)

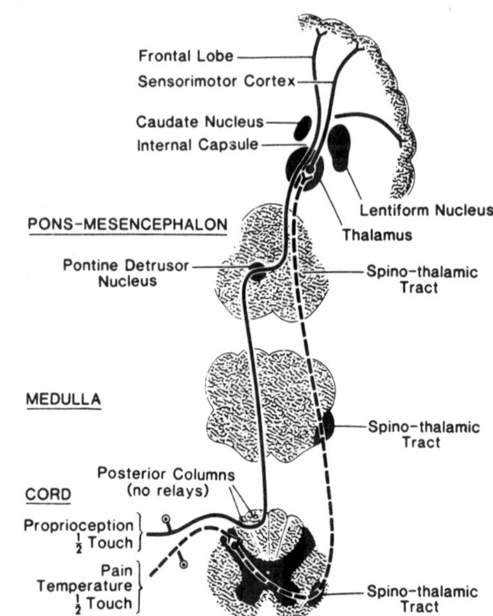

FIG 26.
Afferent neural pathways of exteroceptive and proprioceptive sensory neurons (see text). (From Hald T, Bradley W: *The Urinary Bladder: Neurology and Dynamics.* Baltimore, Williams & Wilkins, 1982. Used with permission.)

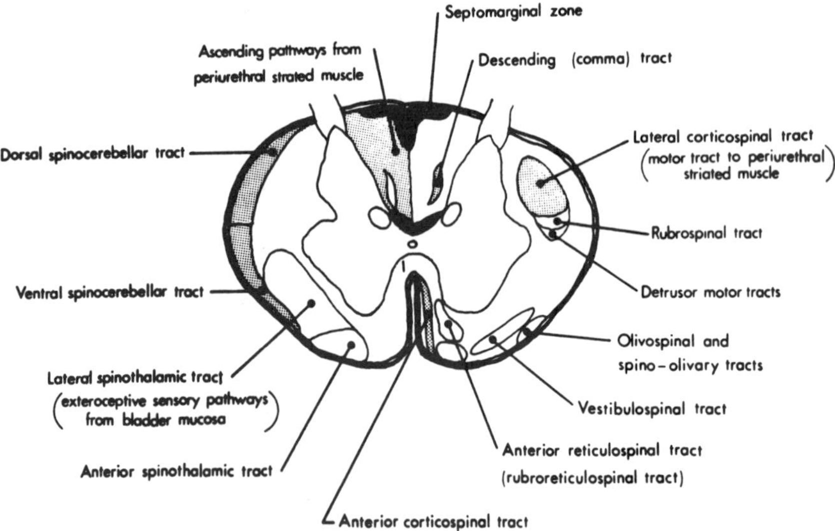

FIG 27.
Spinal cord cross-section (above Fig 27–25) showing relationship of efferent and afferent tracts concerned with lower urinary tract function (see text). (From Bhatia NN, Bradley WE: Neuroanatomy and physiology: Innervation of the urinary tract, in Raz S (ed): *Female Urology*. Philadelphia, WB Saunders, 1983. Used with permission.)

from the detrusor muscle enter the dorsal portion of the gray matter, and turn to travel rostrally to synapse in the area of the pontine-mesencephalic reticular formation designated as the nucleus tegmentolateralis dorsalis tegmentalis of the pons (Hald and Bradley, 1982; Bradley and Sundin, 1982; Bhatia and Bradley, 1983). This exclusive rostral passage of propriospinal afferents is termed "long routing," a concept originally implied by Barrington (1921). This phenomenon certainly occurs in the experimental animal, but awaits confirmation in man (Hald and Bradley, 1982; Bradley and Sundin, 1982; Bhatia and Bradley, 1983). Exteroceptive sensory impulses travel in the spinothalamic tracts and synapse in the thalamus, which projects to the sensorimotor cortex. Whether propriospinal afferents are exclusively "long routed," or whether it simply seems that way with an intact neural axis remains a question. If exclusive long routing occurs, then there can be no true spinal micturition center under any circumstances. If pathways do exist, but are simply vestigial in the normal animal, then there at least exists the potential for spinal reflex pathways to emerge under certain circumstances (such as after spinal cord transsection—see below).

It is agreed, however, that pudendal reflex pathways are organized at a spinal level, although subject to supraspinal influences (Bradley and Sundin, 1982; Hald and Bradley, 1982; Bhatia and Bradley, 1983). Afferent proprioceptive axons that originate in the striated musculature of the pelvic floor enter the sacral spinal cord and divide. One group synapses on pudendal motor neurons in the ventral gray matter of the sacral spinal cord, while another group travels rostrally in the dorsal columns to synapse on neurons in the cerebellum, as well as ascending in the medial lemniscus to synapse on neurons in the nucleus ventralis posterolateralis (thalamus), ending eventually in the sensorimotor cortex (Fig 28).

Brain Stem

Evidence that indicates that the brain stem, specifically the neurons of the pontine-mesencephalic gray matter, contains the nuclei that are the origin of the final common pathway to bladder motor neurons has been summarized by Kuru (1965), Bradley and Teague (1968), deGroat and Ryall (1969), Bradley et al. (1974), deGroat (1975), Carlsson (1978), Bradley and Sundin (1982), Hald and Bradley (1982), and Bhatia and Bradley (1983). The area called Barrington's center (Barrington, 1921) in the anterior pontine region is considered to be the origin of facilitory impulses to the bladder. Destruction of this center or transsection just below it causes a permanent disturbance of bladder emptying (Barring-

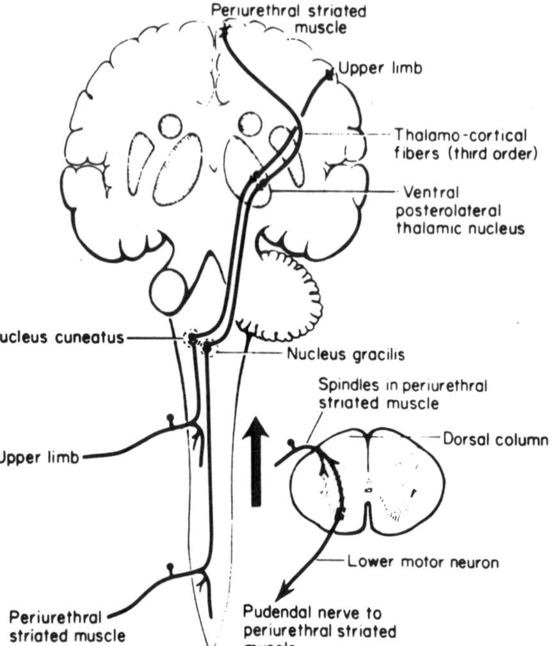

FIG 28.
Spinal and supraspinal organization of pudendal reflex pathways (see text). Connections to cerebellum not pictured. (From Bhatia NN, Bradley WE: Neuroanatomy and physiology: Innervation of the urinary tract, in Raz S (ed): *Female Urology*. Philadelphia, WB Saunders, 1983. Used with permission.)

ton, 1925; Bradley and Conway, 1966; Ruch, 1974). Transsection above this center at the intracollicular level results in detrusor hyperactivity (Ruch, 1974; Carlsson, 1978). Originally, these neurons were described as located in the nucleus locus ceruleus, but subsequent studies have suggested that the location is in the nucleus lateralis dorsalis tegmentalis, which is rostral to the nucleus locus ceruleus (Hald and Bradley, 1982; Bhatia and Bradley, 1983). Input to this area is derived from the cerebellum, basal ganglia, thalamus and hypothalamus, and cerebral cortex (Fig 29). Carlsson (1978) added that experimental stimulation of Barrington's center causes not only bladder contraction, but also a marked decrease in EMG discharge in the periurethral striated musculature.

Cerebellum

The cerebellum serves as a modulator of neural activities that are initiated in other parts of the central nervous system. Insofar as the lower urinary tract is concerned, it receives sensory input from the bladder and from the pelvic floor musculature. Its ultimately efferent

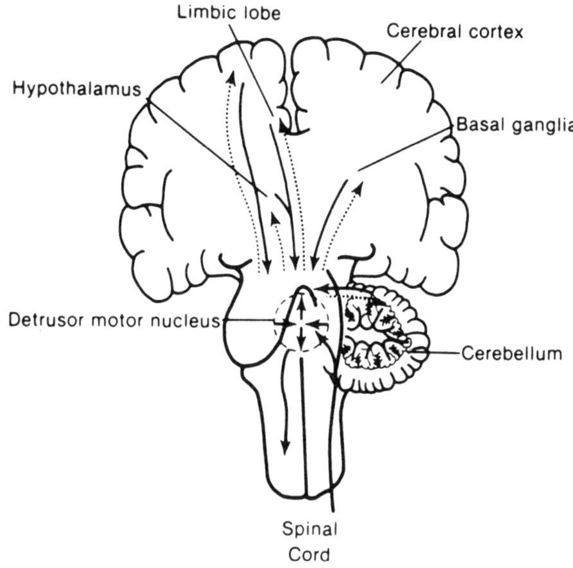

FIG 29.
Pontine detrusor nucleus and its connections (see text). (From Hald T, Bradley W: *The Urinary Bladder: Neurology and Dynamics*. Baltimore, Williams & Wilkins, 1982. Used with permission.)

functions are felt to include maintenance of tone in the pelvic floor striated musculature; an influence on the rate, range, and force of bladder and pelvic floor striated muscle contraction; an influence on the coordination between emptying bladder contraction and periurethral striated muscle relaxation; and a direct effect on the brain stem. Electrical stimulation of the fastigial nucleus in the experimental animal produces suppression of detrusor reflex activity through an inhibitory influence on Barrington's center; ablation of the anterior vermis of the cerebellum produces detrusor hyperactivity (Bradley et al., 1974; Bradley and Sundin, 1982; Hald and Bradley, 1982; Bhatia and Bradley, 1983).

Basal Ganglia

These subcortical nuclei comprise the caudate nucleus, red nucleus, putamen and globus pallidus, and cells of the substantia nigra located in the midbrain. Animal experiments have suggested an inhibitory effect of these nuclei on spontaneous detrusor reflex contractions

(Carlsson, 1978; Hald and Bradley, 1982; Bhatia and Bradley, 1983). This correlates with the detrusor hyperactivity often seen in patients with Parkinson's disease with basal ganglia dysfunction.

Thalamus, Hypothalamus, and Limbic System

The thalamus consists of a collection of nuclei that collectively represent the principal relay nucleus for sensory axons ascending to the cerebral cortex (Bradley and Sundin, 1982; Hald and Bradley, 1982). Splanchnic afferent stimulation has implicated the dorsomedial thalamic nucleus as a relay station, but the precise routing of afferents from the pelvic and pudendal nerves is unknown. The hypothalamus consists of a collection of nuclei at the base of the thalamus, and has a major influence on neuroendocrine function and body water balance. Its function, insofar as the lower urinary tract is concerned, has been little investigated, but bladder distention in the experimental animal has been reported to cause neuronal firing in a posterior group of nuclei (Hald and Bradley, 1982; Bhatia and Bradley, 1983). Carlsson (1978) cited studies that show that the hypothalamus may be involved in the organization of that portion of micturition or defecation mediated by the autonomic nervous system. The limbic system comprises areas that are principally located in the temporal lobe and associated subcortical nuclei considered to be the rostral extensions of the autonomic nervous system. This includes the amygdala, the hippocampal formation, and the neurons of the cingulate gyrus. Electrical stimulation of specific nuclei in the experimental animal has been shown to both facilitate and depress bladder activity, depending on the specific nucleus stimulated (Bradley and Sundin, 1982), but a typical type of bladder dysfunction does not seem to occur in patients with temporal lobe dysfunction (Hald and Bradley, 1982; Bhatia and Bradley, 1983).

Cerebral Cortex

The region of the cerebral hemispheres concerned with bladder muscle innervation consists of the superomedial portion of the frontal lobes and the genu of the corpus callosum (Fig 30) (Andrew and Nathan, 1965; Bradley et al., 1974; Hald and Bradley, 1982; Bhatia and Bradley, 1983). Stimulation of specific areas of the cerebral cortex in the experimental animal can demonstrate either facilitation or inhibition of detrusor muscle contraction (Gjone and Setekleiv, 1963), but transsection experiments seem to indicate that the net effect of these areas is inhibitory (Tang, 1955; Tang and Ruch, 1956; Kuru, 1965; Ruch, 1974;

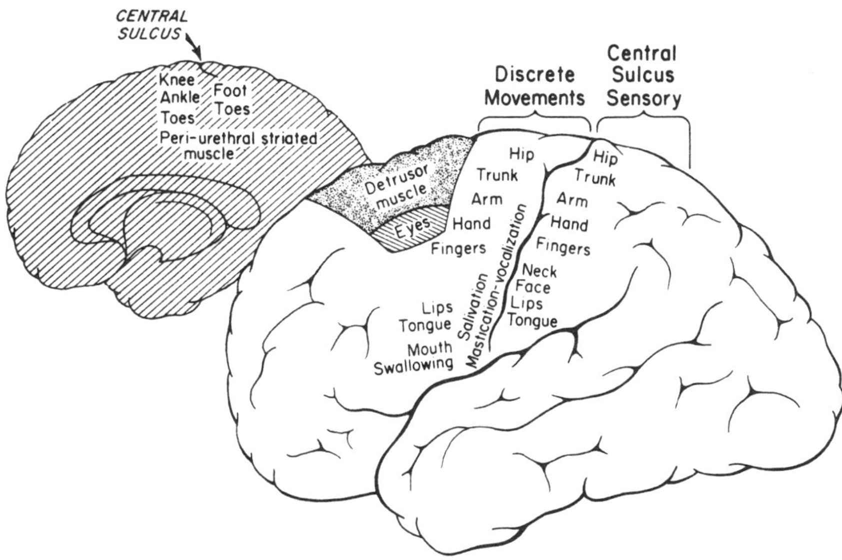

FIG 30.
Areas in the cerebral hemispheres concerned with innervation of the bladder (lateral surface) and periurethral striated muscle (medial surface) (see text). (From Bhatia NN, Bradley WE: Neuroanatomy and physiology: Innervation of the urinary tract, in Raz S (ed): *Female Urology*. Philadelphia, WB Saunders, 1983. Used with permission.)

Nathan, 1976). Voiding dysfunction in patients with functional ablation of cerebral cortical areas is generally characterized by a hyperactive detrusor reflex. The cerebrocortical areas concerned with innervation of the periurethral striated musculature are distinct and geographically separate, located on the medial aspect of the sensorimotor cortex (see Fig 30) (Hald and Bradley, 1982; Bhatia and Bradley, 1983). Axons that originate from neurons in this region pass caudally through the internal capsule and cerebral peduncles in the brain stem, continuing ultimately in the lateral columns of the spinal cord as the còrticospinal tracts. The axons from the detrusor motor area in the frontal lobes traverse the basal ganglia to terminate in the pontine mesencephalic reticular formation. Ascending axons from sensory receptors located in the detrusor muscle and in the periurethral striated muscle terminate in both the detrusor portion of the frontal lobes and the pudendal portion of the sensory motor cortex.

Thus, the prevailing concept regarding central nervous system influences is that of an anterior pontine micturition center, which is considered to be the origin of efferent facilitory impulses in the normal animal or individual. This conclusion, however, has been reached by transsection, destruction, and stimulation experiments only in the laboratory animal, and almost exclusively by inference in the human. Additionally, such experiments have disclosed, at least in cats, alternating inhibitory and facilitory areas rostral to this, each level being capable of functioning in the absence of the more rostral one. The inhibitory areas are found in structures above the transhypothalamic level and in the midbrain; the facilitory areas in the posterior hypothalamus and in the anterior pons (Carlsson, 1978).

CENTRAL TRANSMITTERS AND THE ROLE OF THE ENDOGENOUS OPIOIDS

Although data exist on the location of the central nervous system structures involved in the central regulation of lower urinary tract function, the neurotransmitter mechanisms involved have received little study and are largely unknown. Potential central neurotransmitters are listed in Table 1, and, of these, GABA and glycine have been shown to be inhibitory neurotransmitters. Sillen (1980) has summarized a series of experiments on anesthetized rats, providing certain observations regarding central neurotransmitter mechanisms involved in the control of bladder function in this experimental model. Central adrenergic stimulation was achieved by injection of the amine precursor levodopa, after blockade of its peripheral metabolism, resulting in central accumulation of the metabolites dopamine and noradrenalin, thought responsible for the functional effects of levodopa. Activation of central catecholamine neurons in this fashion resulted in a hyperactive bladder response. This bladder hyperactivity to levodopa seemed to be elicited mainly via stimulation of central dopamine receptors in the pontine-mesencephalic brain region. This hyperactive bladder response occurred even in the presence of maximally inhibited catecholamine neurons, suggesting that impulses to the bladder from these dopamine receptors were propagated via neurons of a noncatecholamine type. Acetylcholine was also reported to serve as a neurotransmitter in the central nervous system as well as in peripheral tissues. Muscarinic receptors predominate in the brain, while nicotinic receptors predominate in the spinal cord. Activation of central muscarinic receptors also (like levodopa) produced a hyperactive bladder response, likewise generated in pontine-mesencephalic structures. Further, there was felt to be an interaction in some instances between dopamine and muscarinic receptors in the generation of the hyperactive bladder response to levodopa. Central GABA receptor activation inhibited the bladder hyperactivity that occurred in response to levodopa. This inhibition was felt to occur at a site postsynaptic to the dopaminergic neurons. Thus, Sillen concluded that excitatory dopaminergic and muscarinic receptors, and inhibitory GABAergic receptors, were involved in the supraspinal modulation of lower urinary tract function, probably by an action on the basic micturition reflex pathways originating in the pontine-mesencephalic area. Further data from other experimental systems are awaited.

There is strong evidence that endogenous opioid peptides influence micturition by a tonic inhibitory effect on detrusor reflex pathways. The evidence for this has been well summarized by deGroat and Kawatani (1986) and by Booth et al. (1985). In cats, systemic administration of naloxone increased the force of bladder contractions at constant bladder volumes, decreased bladder capacity, increased the frequency and magnitude of pressure increases during bladder filling and during micturition, promoted more effective emptying of the bladder, and increased multiunit firing in parasympathetic postganglionic nerves on the surface of the bladder (Roppolo et al., 1983; Hisamitsu and deGroat, 1984; Booth et al., 1985). The inhibitory effects could be mediated at several possible levels, including the peripheral bladder ganglia, the sacral spinal cord, or the brain-stem micturition center (Booth et al., 1985). At each of these sites dense collections of enkephalinergic terminals have been identified (Glazer and Basbaum, 1980; Kawatani et al., 1983; Leger et al., 1983). Also, at each of these sites, local administration of exogenous opioid peptides has produced an inhibition of the micturition reflex (Simonds et al., 1983; Roppolo et al., 1983; Hisamitsu and deGroat, 1984; deGroat and Kawatani, 1985; Booth et al., 1985). In the rat, both intracerebroventricular and systemic morphine inhibited spontaneous bladder contractions, the former effect being reversed by similarly administered naloxone, and the latter by intrathecal naloxone, most effectively in the region of the lumbosacral spinal cord (Dray and Metsch, 1984a, 1984b). Sillen and Rubenson (1986) likewise reported inhibition of the bladder response in rats to central levodopa administration by intracerebroventricular or systemic morphine. Regional (intra-arterial) administration produced an initial weak excitatory effect followed by a slight depression of the bladder reactivity to receptor agonists and peripheral nerve stimulation. Jubelin et al. (1984) showed that the synthetic opiate [D-Ala^2,Me-Phe^4] leu-enkephalin (DAMLE) inhibited bladder contractions and voiding in acutely decerebrate cats (intercollicular transsection of the brain stem). However, there was no effect on the bladder contraction of acute spinal cats (C5–6) or on electrically induced contraction of in vitro bladder strips. Naloxone antagonized this inhibitory effect and per se induced a bladder contraction. The conclusion from this set of experiments was that the inhibitory effect was exerted either at the level of ascending spinal pathways (spinobulbar or spinopontine) or in the pontine micturition center, probably the latter. Murray and Feneley (1982), using cystometric recordings, showed that naloxone increased intravesical pressure throughout filling in a group of normal men and women, and reduced bladder capacity. Maximum urethral closure pressure was reduced in females, but not in males. Vaidyanathan et al. (1981b) showed that intravenous naloxone resulted in a rapid and evanescent enhancement of detrusor reflex activity in five patients with neurogenic bladder dysfunction secondary to incomplete suprasacral spinal cord lesions. No effect was seen in two patients with complete suprasacral lesions. Thor et al. (1983) noted that naloxone did not alter bladder function in acute spinal cats (before the development of reflex bladder contractions) but, in large doses, did enhance reflex bladder activity and promote micturition in chronic spinal cats after reflex bladder activity had developed.

Different mechanisms and different opioid receptors seem to be involved in mediating these inhibitory effects at each level of the nervous system. In bladder ganglia, agents that selectively activate δ receptors are effective in blocking transmission, whereas μ and κ agonists are relatively ineffective, indicating that the δ receptors present on preganglionic nerve terminals are primarily responsible for enkephalinergic inhibition at this level (deGroat and Kawatani, 1985). These authors proposed that the mechanism of inhibition in bladder parasympathetic ganglia by endogenous enkephalins is by depression of the release of acetylcholine from the preganglionic nerve. They hypothesized that enkephalins are co-released with acetylcholine at this level and likely mediate a negative feedback or presynaptic inhibitory action in these ganglia. Summarizing a large amount of data from their laboratory, deGroat and Kawatani (1985) and Booth et al. (1985) theorized that μ receptors in the brain stem primarily are concerned with the alteration of bladder capacity, while δ receptors in the spinal cord are primarily involved in the modulation of the magnitude and duration of bladder contraction. The μ brain-stem receptors are thought also to be possibly involved in the control of bladder stability during urine storage, since small doses of naloxone in the cat also increased the frequency and magnitude of uninhibited pressure rises during the tonus limb of the cystometrogram. Equally intriguing is the fact that sphincter motor neurons in the nucleus of Onuf (supplying the periurethral striated muscle) are also densely innervated by enkephalingeric terminals (Glazer and Basbaum, 1980; deGroat et al., 1983). Booth et al. (1985) cited further work in their laboratory that shows that sphincter reflexes in the cat can be inhibited by κ opiate agonists. The κ receptors seem to have little effect on bladder reflex activity at any level.

Thus, enkephalinergic mechanisms may have an important influence on bladder capacity and stability during filling, on bladder contractility during emptying, and on reflex-induced sphincter activity. These mechanisms may be predominantly mediated at different sites by different opiate receptors, raising the very interesting possibility of the development of specific opioid drugs to selectively alter different components of the lower urinary tract during the micturition cycle (deGroat et al., 1985; Booth et al., 1985).

ORGANIZATION OF THE MICTURITION REFLEX

Sacral vs. Supraspinal Micturition Center

The pelvic nerves contain major afferent pathways from the lower urinary tract and also the preganglionic parasympathetic fibers responsible for the bladder contraction of normal micturition. It has long been recognized that the sacral spinal cord, the origin of this nerve, contains neural pathways involved in the micturition reflex (Langley and Anderson, 1895, 1896; Learmoth, 1931; Gruber, 1933). Originally, controversy existed regarding the location of the primary neurologic organizational center for the micturition reflex. Denny-Brown and Robertson (1933), McClellan (1939), and Lapides (1970) all have implied that the micturition reflex is primarily a sacral reflex mediated by the pelvic and pudendal nerves, and subject to facilitation or inhibition by descending central nervous system pathways (Fig 31). Much evidence has been presented in this chapter that in fact the actual organizational center for micturition is localized in the pontine-mesencephalic reticular formation. A full synthesis of data supporting the existence of a pontine-mesencephalic micturition center was more or less concurrently published by Bradley (1974) and by deGroat (1975), but the concept of a supraspinal organization of the basic reflex arc responsible for micturition was originally implied by Barrington in 1914. The theories popularized by Bradley and by deGroat, both of which incorporate the concept of the pontine-mesencephalic micturition center, differ somewhat, and the differences will be pointed out. Over the years, Bradley's

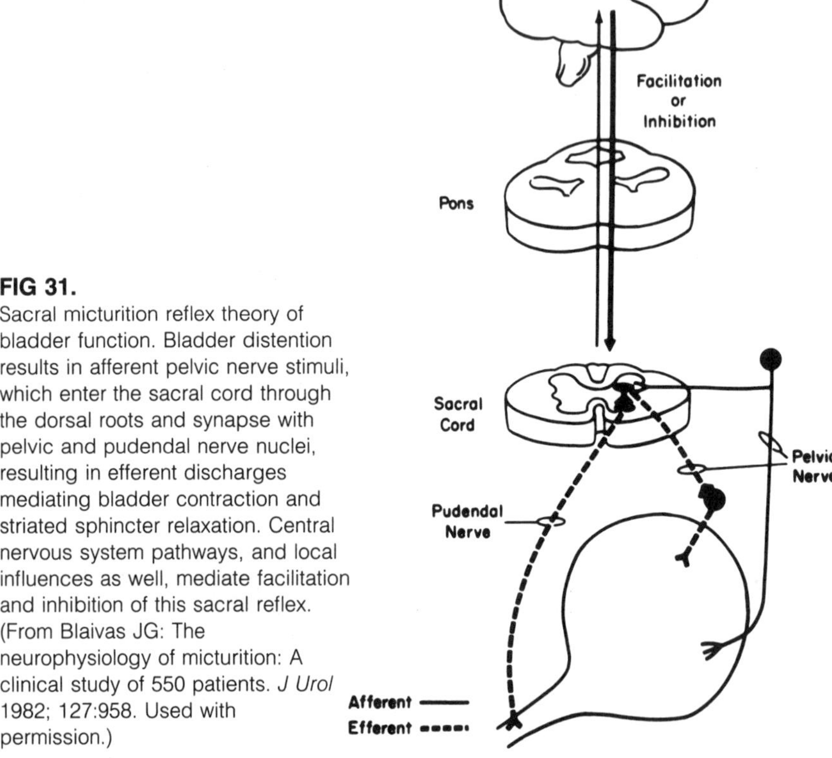

FIG 31.
Sacral micturition reflex theory of bladder function. Bladder distention results in afferent pelvic nerve stimuli, which enter the sacral cord through the dorsal roots and synapse with pelvic and pudendal nerve nuclei, resulting in efferent discharges mediating bladder contraction and striated sphincter relaxation. Central nervous system pathways, and local influences as well, mediate facilitation and inhibition of this sacral reflex. (From Blaivas JG: The neurophysiology of micturition: A clinical study of 550 patients. *J Urol* 1982; 127:958. Used with permission.)

theory has evolved into his defining several neurophysiologic "loops" (described below), which now constitute an overall theory of micturition and its dysfunction.

In the writings of deGroat (deGroat, 1975; deGroat and Booth, 1984; deGroat and Kawatani, 1985), one finds a continuously evolving synthesis of the sacral vs. supraspinal organizational theories, and finds further that these are not mutually exclusive, but complementary. According to deGroat's initial studies of cats with an intact neural axis, bladder distention caused a reflex firing of the preganglionic parasympathetic fibers with a subsequent micturition contraction. The electrophysiologic characteristics of the entire reflex pathway, however, were those of a supraspinal reflex rather than a sacral reflex. In chronic animals (cats) with transsected spinal cords, most ultimately develop reflex contractions of the bladder in response to bladder distention. The

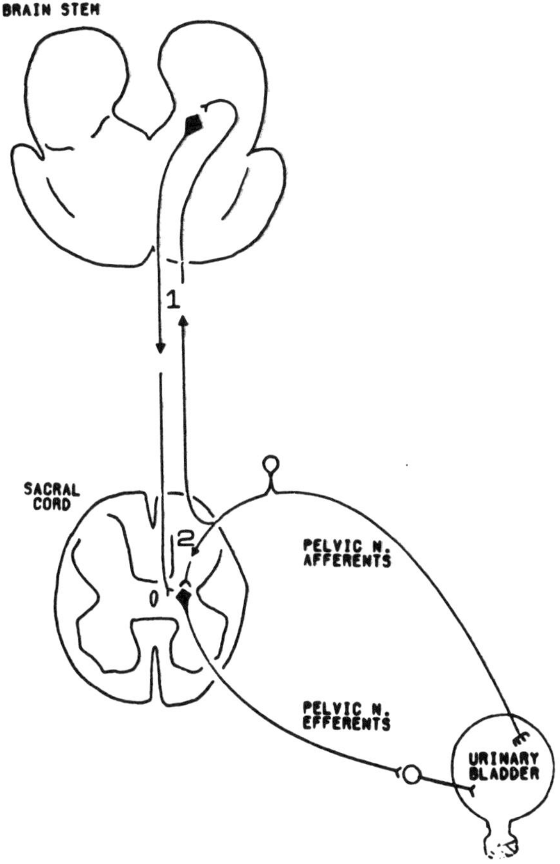

FIG 32.
Reflex micturition pathways involved in micturition in normal (1-supraspinal reflex pathway) and chronic spinal (2-spinal reflex pathway) cats. (From deGroat WC: Nervous control of the urinary bladder of the cat. *Brain Res* 1975; 87:201. Used with permission.)

electrophysiologic properties of this neural circuit were those of a spinal reflex, i.e., a reflex organized in the area of the sacral spinal cord. Figure 32 shows deGroat's initial conceptualization of these data. The so-called reflex neurogenic bladder that develops in patients with spinal cords that have been transsected or severely injured above the sacral level provides an analogy to the bladder contractions during filling that develop in the chronic spinal cat. Whether the appearance of this reflex voiding pattern after spinal transsection results from the formation of new neural pathways by "collateral sprouting" (Liu and

Chambers, 1958; Guth, 1974), or from the removal of an inhibitory influence on an existing pathway, or by the emergence of a vestigial reflex pathway is still speculative, although deGroat and co-workers (deGroat et al., 1981; deGroat and Booth, 1984; deGroat and Kawatani, 1985) have provided compelling evidence to support the latter theory. Their later electrophysiologic studies not only have confirmed the existence of a supraspinal reflex pathway to the bladder in cats, but have provided evidence for the existence of a spinal reflex pathway as well. In animals with an intact neural axis the supraspinal reflex mechanism was the most prominent. Recordings from postganglionic nerves on the surface of the urinary bladder showed that reflex firing occurred with a long latency (mean of 100 msec) following stimulation of myelinated afferent fibers in the pelvic nerve from the bladder. The supraspinal reflex was present in decerebrate animals, but absent in acute or chronic spinal animals. A second reflex, less prominent and noted in only 60% of animals with an intact neural axis, occurred with a considerably longer latency (180–200 msec) following stimulation of vesical afferents. This second reflex occurred only at intensities of stimulation that were sufficient to activate unmyelinated afferent fibers. This reflex was abolished by transsection of the spinal cord at lower thoracic or upper lumbar levels, but was again detectable 3–7 days after transsection in chronic spinal animals. For several weeks this second reflex continued to increase in magnitude in conjunction with the development of reflex micturition. Thus, deGroat's data synthesize the two theories regarding micturitional reflex organization. Both a spinal and supraspinal central pathway appear to exist, each with different afferent limbs for the mediation of detrusor to detrusor reflexes. The supraspinal reflex pathway appears to have the major role in the initiation of bladder contractions in animals with an intact neural axis. The function of the spinal reflex pathway in normal animals is unknown, but appears to be responsible for the development of reflex bladder contractions in the chronic spinal animals, which it may, by inference, in the human clinical counterpart as well. Figure 33 illustrates this concept. deGroat's theory of the reflex pathways involved in micturition (Fig 34) (deGroat and Booth, 1980; deGroat and Booth, 1984; deGroat and Kawatani, 1985) differs from that of Bradley (Bradley et al., 1974; Bradley and Sundin, 1982; Hald and Bradley, 1982; Bhatia and Bradley, 1983) in a few respects. deGroat and associates stressed the importance of the sympathetic nervous system in modulating lower urinary tract function to facilitate urine storage, while Bradley and associates ascribed minimal significance to this. deGroat postulated a synapse between efferent fibers from the brain-stem center and the nuclei of the preganglionic parasympathetic fibers in the sacral spinal cord; Bradley

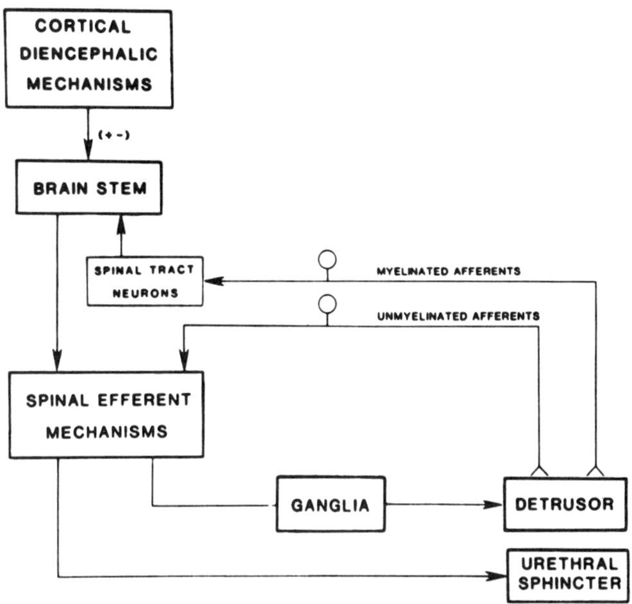

FIG 33.
Central micturition reflex pathways in the cat. With an intact neural axis, micturition is initiated by a supraspinal reflex pathway centered in the pontine-mesencephalic reticular formation. The reflex is triggered by myelinated afferents (A-δ) subserving tension receptors in the bladder wall. In chronic spinal animals, micturition is initially blocked as connections between the brain stem and sacral cord are interrupted. A spinal reflex emerges that is triggered by unmyelinated C-fiber vesical afferents. This reflex is usually weak or undetectable in animals with an intact neural axis. (From deGroat WC, Kawatani M: Neural control of the urinary bladder: Possible relationship between peptidergic inhibitory mechanisms and detrusor instability. *Neurourol Urodynamics* 1985; 4:285. Used with permission.)

and associates did not originally picture such a synapse (1974), although subsequent conceptualizations have included an efferent synapse in the sacral spinal cord (Bradley and Sundin, 1982; Hald and Bradley, 1982; Bhatia and Bradley, 1983). deGroat implied that striated sphincter integration is primarily a sacral spinal cord phenomenon, while Bradley and associates have provided data that separate neural pathways govern voluntary control of the striated sphincter and the bladder (see below).

The Loop Concept

Bradley has extended his original concept of a pontine-mesencephalic micturition center to include a conceptualization of central nervous system control of the lower urinary tract that identifies four neu-

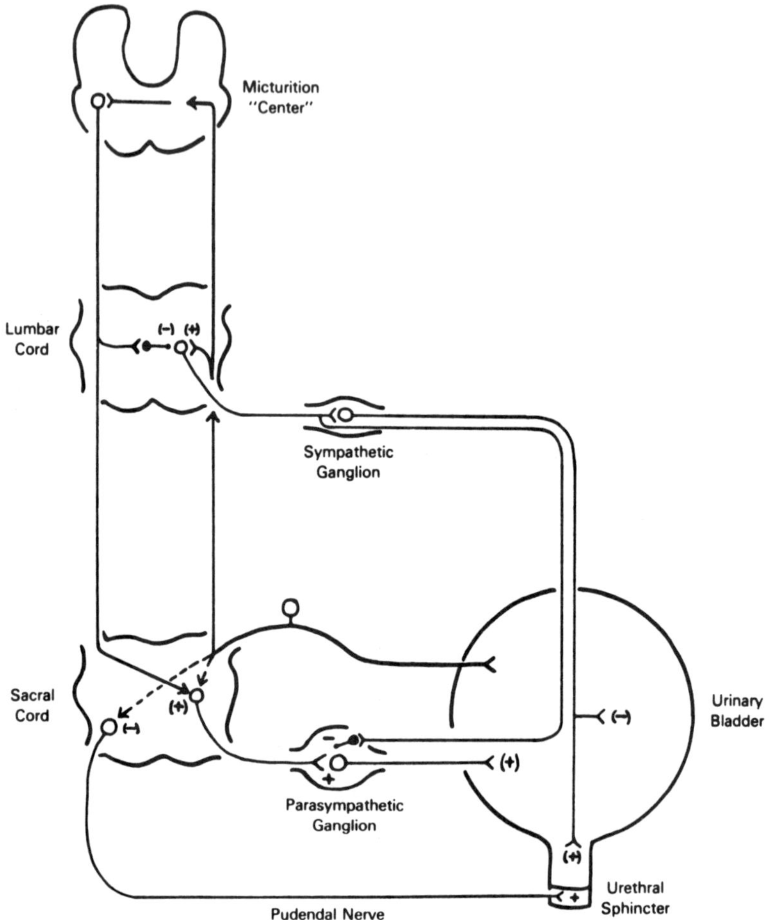

FIG 34.
deGroat's diagram of the reflex pathways involved in micturition. Plus and minus signs indicate excitatory and inhibitory synaptic actions. Voluntary control is accomplished by connection (not pictured) between the frontal cortex and pontine micturition center. Note the prominent role of the sympathetic nervous system and the synapse between the descending fibers from the micturition center (excitatory) and the preganglionic parasympathetic fibers in the sacral spinal cord. (From deGroat WC, Booth AM: Physiology of the urinary bladder and urethra. *Ann Intern Med* 1980; 92(pt 2):321. Used with permission.)

rologic "loops." This concept has evolved over the years (Bradley et al., 1974; Bradley and Sundin, 1982; Hald and Bradley, 1982; Bhatia and Bradley, 1983) and represents a very coherent theory of micturition, consistent with which Bradley has developed one of the popular classification systems of voiding dysfunction. Close interaction exists among all four loops and successful function of one loop depends on the integrity of the remaining loops. Successful integration of the micturition reflex requires a balanced contribution by all loops.

Loop 1 (Fig 35) consists of neuronal connections between the specific areas of the frontal lobes of the cerebral cortex and the micturition center in the pontine-mesencephalic reticular formation. The cerebellum and basal ganglia provide additional input. Loop 1 coordinates voluntary control of the detrusor reflex. Maturation of loop 1 may account for the attainment of voluntary control over the micturition reflex during infancy, and interruption of this loop may cause involuntary bladder contractions. Loop 2 (Fig 36) consists of the routing of bladder sensory afferents in the spinal cord and brain stem and descending pathways from the micturition center to the detrusor motor neurons in the sacral gray matter. Loop 2 includes the intraspinal pathway of detrusor muscle afferents to the brain-stem micturition center and the motor impulses from this center to the sacral spinal cord. Strictly speaking, it does not include peripheral sensory or motor pathways (Hald and Bradley, 1982), and so is not a true "loop," but does include the long routed portion of the sensory afferent fibers that originate in the bladder musculature and synapse in the brain stem. Loop 2 is thought to coordinate and provide for a detrusor reflex of adequate temporal duration to allow total evacuation of intravesical contents. Partial interruption of this loop by spinal cord injury is felt to result in a detrusor reflex of low threshold and in poor emptying, as manifested by residual urine. Spinal cord transsection of this circuit produces detrusor arreflexia and urinary retention, the urinary tract correlates of "spinal shock," which refers to the loss of detrusor reflex activity response of the detrusor and periurethral striated muscle seen following

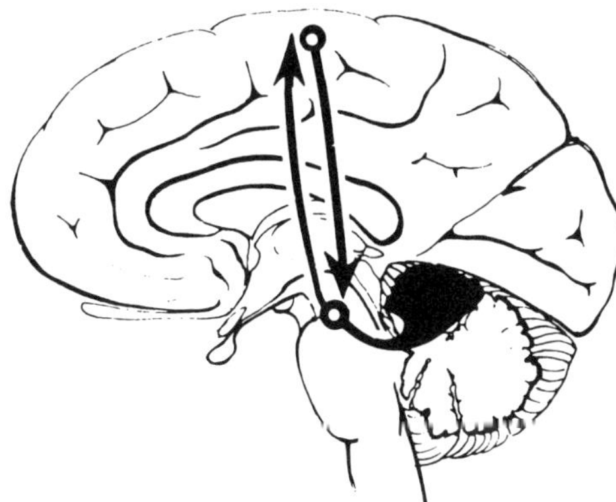

FIG 35.
Bradley's loop 1. See text for description. (From Bhatia NN, Bradley WE: Neuroanatomy and physiology: Innervation of the urinary tract, in Raz S (ed): *Female Urology*. Philadelphia, WB Saunders, 1983. Used with permission.)

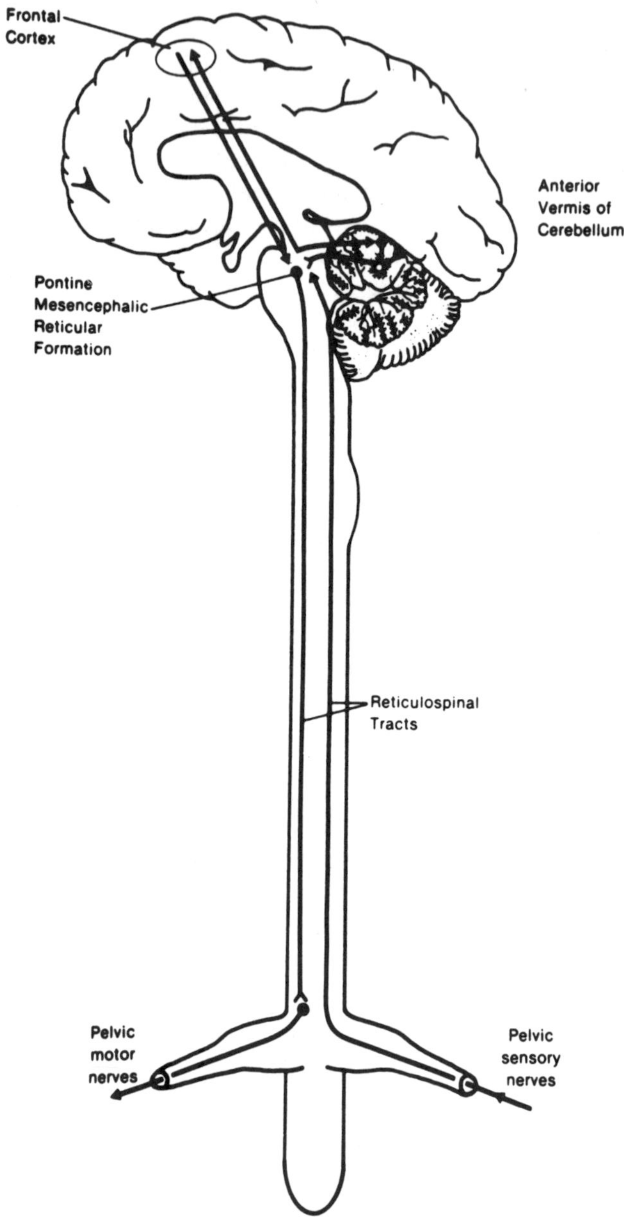

FIG 36.
Bradley's loops 1 and 2. See text for description. (From Bhatia NN, Bradley WE: Neuroanatomy and physiology: Innervation of the urinary tract, in Raz S (ed): *Female Urology*. Philadelphia, WB Saunders, 1983. Used with permission.)

acute spinal cord transsection. The development of reflex bladder activity following suprasacral spinal cord transsection, according to this theory, occurs subsequent to the development of neuroma formation and "ephaptic interaction between neurites and axons at the level of spinal cord transsection" (Hald and Bradley, 1982)—conceptually similar to but not exactly the same as collateral sprouting.

Loop 3 consists of the peripheral detrusor afferent axons and their pathway in the spinal cord, which terminates by synapsing on pudendal motor neurons that ultimately innervate the periurethral striated muscle (Fig 37). This loop provides the neurological substrate whereby impulses from detrusor afferents can inhibit pudendal motor efferents, and thus allow the contracted striated sphincter (during bladder filling and urine storage) to relax in synchrony with bladder contraction during the emptying phase of micturition. Dysfunction of this loop may be responsible for detrusor striated sphincter dyssynergia or for voluntary sphincter relaxation. Loop 4 (Fig 38) consists of two components. Loop 4A consists of the suprasacral afferent and efferent innervation of the pudendal motor neurons to the periurethral striated musculature. Loop 4B (see Fig 37) consists of afferent fibers from the periurethral striated musculature, which synapse on pudendal motor neurons, i.e., the segmental innervation of the periurethral striated muscle. In contrast to stimulation of detrusor afferent fibers, which produce inhibitory postsynaptic potentials in pudendal motor neurons

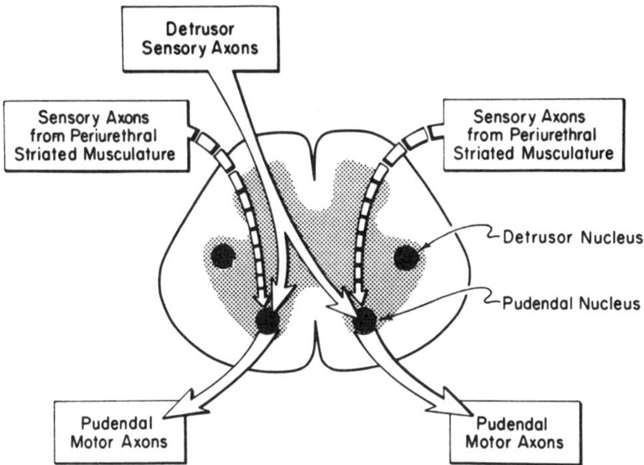

FIG 37.
Bradley's loops 3 and 4B. See text for description. (From Hald T, Bradley W: *The Urinary Bladder: Neurology and Dynamics*. Baltimore, Williams & Wilkins, 1982. Used with permission.)

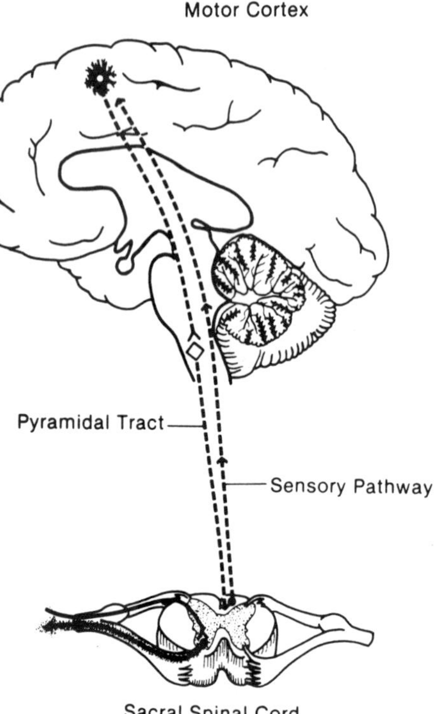

FIG 38.
Bradley's loop 4A. See text for description. (From Hald T, Bradley W: *The Urinary Bladder: Neurology and Dynamics*. Baltimore, Williams & Wilkins, 1982. Used with permission.)

through loop 3, pudendal nerve afferents produce excitatory postsynaptic potentials in these motor neurons through loop 4B. This provides for contraction of the periurethral striated muscle during bladder filling and urine storage. The sensory impulses concerned arise from muscle spindles and tendon organs in the pelvic floor musculature. Loop 4 provides for volitional control of the striated sphincter. Abnormalities of the suprasacral portion result in abnormal responses of the pudendal motor neurons to bladder filling and emptying, which may be manifested as detrusor striated sphincter dyssynergia or/and loss of voluntary contraction of the striated sphincter on command.

Injury or Disease of the Neural Axis

Blaivas (1982) has made a nice attempt to correlate the clinical and urodynamic data from 550 patients with voiding dysfunction with current theories of micturition. He has made the following observations. In 155 patients with suprasacral neurologic lesions (complete and incomplete), physiologically normal voiding was seen in only 41%. Detrusor-striated sphincter dyssynergia was demonstrated in 34% and, surprisingly (and paradoxically), detrusor areflexia was noted in 25%. These data suggest that coordinated voiding is not a simple segmental sacral reflex, but requires higher neurologic integration. Detrusor striated sphincter dyssynergia was found in 45% of 119 patients with suprasacral spinal cord lesions. However, none of 36 patients with supraspinal neurologic lesions (nor none of 213 patients without neurologic disease) had striated sphincter dyssynergia. These data support the view that coordinated voiding is regulated by neurologic centers above the spinal cord, and suggest that a clinical diagnosis of striated sphincter dyssynergia implies a neurologic lesion that interrupts the neural axis between the pontine-mesencephalic reticular formation and the sacral spinal cord. All 27 patients with neurologic lesions above the pons and who were able to void, did so synergistically (with relaxation of the striated sphincter preceding detrusor contraction). Twenty of these patients had involuntary bladder contractions, but 12 of these 20 had voluntary control of the striated sphincter. This supports Bradley's concept of separate neural pathways governing voluntary control of the bladder and the periurethral striated musculature. Most of Blaivas' patients with involuntary bladder contractions secondary to neurologic lesions above the pons were able to voluntarily contract their striated sphincter without abolishing bladder contraction. This would seem to suggest that the inhibition of bladder contraction by pudendal motor activity is not merely a simple sacral reflex, but that such inhibition is a complex neurologic event. Twenty-two of Blaivas' patients had evidence of sacral or infrasacral neurologic impairment of bladder function but had suprasacral control of striated sphincter function, or vice versa, providing a clinical correlate to the distinct anatomical locations of the parasympathetic motor nucleus and the pudendal nucleus of the sacral spinal cord.

Component Reflexes of Micturition

Preceding discussions give some idea of the complexity and diversity of the experimental data and resulting hypotheses relating to the component functions thought to be important for normal filling/storage and emptying of the lower urinary tract. Historically, based on what information was available at the time, authors have been tempted to divide micturition into various "reflexes" related to its initiation, continuation and completion, and cessation. In a series of experiments in the cat reported between 1914 and 1941 Barrington (1914 and cited by

Kuru, 1965) originally described seven component reflexes of micturition (Table 3). Kuru (1965) classified all "reflexes" related to micturition according to whether they were concerned primarily with the storage of urine or the initiation, continuation, and cessation of micturition. Kuru's initial scheme has been used by others (Mahoney et al., 1977; Wein and Raezer, 1979; Schmidt, 1983) to include additional "reflexes" affecting micturition (Tables 4 through 7). Although it is impressive to list these, and quite interesting from a historical standpoint, close inspection will readily reveal that some of these reflexes are contradictory, some are without much experimental or any clinical correlation, and some seem to be based on an attempt to explain a particular event in simple terms rather than to physiologically investigate it. In other words, some are consistent with neuromorphologic, neurophysiologic, neuropharmacologic, and clinical data and make sense in this respect, and others are inconsistent with such data, and therefore do not.

TABLE 3.
Component Reflexes of Micturition According to Barrington*

Reflex	Afferent Pathway	Efferent Pathway	Center
Strong vesical contraction following bladder distention (I)	Pelvic nerve	Pelvic nerve	Supraspinal
Strong vesical contraction evoked by running liquid in the urethra (II)	Pudendal nerve	Pelvic nerve	Supraspinal
Transient, slight vesical contraction following distention of proximal urethra (III)	Hypogastric nerve	Hypogastric nerve	Spinal
Relaxation of urethra following running of liquid through the urethra (IV)	Pudendal nerve	Pudendal nerve	Spinal
External sphincter relaxation evoked by bladder distention (V)	Pelvic nerve	Pudendal nerve	Spinal
Relaxation of smooth musculature of proximal urethra following bladder distention (VI)	Pelvic nerve	Pelvic nerve; hypogastric nerve	Spinal
Transient, slight vesical contraction evoked by running liquid through the urethra (VII)	Pelvic nerve	Pelvic nerve	Spinal

*Adapted from Kuru M: Nervous control of micturition. *Physiol Rev* 1965; 45:425.

TABLE 4.
Reflexes Related to Urine Storage*

Reflexes	Afferent Pathway	Efferent Pathway	Center
Inhibition of vesical contraction during bladder filling	Pelvic nerve; dorsal funiculus; lateral funiculus	Ventral reticulospinal tract (?), pelvic nerve	Bulbar
Increased external sphincter (sacral) contraction evoked by bladder filling	Pelvic nerve	Pudendal nerve	Spinal
Increased external sphincter (sacral) contraction evoked by urine involuntarily entering the proximal urethra	Pudendal nerve	Pudendal nerve	Spinal
Inhibition of vesical contraction during bladder filling†	Pelvic nerve	Hypogastric nerve	Spinal (thoracolumbar)
Increased contraction (closure) of bladder neck and proximal urethra during bladder filling	Pelvic nerve	Hypogastric nerve	Spinal (thoracolumbar)

*After Kuru M: Nervous control of micturition. *Physiol Rev* 1965; 45:425. Original references cited by Kuru (1965) and Mahoney et al. (1977).
†Directly by an inhibitory effect on bladder muscle cells, and indirectly by an inhibitory effect on bladder parasympathetic ganglia (see text).

TABLE 5.
Reflexes Related to Initiation of Micturition*

Reflexes	Afferent Pathway	Efferent Pathway	Center
Vesical contraction and proximal urethral relaxation evoked by bladder distention	Pelvic nerve; hypogastric nerve	Pelvic nerve; hypogastric nerve	Spinal
Vesical contraction evoked by bladder distention†	Pelvic nerve; dorsal funiculus; lateral funiculus	Lateral reticulospinal tract (?); pelvic nerve	Bulbar
Relaxation of pelvic musculature evoked by bladder distention and subsequent contraction	Pelvic nerve; lateral funiculus	Corticospinal tract (?); pudendal nerve	Bulbar

*After Kuru M: Nervous control of micturition. *Physiol Rev* 1965; 45:425. Original references cited by Kuru (1965) and Mahoney et al. (1977).
†Also central inhibition of bulbar relaxer center and thereby of the first reflex listed in Table 4.

TABLE 6.
Reflexes Related to Continuation and Completion of Micturition*

Reflex	Afferent Pathway	Efferent Pathway	Center
Continued vesical contraction during voiding† evoked by receptors in detrusor muscle	Pelvic nerve; lateral funiculus; juxtasolitariothalamic tract	Lateral reticulospinal tract (?); pelvic nerve	Pontine
Promotion of vesical contraction during voiding‡ evoked by receptors in detrusor muscle	Pelvic nerve; lateral funiculus; juxtasolitariothalamic tract	Tectobulbar, mesencephalobulbospinal, lateral reticulospinal tract (?); pelvic nerve	Bulbar
Continued vesical contraction during voiding evoked by running liquid through the urethra	Pudendal nerve; lateral funiculus; juxtasolitariothalamic tract	Lateral reticulospinal tract (?); pelvic nerve	Pontine; bulbar; mesencephalic
Continued vesical contraction during voiding evoked by running liquid through the urethra	Pelvic nerve	Pelvic nerve	Spinal
Continued vesical contraction during voiding evoked by receptors in detrusor muscle	Pelvic nerve	Pelvic nerve	Spinal

* After Kuru M: Nervous control of micturition. *Physiol Rev* 1965; 45:425. Original references cited by Kuru (1965) and Mahoney et al. (1977).
†Also centrally based (probably pontine) reflex inhibition of external urethral sphincter tone.
‡By inhibition of bulbar relaxer center.

TABLE 7.
Reflexes Related to Cessation of Micturition*

Reflex	Afferent Pathway	Efferent Pathway	Center
Vesical relaxation following cessation of stream in urethra†	Pelvic and/or pudendal nerve; dorsal funiculus; lateral funiculus	Ventral reticulospinal tract (?); pelvic nerve	Bulbar‡
Recovery of external sphincter tone following cessation of stream in urethra	Pelvic and/or pudendal nerve	Pudendal nerve	Spinal§

*After Kuru M: Nervous control of micturition. *Physiol Rev* 1965; 45:425. Original references cited by Kuru (1965) and Mahoney et al. (1977).
†Similar reflex probably exists with afferent limb from cessation of stimuli on receptors in series with detrusor muscle fibers.
‡Similar reflex probably exists at spinal level.
§Similar reflex probably exists at central (most likely pontine) level.

Important Functional Questions

Based on the preceding experimental and clinical data, and the various theories and hypotheses that have been proposed relative to these, we can now at least address, and in some cases answer, certain important questions that relate to the activity of the bladder and the outlet during the filling/storage and emptying phases of micturition. Further, we can now also look at at least some of the alterations of lower urinary tract function produced by a variety of experimental and clinical conditions and try to provide neuromorphologic, neurophysiologic, and neuropharmacologic correlates, based on these data, theories, and hypotheses. Most of the material in this section is strictly based on references previously cited in this chapter. However, some of the viewpoints expressed, though based on selected data, reflect our own personal prejudices, consistent with our own experimental and clinical experience.

WHAT DETERMINES BLADDER RESPONSE DURING FILLING?

It is clear that the normal bladder response to filling at a physiological rate is an almost imperceptible change in intravesical pressure. During at least the initial stages of bladder filling, there is little question that this very high compliance is due to purely passive properties of the bladder wall. These passive properties have been described by various authorities (see Zinner et al. [1983], Coolsaet [1984], and Griffiths [1984] for summaries and references). The definition employed and the graphs and formulas used by these authors may be somewhat different, but the implied conclusions are the same. The elastic properties of the bladder wall allow it to stretch to a certain degree without any increase in tension, thus allowing intravesical pressure to remain virtually unchanged within certain limits. The viscoelastic properties of the bladder wall allow for an increase in intravesical pressure when the rate of stretch (filling volume) exceeds the rate of stress relaxation. They also allow for a decrease in this tension when this rapid filling slows or stops. Although the mathematical descriptions and terminologies may be relatively new, the concept of nonneurogenic tonus during filling is not, and was clearly implied and supported by Nesbit and Lapides (1947, 1948) and by Tang and Ruch (1955). Filling cystometry, in the usual clinical setting, seems to show a slight increase in intravesical pressure during infusion of the medium employed. However, Klevmark (1974, 1977, 1980) has shown, in an elegant series of experiments on cats, that this pressure rise during filling is a function of the fact that the filling is carried out at a greater than physiologic rate, and that, at physiologic filling rates, there is essentially no rise in bladder pressure until bladder capacity is reached. During filling, if an acute increase in volume introduction occurs, the bladder wall will respond with an increase in intravesical pressure, which is a combination of the elastic and viscoelastic properties of the bladder wall and the inherent response of smooth muscle to stretch. Clinically, loss of the elastic fibers of the bladder wall and their replacement by fibrous tissue is most commonly observed in patients with chronic pancystitis, especially those who have had an indwelling catheter present for some time. The effect of the loss of elastic and viscoelastic properties of the bladder wall is clearly seen in these patients, whose filling cystometrograms exhibit a decrease in compliance at low filling rates. Such decreased compliance, secondary to loss of the passive properties of the bladder wall, is generally unresponsive to pharmacologic manipulation, hydrodistention, or nerve section, and most often requires augmentation cystoplasty to achieve satisfactory bladder reservoir function.

A small fraction of our previous discussions has mentioned the possibility of substances released from the bladder muscle or epithelium during filling (primarily prostaglandins), which contribute to the small rise in bladder wall tension that occurs. A much larger fraction of our discussion has considered the question of inhibitory neural mechanisms that are operative during the filling/storage phase of micturition. It is certainly clear that in animals a spinal sympathetic reflex, which is evoked by bladder filling, exists. One arm of this seems to involve direct neurally mediated stimulation of β-adrenergic receptors located predominantly in the bladder body smooth musculature. Evidence for a major such inhibitory influence in humans is sparse, but a minor such role could conceivably exist. It is quite clear that the "normal" bladder response during filling is most vividly disrupted by efferent activity in the pelvic nerve excitatory tract, causing involuntary bladder contraction. Most discussions of neural reflex mechanisms causing an inhibitory influence on bladder activity during the filling/storage phase of micturition have centered on indirect inhibitory mechanisms of this parasympathetic efferent activity. Such an inhibitory role at the level of the bladder parasympathetic ganglia has clearly been confirmed by deGroat (deGroat and Saum, 1971 and 1972; deGroat and Theoblad, 1976; deGroat and Booth, 1984) as a part of the spinal sympathetic reflex that occurs during bladder filling in cats. Compelling, although indirect, evidence exists to support such a role in humans. The afferent stimuli that initiate this reflex are mediated primarily through the pelvic nerves, but there is evidence to support inhibitory reflex mechanisms that are activated through pudendal nerve stimuli as well. McGuire (1978, 1983, 1984a) implies a direct inhibition of the detrusor motor neurons in the sacral spinal cord due to increased afferent pudendal nerve activity generated by receptors in the striated sphincter. Such a reflex was first described in man by Kock and Pompeius (1963), who showed an inhibition of bladder contractile activity initiated by anal distention. Sundin et al. (1974) have proposed a similar pudendal nerve–mediated inhibition of bladder activity during stimulation, but one that is mediated through hypogastric nerve activity.

Good evidence also seems to exist to support a strong tonic inhibitory effect of endogenous opioids on bladder activity at at least two levels, the spinal cord and the brain stem (Hisamitsu and deGroat, 1984; deGroat and Booth, 1984; deGroat and Kawatani, 1984). Such activity likely affects the bladder response (or lack of it) during filling, and may affect contractility during emptying as well.

The presence and functional significance (if any) of spontaneous activity during filling in the normal urinary bladder is a very controversial subject that certainly bears on the question of what determines the bladder response during filling. In the anesthetized cat, intravesical pressure recordings have revealed marked "spontaneous" rhythmic bladder activity (Klevmark, 1974, 1977, 1980). Rhythmic activity, however, was unable to be elicited in the awake state in this animal. In the deeply relaxed or anesthetized animals, when rhythmic bladder contractions were demonstrated during filling, they were demonstrated at physiologic filling rates, as opposed to other experiments (Plum and Colfelt, 1960), where more rapid and unphysiologic rates of filling were utilized. Klevmark (1980) found that these spontaneous bladder contractions in deeply asleep or anesthetized cats during filling were not affected by spinal cord transsection above the T10 level, but were either abolished or converted to an irregular, dissimilar pattern by partial or complete peripheral denervation, supporting the notion that such spontaneous rhythmic activity in response to distention was dependent on intact bladder innervation from the spinal cord. Plum and Colfelt (1960) maintained that the rhythmic contractions of the cat urinary bladder were nonneurogenic and, further, that the rhythmic waves were a fundamental and necessary component of normal micturition, a micturition contraction developing as a rapid summation and fusion of smaller waves. They suggested that an increase in such contractions followed sacral rhizotomy or distal cordectomy, implying that the sacral spinal cord segments tonically inhibited bladder rhythmicity.

Older reports (Plum, 1960; Kock and Pompeius, 1963) cite the occurrence of rhythmic bladder activity in awake humans with neurologically intact bladders. It is difficult to correlate this information with, and integrate it into, current urodynamic doctrine, which suggests that phasic increases in intravesical pressure that occur during bladder filling are always abnormal, regardless of whether there is any sensory perception of these increases. Any contemporary description of filling cystometry (see Abrams [1984]) will be found to state quite conclusively that "in the normal bladder no detrusor activity is evident during the filling phase of cystometry; therefore, strictly speaking, any detrusor contractions occurring during the filling phase should be regarded as abnormal." In the anesthetized rabbit, bladder activity during filling is absent at low intravesical volumes and pressures, and develops only on reaching a critical pressure, this activity being completely inhibited by ganglionic blockade. In the presence of ganglionic blockade, the in vivo bladder is devoid of activity at any volume or pressure, suggesting that this activity is not really "spontaneous," but occurs in response to bladder filling and is in fact a neuronal reflex phenomenon (Levin et al., 1986). In the rabbit, the in vitro whole bladder preparation is totally devoid of any spontaneous phasic contractile activity at any volume or pressure during filling unless longitudinal tension is applied to the preparation (Levin et al., 1986). This study further suggested that the "spontaneous" activity commonly observed in isolated urinary bladder strip preparations is in fact a simple myogenic response to stretch, and has little physiologic significance under normal conditions. Klevmark (1980) wisely commented on the term "spontaneous," pointing out that this term generally applies only to contractions due to membrane potential variations that occur either spontaneously in pacemaker regions or following chemical or mechanical stimulation of smooth muscle. Thus, the type of "spontaneous" activity seen in bladder smooth muscle strips (invariably under some stretch) would seem to have little functional significance insofar as the emptying contraction of a normal micturition is concerned. It is possible, however, that localized contractile activity in response to various types of pathology might be sufficient to generate a rise in intravesical pressure, causing pathologic symptomatology during the filling phase of micturition (urgency, frequency, and, perhaps, urge incontinence), irrespective of the emptying ability of such activity.

WHAT DETERMINES OUTLET RESPONSE DURING FILLING?

Virtually all authorities would agree that there is a gradual increase in urethral pressure during bladder filling (see references at the beginning of this chapter, and also Tanagho and Smith, 1966; Jonas and Tanagho, 1975; Ghonheim et al., 1975; Khalaf et al., 1979; and Abdel-Rahman et al., 1981, 1983). Urethral pressure is an ill-defined phenomenon, measurement of which is far from standardized. It is clear that, whatever definition one accepts, this is not equivalent to urethral resistance, nor are increases or decreases in either "pressure" or "resistance" reproducibly correlated with urinary continence and incontinence. Experiments and discussions that have attempted to delineate the various components of urethral "pressure," "resistance," and continence/incontinence are flawed by the lack of a definitive method to separate even active from passive characteristics of the urethral wall. Moreover, in our opinion, there is no truly reliable way to separate the smooth from the striated muscular contribution to urethral pressure by strictly pharmacologic means, as long as significant disagreement exists regarding the innervation and receptor content of the smooth muscle of the wall of the urethra, of the intramural striated muscle, and of the extramural striated muscle. Various estimates of the contribution of components of the urethral wall to urethral "pressure" are given in Table 8. It must be recognized that these estimates were derived from different experimental animals (and man), under totally different experimental and clinical conditions and with totally different rationales. However, it is clear that most authors at least recognize the presence of relatively passive elements in the urethral wall, as opposed to active elements, in which the tension can change in response to neural or humoral mechanisms.

The rise in urethral pressure that is seen during the filling phase

TABLE 8.
Estimates of Urethral Pressure Components (Percentage)

Author(s)	Striated Muscle*	Smooth Muscle	Connective Tissue†	Vasculature
Tanagho et al., (1969a, 1969b, 1978)	50	50	. . .	. . .
Donker et al. (1972)	Minimal	. . .	. . .	. . .
Raz et al. (1972b)	. . .	. . .	. . .	30
Awad and Downie (1976b)	16(F)	40	41	
	31(M)	45	24	
Koff (1977)	43	. . .	. . .	. . .
Rud et al. (1980)	33	33		33
Rossier et al. (1982)	60	. . . 30	. . .	. . .

*Includes (and does not differentiate between) extramural and intramural.
†Includes elastic, collagenous, and fibrous tissue within or outside urethral wall.

of micturition can be correlated with an increase in efferent pudendal nerve and hypogastric nerve impulse frequencies, at least in cats (deGroat and Booth, 1980, 1984). This, and the well-known phenomenon of a gradual increase in pelvic EMG activity during bladder filling, make it certain that a reflex increase in striated sphincter activity contributes significantly to this urethral response. Neurophysiologic, neuromorphologic, and neuropharmacologic data are all consistent with this. However, it should be recognized that most of these data are based on the "classic" model of a striated sphincter innervated by the pudendal nerve, and do not include the possibility of the contribution of efferent pelvic nerve impulses. Furthermore, if the possibility of a different innervation of the intramural vs. the extramural striated sphincter is considered, it is not quite clear to us exactly how one goes about discretely separating the contribution of the intramural vs. the extramural striated component to the urethral response during bladder filling.

Although it seems logical (and compatible with neuropharmacologic, neurophysiologic, and neuromorphologic data) to assume that the urethral smooth muscle component also contributes to the change in urethral response during bladder filling, it is extremely difficult to prove this either experimentally or clinically. Those, like ourselves, who intuitively believe that an increase in smooth sphincter activity contributes to urethral response during bladder filling should not ignore significant questions that inevitably arise during consideration of this subject. To say that the urethral smooth muscle possesses a tonus, and that this tonus itself is sufficient to maintain continence, is certainly not equivalent to saying that this tonus is neurologically mediated or that it changes during bladder filling. Abdel-Rahman et al. (1981) failed to demonstrate a change in proximal urethral smooth muscle activity in the cat during bladder filling, but did, however, feel that the intrinsic tone of this area was what maintained urinary continence. It is difficult to prove that the increases in hypogastric nerve activity seen during bladder filling in experimental animals affect urethral smooth sphincter tone. In other words, these efferent impulses may not terminate on the smooth musculature of the urethra or on ganglion cells affecting urethral motility, but may simply be terminating only on parasympathetic ganglion cells relaying to the smooth musculature of the bladder.

There is also a potential for substances, such as prostaglandins, released either from the bladder mucosa or bladder musculature during filling, to raise urethral resistance by a humoral effect on the urethral wall, and without any neurologic mediation.

Finally, it is certainly possible, if one believes that there is a continuity of smooth musculature from the bladder base into the proximal urethra, that bladder filling increases mural tension in the bladder neck area, and that this may be transmitted to the urethra and reflected by tension changes in its wall.

The passive properties of the urethral wall certainly deserve mention, as these undoubtedly play a large role in the maintenance of continence (see Zinner et al. [1983] and references contained therein). To maintain urinary continence, the urethral lumen must be completely sealed. Urethral wall tension develops within the outer layers of the urethra and is a product not only of the active characteristics of smooth and striated muscle, but of the passive characteristics of the elastic and collagenous tissue as well. This tension must be exerted on a soft or plastic inner layer capable of being compressed to a closed configuration. This region of compression full of "filler material" (Zinner et al., 1980, 1983) represents the submucosal portion of the urethra. The softer and more plastic this area is, the less pressure is required by the tension-producing area to produce continence. Finally, whatever the compressive forces, the lumen must be capable of being obliterated by a watertight seal. This mucosal seal mechanism (the term seems to have been originated by Caine and Raz [1973]) explains why a very thin-walled rubber tube requires less pressure to close an open end when the inner layer is coated with a fine layer of grease than when it is not, the latter case being much like a scarred or atrophic urethral mucosa. Also, this explains why one can pass a pair of small clamped catheters through a normal urethra into the bladder with no leakage around the catheters (Zinner et al., 1983).

WHY DOES URINARY LEAKAGE NOT OCCUR WITH INCREASES IN INTRA-ABDOMINAL PRESSURE?

Outlet resistance to the flow of urine from the bladder is maintained by the passive and active factors mentioned above. During voluntarily initiated micturition, the bladder pressure becomes higher than the outlet pressure, certain adaptive changes occur in the shape of the bladder outlet, and urine pases into and through the proximal urethra. One could reasonably ask why such changes do not occur with increases in intravesical pressure, which are similar in magnitude, but which are produced only by changes in intra-abdominal pressure, such as straining and coughing. First of all, a coordinated bladder contraction does not occur in response to such stimuli, and this fact clearly points out that increases in intravesical pressure are by no means equivalent to emptying ability. For urine to flow into the proximal urethra, not only must an increase in intravesical pressure occur, but it must be a product of a coordinated bladder contraction, occurring through a neurally mediated reflex mechanism, and associated with characteristic changes in the bladder neck and proximal urethral area, themselves either directly or indirectly a part of this reflex mechanism. A decrease in tension in the striated sphincter is reflexly coordinated with this type of bladder contraction, and so is, most probably, a decrease in smooth sphincter tension as well.

A major factor in the prevention of urinary leakage during increases in intra-abdominal pressure is the location of the sphincter unit (the bladder neck and proximal urethra). Normally, this is situated within the abdominal cavity to allow at least equal pressure transmission of any increase in intra-abdominal pressure to the bladder neck and proximal urethra. This phenomenon was first extensively described by Enhorning (1961), has been confirmed in virtually every urodynamic laboratory that has studied stress urinary incontinence, and is illustrated in Figure 39. The structures that normally support the female bladder neck and proximal urethra, and that prevent the descent of this sphincteric area into a position where intra-abdominal pressure increases are not transmitted at least equally to it, are the pubourethral ligaments, the pubocervical fascia, and the levator ani muscles (Stanton, 1984). Alteration of these structures such that pathologic descent does occur with abdominal straining occurs secondary to many etiologic factors, and stress incontinence is the result. To correct this, it is necessary only to substitute a mechanism to prevent this descent and to restore the normal resting position of the bladder neck and proximal

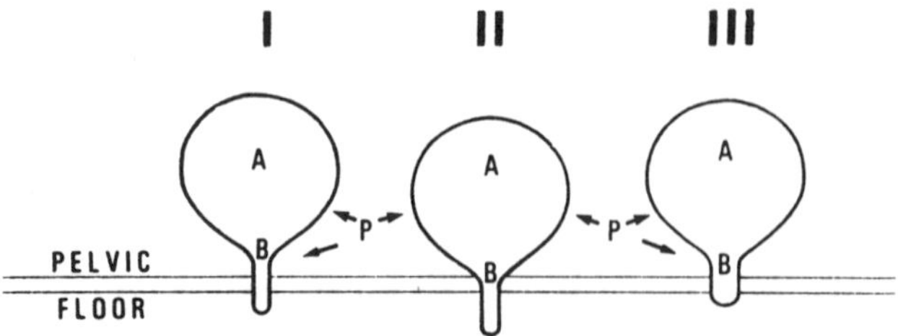

FIG 39.
Transmission of increases in intra-abdominal pressure to bladder neck and proximal urethra. "I" represents the normal state. Intra-abdominal pressure increases are transmitted at least equally to the bladder neck/proximal urethral area (P + B ≥ P + A). "II" illustrates the genesis of stress urinary incontinence. During increases in abdominal pressure, the bladder neck/proximal urethra area exhibits abnormal descent to a position in which a positive pressure gradient no longer occurs (P + B < P + A). In "III" the support of the bladder neck/proximal urethra is adequate, but the bladder neck and proximal urethra are nonfunctional. They exhibit essentially no closure pressure and are isobaric with the bladder. P + B is never greater than P + A. Restoring a support mechanism to check descent will correct the incontinence resulting from "II" but not from "III." Correction of "III" requires, assuming the support mechanism is satisfactory, reconstruction or compression of the bladder neck/proximal urethra (urethral sling, artificial sphincter, periurethral polytef injection). (From Stanton SL: Urethral sphincter incompetence (stress incontinence), in Mundy AR, et al (eds): *Urodynamics: Principles, Practice, Application.* New York, Churchill Livingstone, 1984. Used with permission.)

urethra. This is accomplished by any of the standard vesicourethral suspension procedures.

There is evidence (Tanagho, 1978) to show that the increase in urethral closure pressure seen with increments in extrinsic pressure applied to the abdomen actually exceeds the extrinsic pressure increase, indicating that active muscular function, in addition to simple transmission of pressure, is involved. Tanagho (1978) cogently summarized evidence that the increment in urethral closure pressure involves a reflex increase in sphincter activity, primarily of the striated sphincter, but involving the smooth sphincter as well.

WHY DOES VOIDING ENSUE WITH A NORMAL BLADDER CONTRACTION?

As previously indicated, there is a reflex coordination between a voluntarily induced bladder contraction of adequate magnitude and active responses of the proximal urethra. Most would agree with the observations cited and reconfirmed by Tanagho (1978) and McGuire

(1983, 1984a) that urethral pressure actually decreases prior to bladder contraction, although some (Khalaf et al., 1979) would disagree. The decrease in pelvic floor striated muscle EMG activity prior to voluntary bladder contraction would strongly suggest that at least a portion of this decrease in urethral response is secondary to a reflex mechanism involving the striated sphincter and mediated through the pudendal nerves (Tanagho, 1978; McGuire, 1983, 1984a; deGroat, 1984). It is certainly tempting to speculate that a similar coordination of smooth sphincter activity exists, reflected by a decrease in efferent hypogastric nerve activity that occurs with the onset of bladder contraction (deGroat and Booth, 1980, 1984). Although there is much indirect evidence to support a reflex inhibition of smooth sphincter activity during bladder contraction, it is very difficult to accrue direct evidence to confirm this. McGuire (1984a) seems to agree that there is indeed an active mechanism that occurs that decreases urethral smooth muscle activity during bladder contraction, but postulates, on the basis of data previously cited, that this is an active mechanism involving stimulation of β-adrenergic receptors, a concept supported by El Badawi (1982, 1983) and Khanna (1983).

Tanagho (see 1978 for summary) originated the ingenious bipartite animal bladder, where the detrusor compartment was separated from the sphincter compartment. This effectively excludes vesicourethral smooth muscle continuity as a mechanism contributing to bladder neck and proximal urethral pressure changes during bladder filling and bladder contraction. The bipartite model in the dog clearly showed that there was indeed a rise in urethral pressure with bladder filling, and active contraction of the bladder was still preceded by a drop in urethral closure pressure. However, this by no means excludes a contributory mechanistic effect on the bladder neck and proximal urethra by virtue of smooth muscle continuity between the bladder base and proximal urethra in the intact animal or in man. There is clearly a difference between the type of tension developed in the bladder wall smooth musculature during filling and that seen during active contraction. Some contribution to the architectural changes seen in the area of the bladder neck and proximal urethra during bladder emptying may very likely be a result of mural continuity.

Finally, consistent with the observation of Anderson et al. (1983) and Klarskov et al. (1983), we cannot eliminate the possibility that some of the changes that occur in the bladder neck/proximal urethral area during active bladder contraction are wholly or in part neurologically mediated, but through a noncholinergic and nonadrenergic postganglionic neurotransmitter mechanism.

Normal Lower Urinary Tract Filling/ Storage and Emptying: Simple Overview, Extrapolation, and Application of the Two-Phase Concept

It is obvious that a discussion of any magnitude regarding the central and peripheral factors involved in micturition is bound to engender at least some disagreement. What follows is a concise and simplified description of the normal processes involved in lower urinary tract function, which seems to us to be consistent with the data and opinions presented.

The two functions of the lower urinary tract are the storage and the active expulsion of the urine. During bladder filling at physiological rates, intravesical pressure initially rises slowly despite large increases in volume. This phenomenon is due primarily to the passive elastic and viscoelastic properties of the smooth muscle and connective tissue of the bladder wall. There is little neural efferent activity to the lower urinary tract until a certain critical intravesical pressure is reached, following which there is a gradual reflex increase in somatic nerve efferent activity through the pudendal nerve, and perhaps the pelvic nerve, which causes increased activity in the striated sphincter. In animals, and perhaps in humans as well, an additional spinal sympathetic reflex also results from pelvic nerve afferents. The efferent limb of this reflex is through the hypogastric nerve, resulting in inhibition of bladder contractile activity by an inhibitory effect on parasympathetic ganglionic transmission, and also in an increase in outlet resistance because of active stimulation of the predominantly α-adrenergic receptors of the smooth muscle of the bladder neck and proximal urethra. A decrease in bladder body contractility, because of active stimulation through this reflex of the predominantly β-adrenergic receptors in that area, may also play a role. The net effect of all these actions is filling of the bladder cavity, but with a low increase in intravesical pressure relative to volume, and without any evidence of active coordinated bladder contractile activity. A tonic inhibitory influence exerted by endogenous opioids very likely plays a contributory role in maintaining this stability.

Intraurethral pressure is always greater than intravesical pressure, and this relationship is maintained during increases in intra-abdominal pressure because of the anatomic localization of the "sphincter unit" and the positive pressure transmission ratio to this area with respect to intravesical contents.

Although many factors are involved in the micturition reflex, it is intravesical pressure producing the sensation of distention that is primarily responsible for the initiation of voluntarily induced emptying of the lower urinary tract. The origin of the parasympathetic neural outflow to the bladder, the pelvic nerve, is in the sacral spinal cord. However, the actual organizational center for the micturition reflex in an intact neural axis is in the brain stem, and the complete neural circuit for normal micturition includes the ascending and descending spinal cord pathways to and from this area and the facilitory and inhibitory influences from other parts of the brain.

The final step in voluntarily induced micturition involves inhibition of the somatic neural efferent activity to the striated sphincter and an inhibition of all aspects of the spinal sympathetic reflex evoked during filling. Efferent parasympathetic pelvic nerve activity is ultimately what is responsible for a highly coordinated contraction of the bulk of the bladder smooth musculature. A decrease in outlet resistance occurs, with adaptive shaping or funneling of the relaxed bladder outlet. This may involve reflex inhibition of both the striated sphincter and of α-adrenergically mediated smooth sphincter tone. It may also involve active β-adrenergic–induced smooth muscle relaxation or smooth muscle relaxation through a noncholinergic, nonadrenergic mechanism. The adaptive changes are also due at least in part to the anatomic interrelationships of the smooth muscle of the bladder base and proximal urethra. Other reflexes that are elicited by bladder contraction and by the passage of urine through the urethra may reinforce and facilitate complete bladder emptying. Superimposed on these autonomic and somatic reflexes are complex modifying supraspinal inputs from other central neuronal networks. These facilitory and inhibitory impulses, which originate from several levels of the nervous system, including the brain stem, cerebellum, and cerebral cortex, allow for the full conscious control of micturition.

Whatever disagreements exist, it is extremely important to note that all "experts" would agree, however, on certain points. The micturition cycle involves two relatively discrete processes: (1) bladder filling and urine storage, and (2) bladder emptying. Whatever the neuromorphologic, neurophysiologic, neuropharmacologic, and mechanical details involved, the following summary must apply for these processes to occur normally.

BLADDER FILLING AND URINE STORAGE

1. Accommodation of increasing volumes of urine at a low intravesical pressure and with appropriate sensation.
2. The bladder outlet must be closed at rest and remain so during increases in intra-abdominal pressure.
3. There must be no involuntary bladder contractions.

BLADDER EMPTYING

1. There must be a coordinated contraction of the bladder smooth musculature of adequate magnitude.
2. A concomitant lowering of resistance must occur at the level of the smooth sphincter and the striated sphincter.
3. There must be no anatomic obstruction.

Further extrapolating this concept, one recognizes that any type of voiding dysfunction *must* result from an abnormality of one of the factors listed above. Thus, any abnormality of bladder filling and/or urine storage must result from a problem related to one of three simple factors or from some combination thereof. Any problem with bladder emptying must occur on a similar basis. One may reasonably argue about the anatomic, physiologic, and pharmacologic factors involved in these two relatively discrete phases of micturition, but one cannot argue about the conceptual simplicity of component contributions involved in each phase. This division, with its implied subdivisions under each category into causes related to the bladder and causes related to the outlet, provides a perfect rationale for the classification of all types of voiding dysfunction into disorders related to bladder filling or urine storage, and disorders related to bladder emptying. There are indeed some types of voiding dysfunction that represent combinations of filling/storage and emptying disorders. Within this scheme, these become readily understandable. Further, one may take all aspects of urodynamic and videourodynamic evaluation and classify the individual component studies as to exactly what they evaluate, in terms of either bladder or outlet (smooth and striated sphincter) activity during bladder filling/storage, or during bladder emptying. Urodynamics thus become readily understandable. Finally, one can then easily classify all known treatments for voiding dysfunction under the broad categories of whether they facilitate bladder filling/storage or bladder emptying, and whether they do so by an action primarily on the bladder or on the components of the bladder outlet. These clinical considerations are fully expanded in the next chapter.

ACKNOWLEDGMENT

The authors wish to thank Karl Erik Andersson and David M. Jacobowitz for reviewing the manuscript of this section and for providing valuable advice for its final form.

REFERENCES

1. Abdel-Hakim A, Hassouna M, Rioux F, et al: Response of urethral smooth muscles to pharmacological agents. II. Non-cholinergic non-adrenergic agonists and antagonists. *J Urol* 1983; 130:988.
2. Abdel-Rahman M, Galeano C, Elhilali M: New approach to study of voiding cycle in cat: Preliminary report on pharmacologic studies. *Urology* 1983; 22:91.
3. Abdel-Rahman M, Galeano C, Lamarch J, et al: A new approach to the study of the voiding cycle in the cat. *Invest Urol* 1981; 18:475.
4. Abrams P: The practice of urodynamics, in Mundy AR, Stephenson TP, Wein AJ (eds): *Urodynamics: Principles, Practice and Applications.* New York, Churchill Livingstone, 1984, pp 76–92.
5. Abrams PH, Feneley RCL: The actions of prostaglandins on the smooth muscle of the human urinary tract in vitro. *Br J Urol* 1976; 47:909.
6. Adami M, Bertaccini G, Coruzzi C, et al: Characterization of cholinoreceptors in the rat urinary bladder by the use of agonists and antagonists of the cholinergic system. *J Auton Pharmacol* 1985; 5:197.

7. Alm P, Alumets J, Hakonson P, et al: Peptidergic nerves in the genitourinary tract. *Neuroscience* 1977; 2:751.
8. Alm P, Alumets J, Broden E, et al: Peptidergic (substance P) nerves in the genitourinary tract. *Neuroscience* 1978; 3:419.
9. Alm P, Elmer M: Adrenergic and cholinergic innervation of the rat urinary bladder. *Acta Physiol Scand* 1975; 94:36.
10. Ambache N: The use and limitation of atropine for pharmacological studies on autonomic effectors. *Pharmacol Rev* 1955; 7:467.
11. Ambache N, Zar MA: Non-cholinergic transmission by post-ganglionic motor neurones in the mammalian bladder. *J Physiol Lond* 1970; 210:761.
12. Anderson GF, Marks BH: Spare cholinergic receptors in the urinary bladder. *J Pharmacol Exp Ther* 1982; 221:598.
13. Anderson GF, Marks BH: Beta adrenoceptors in the rabbit detrusor muscle. *J Pharmacol Exp Ther* 1984; 228:283.
14. Anderson GF, Pierce JM, Fredericks CM, et al: A pharmacologic evaluation of the adrenergic receptors of the rabbit detrusor muscle. *Arch Int Pharmacodyn Ther* 1971; 191:220.
15a. Andersson KE: Classification and function of peripheral vascular α-adrenoreceptors, in Refsum H, Mjøs O (eds): *α-Adrenoreceptor Blockers in Cardiovascular Disease.* New York, Churchill Livingstone, 1985, pp 3–18.
15. Andersson KE: New trends in lower urinary tract pharmacology. *Trends Pharmacol Sci* 1984; 5:521.
16. Andersson KE, Ek A, Persson CGA: Effects of prostaglandins on the isolated human bladder and urethra. *Acta Physiol Scand* 1977; 100:165.
17. Andersson KE, Husted S, Sjogren C: Contribution of prostaglandins to the adenosine triphosphate induced contraction of rabbit urinary bladder. *Br J Pharmacol* 1980; 70:443.
18. Andersson KE, Larsson B, Sjogren C: Characterization of the adrenoceptors in the female rabbit urethra. *Br J Pharmacol* 1984; 81:293.
19. Andersson KE, Mattiasson A, Sjogren C: Electrically induced relaxation of the noradrenaline contracted isolated urethra from rabbit and man. *J Urol* 1983; 129:210.
20. Andersson KE, Sjogren C: Aspects on the physiology and pharmacology of the bladder and urethra. *Prog Neurobiol* 1982; 19:71.
21. Andrew J, Nathan PW: The cerebral control of micturition. *Proc R Soc Med* 1965; 58:553.
22. Appenzeller O: Anatomy and histology; Autonomic hyperreflexia, in Appenzeller O (ed): *The Autonomic Nervous System.* Elsevier Biomedical Press, 1982, pp 1–30, 406–407.
23. Atta MA, El Badawi A: Intrinsic neuromuscular defects in the neurogenic bladder: IV. Loss of somato-motor and preservation of autonomic innervation of the male feline rhabdosphincter following bilateral sacral ventral rhizotomy. *Neurourol Urodynamics* 1985; 4:219.
24. Awad SA, Bruce AE, Carro-Ciampi G, et al: Distribution of alpha and beta adrenoreceptors in human urinary bladder. *Br J Pharmacol* 1974; 50:525.

25. Awad SA, Downie JW: The effect of adrenergic drugs and hypogastric nerve stimulation on the canine urethra. *Invest Urol* 1976a; 13:298.
26. Awad SA, Downie JW: Relative contribution of smooth and striated muscles to the canine urethral pressure profile. *Br J Urol* 1976b; 48:347.
27. Awad SA, Downie JW: The adrenergic component in the proximal urethra. *Urol Int* 1977; 32:192.
28. Barrington FJF: The nervous mechanism of micturition. *Q J Exp Physiol* 1914; 8:33.
29. Barrington FJF: The relation of the hindbrain to micturition. *Brain* 1921; 44:23.
30. Barrington FJF: The effect of lesions of the hind- and mid-brain on micturition in the cat. *Q J Exp Physiol* 1925; 15:81.
31. Bazeed MA, Thuroff JM, Schmidt RA, et al: Histochemical study of urethral striated musculature in the dog. *J Urol* 1982; 128:406.
32. Benson GS: Mechanisms of autonomic drug action on the bladder outlet, in Hinman F Jr (ed): *Benign Prostatic Hypertrophy.* Berlin, Springer-Verlag, 1983, pp 373–382.
33. Benson GS, Jacobowitz D, Raezer DM, et al: Adrenergic innervation and stimulation of canine urethra. *Urology* 1976; 7:337.
34. Benson GS, McConnell JA, Wood JG: Adrenergic innervation of the human bladder body. *J Urol* 1979; 122:189.
35. Benson GS, Wein AJ, Raezer DM, et al: Adrenergic and cholinergic stimulation and blockade of the human bladder base. *J Urol* 1976; 116:174.
36. Berridge MJ, Irvine RF: Inositol triphosphate, a novel second messenger in cellular signal transduction. *Nature* 1984; 312:315.
37. Berthelson S, Pettinger WA: A functional basis for classification of alpha adrenergic receptors. *Life Sci* 1977; 21:595.
38. Bhatia NN, Bradley WE: Neuroanatomy and physiology: Innervation of the urinary tract, in Raz S (ed): *Female Urology.* Philadelphia, WB Saunders Co, 1983, pp 12–32.
39. Blaivas JG: The neurophysiology of micturition: A clinical study of 550 patients. *J Urol* 1982; 127:958.
40. Booth AM, Hisamitsu T, Kawatani M, et al: Regulation of urinary bladder capacity by endogenous opioid peptides. *J Urol* 1985; 133:339.
41. Bors E, Comarr AE: *Neurological Urology.* Baltimore, University Park Press, 1971.
42. Bowen JM, Timm GW, Bradley WE: Some contractile and electrophysiologic properties of the periurethral striated muscle of the cat. *Invest Urol* 1976; 13:327.
43. Bozler E: Action potentials and conduction of excitation in smooth muscle. *Biol Symp* 1941; 3:95.
44. Bradley WE, Conway CJ: Bladder representation in the pontine-mesencephalic reticular formation. *Exp Neurol* 1966; 16:237.
45. Bradley WE, Sundin T: The physiology and pharmacology of urinary tract dysfunction. *Clin Neuropharmacol* 1982; 5:131.

46. Bradley WE, Teague CT: Spinal cord organization of micturition reflex afferents. *Exp Neurol* 1968; 22:504.
47. Bradley WE, Timm GW, Scott FB: Innervation of the detrusor muscle and urethra. *Urol Clin North Am* 1974; 1:3.
48. Bro-Rasmussen F, Sorensen AH, Bredahl E, et al: The structure and function of the urinary bladder. *Urol Int* 1965; 19:280.
49. Bruschini H, Schmidt RA, Tanagho EA: The male genitourinary sphincter mechanism in the dog. *Invest Urol* 1978; 15:284.
50. Bulbring E, Brading AF, Jones AW, et al: *Smooth Muscle: An Assessment of Current Knowledge.* Austin, University of Texas Press, 1981.
51. Bultitude MI, Hills NH, Shuttleworth KED: Clinical and experimental studies on the action of prostaglandins and their synthesis inhibitors on detrusor muscle in vitro and in vivo. *Br J Urol* 1976; 48:631.
52. Burnstock G: Purinergic nerves. *Pharmacol Rev* 1972; 24:509.
53. Burnstock G: Cholinergic, adrenergic, and purinergic transmission. *Fed Proc* 1977; 36:2434.
54. Burnstock G: Nervous control of smooth muscle by transmitters, cotransmitters and modulators. *Experientia* 1985; 41:869.
55. Burnstock G: The changing face of autonomic neurotransmission. *Acta Physiol Scand* 1986; 126:67.
56. Burnstock G, Bell C: Peripheral autonomic transmission, in Hubbard JI (ed): *The Peripheral Nervous System.* New York, Plenum, 1974, pp 277–327.
57. Burnstock G, Cocks T, Grave R, et al: Purinergic innervation of the guinea pig urinary bladder. *Br J Pharmacol* 1978a; 63:125.
58. Burnstock G, Cocks T, Kasakov L, et al: Direct evidence for ATP release from non-adrenergic non-cholinergic ('purinergic') nerves in the guinea pig *Taenia coli* and bladder. *Eur J Pharmacol* 1978b; 49:145.
59. Burnstock G, Dumsday B, Smythe A; Atropine resistant excitation of the urinary bladder: The possibility of transmission via nerves releasing a purine nucleotide. *Br J Pharmacol* 1972; 44:451.
60. Caine M: *The Pharmacology of the Urinary Tract.* Berlin, Springer-Verlag, 1984, pp 5–29, 31–47.
61. Caine M, Raz S: The role of female hormones in stress incontinence. Presentation at Societe Internationale d'Urologie, 16th Congress, Amsterdam, 1973.
62. Caine M, Raz S, Zeigler M: Adrenergic and cholinergic receptors in the human prostate, prostatic capsule and bladder neck. *Br J Urol* 1975; 47:193.
63. Carlsson CA: The supraspinal control of the urinary bladder. *Acta Pharmacol Toxicol* 1978; 43:8.
64. Carpenter FG: Atropine resistance and muscarinic receptors in the rat urinary bladder. *Br J Pharmacol* 1977; 59:43.
65. Conway CJ, Bradley WE: Measurement of the spread of excitation in the urinary detrusor muscle during reflex induction. *J Urol* 1969; 101:533.

66. Coolsaet BLRA: Cystometry, in Stanton SL (ed): *Clinical Gynecologic Urology*. St Louis, CV Mosby Co, 1984, pp 59–81.
67. Cooper JR, Meyer EM: Possible mechanisms involved in the release and modulation of release of neuroactive agents. *Neurochem Int* 1984; 6:419.

67a. Cowan WD, Daniel EE: Human female bladder and its noncholinergic contractile function. *Can J Physiol Pharmacol* 1983; 61:1236.

68. Creed K: The role of the hypogastric nerve in bladder and urethral activity of the dog. *Br J Pharmacol* 1979; 65:367.
69. Daniel EE, Cowan W, Daniel VP: Structural basis for neural and myogenic control of human detrusor muscle. *Can J Physiol Pharmacol* 1983; 61:1247.
70. Dean DM, Downie JW: Contribution of adrenergic and 'purinergic' neurotransmission to contraction in the rabbit detrusor. *J Pharmacol Exp Ther* 1978; 207:431.
71. deGroat WC: Nervous control of the urinary bladder of the cat. *Brain Res* 1975; 87:201.
72. deGroat WC, Booth AM: Autonomic systems to the urinary bladder and sexual organs, in Dyck PJ, Thomas PK, Lambert EH, et al (eds): *Peripheral Neuropathy*. Philadelphia, WB Saunders Co, 1984, pp 285–299.
73. deGroat WC, Booth AM: Physiology of the urinary bladder and urethra. *Ann Intern Med* 1980; 92(pt 2):321.
74. deGroat WC, Kawatani M: Neural control of the urinary bladder: Possible relationship between peptidergic inhibitory mechanisms and detrusor instability. *Neurourol Urodynamics* 1985; 4:285.
75. deGroat WC, Kawatani M, Hisamitsu T, et al: The role of neuropeptides in the sacral autonomic reflex pathways of the cat. *J Auton Nerv Syst* 1983; 7:339.
76. deGroat WC, Nadelhaft I, Milner J, et al: Organization of the sacral parasympathetic reflex pathways to the urinary bladder and large intestine. *J Auton Nerv Syst* 1981; 3:135.
77. deGroat WC, Ryall RW: Reflexes to sacral parasympathetic neurons concerned with micturition in the cat. *J Physiol* 1969; 200:87.
78. deGroat WC, Saum WR: Adrenergic inhibition in mammalian parasympathetic ganglia. *Nature* 1971; 231:188.
79. deGroat WC, Saum WR: Sympathetic inhibition of the urinary bladder and of pelvic ganglionic transmission in the cat. *J Physiol Lond* 1972; 220:297.
80. deGroat WC, Saum WR: Synaptic transmission in parasympathetic ganglia in the urinary bladder of the cat. *J Physiol Lond* 1976; 256:137.
81. deGroat WC, Theobald RJ: Reflex activation of sympathetic pathways to vesical smooth muscle and parasympathetic ganglia by electrical stimulation of vesical afferents. *J Physiol Lond* 1976; 259:223.
82. Denny-Brown D, Robertson EG: On the physiology of micturition. *Brain* 1933; 56:149.
83. Dixon JS, Gilpin SA, Gilpin CT, et al: Intramural ganglia of the human urinary bladder. *Br J Urol* 1983; 55:195.

84. Dixon JS, Gosling JA: Histology and fine structure of the muscularis mucosae of the human urinary bladder. *J Anat* 1983; 136:265.
85. Donker PJ, Droes JTPM, Van Ulder BM: Anatomy of the musculature and innervation of the bladder and urethra, in Chisholm GD, Williams DI (eds): *Scientific Foundations of Urology*. Chicago, Year Book Medical Publishers, 1982, pp 404–411.
86. Donker PJ, Ivanovici F, Noach EL: Analyses of the urethra pressure profile by means of electromyography and the administration of drugs. *Br J Urol* 1972; 44:180.
87. Douglas WW: Polypeptides—angiotensin, plasma kinins, and others, in Gilman AG, Goodman LS, Rall TW, (eds): *The Pharmacological Basis of Therapeutics*. New York, Macmillan Publishing Co, 1985, pp 639–659.
88. Downie JW, Dean DM: The contribution of cholinergic postganglionic neurotransmission to contractions of rabbit detrusor. *J Pharmacol Exp Ther* 1977; 203:417.
89. Downie JW, Karmazyn M: Mechanical trauma to bladder epithelium liberates prostanoids which modulate neurotransmission in rabbit detrusor muscle. *J Pharmacol Exp Ther* 1984; 230:445.
90. Downie JW, Larsson C: Prostaglandin involvement in contractions evoked in rabbit detrusor by field stimulation and by adenosine 5-triphosphate. *Can J Physiol Pharmacol* 1981; 59:253.
91. Dray A, Metsch R: Opioid receptor subtypes involved in the central inhibition of bladder motility. *Eur J Pharmacol* 1984a; 104:47.
92. Dray A, Metsch R: Inhibition of urinary bladder contractions by a special action of morphine and other opioids. *J Pharmacol Exp Ther* 1984b; 231:254.
93. Droogmans G, Himpens B, Casteels R: Co-exchange, co-channels and co-antagonists. *Experientia* 1985; 41:895.
94. Edvardsen P: Nervous control of the urinary bladder in cats: I. The collecting phase. *Acta Physiol Scand* 1968a; 72:157.
95. Edvardsen P: Nervous control of the urinary bladder in cats: II. The expulsion phase. *Acta Physiol Scand* 1968b; 72:172.
96. Edvardsen P: Nervous control of the urinary bladder in cats: III. Effects of autonomic blocking agents in the intact animal. *Acta Physiol Scand* 1968c; 72:183.
97. Edvardsen P: Nervous control of the urinary bladder in cats: IV. Effects of autonomic blocking agents on responses to peripheral nerve stimulation. *Acta Physiol Scand* 1968d; 72:234.
98. Edvardsen P, Setekleiv J: Distribution of adrenergic receptors in the urinary bladder of cats, rabbit, and guinea pigs. *Acta Pharmacol Toxicol* 1968; 26:437.
99. Ek A, Alm P, Andersson KE, et al: Adrenergic and cholinergic nerves of the human urethra and urinary bladder: A histochemical study. *Acta Physiol Scand* 1977a; 99:345.
100. Ek A, Alm P, Andersson KE, et al: Adrenoreceptor and cholinoceptor

mediated responses of the isolated human urethra. *Scand J Urol Nephrol* 1977b; 11:97.
101. Eglen RM, Whiting RL: Muscarinic receptors' subtypes: Problems of classification. *Trends Pharmacol Sci* 1985; 6:357.
102. Ekstrom J, Malmberg L: On a cholinergic motor innervation of the rat urethra. *Acta Physiol Scand* 1984; 120:237.
103. El Badawi A: Neuromorphologic basis of vesicourethral function. I. Histochemistry, ultrastructure, and function of intrinsic nerves of the bladder and urethra. *Neurourol Urodynamics* 1982; 1:3.
104. El Badawi A: Autonomic muscular innervation of the vesical outlet and its role in micturition, in Hinman F Jr (ed): *Benign Prostatic Hypertrophy.* Berlin, Springer-Verlag, 1983, pp 330–348.
105. El Badawi A: Ultrastructure of vesicourethral innervation: II. Postganglionic axoaxonal synapses in intrinsic innervation of the vesicourethral lissosphincter: A new structural and functional concept in micturition. *J Urol* 1984; 131:781.
106. El Badawi A: Ultrastructure of vesicourethral innervation: III. Anoaxonal synapses between postganglionic cholinergic axons and probably SIF-cell derived processes in the feline lissosphincter. *J Urol* 1985; 133:524.
107. El Badawi A, Atta MA: Ultrastructure of vesicourethral innervation: IV. Evidence for somatomotor plus autonomic innervation of the male feline rhabdosphincter. *Neurourol Urodynamics* 1985; 4:23.
108. El Badawi A, Schenk EA: Dual innervation of the mammalian urinary bladder: A histochemical study of the distribution of cholinergic and adrenergic nerves. *Am J Anat* 1966; 119:405.
109. El Badawi A, Schenk EA: A new theory of the innervation of bladder musculature: I. Morphology of the intrinsic vesical innervation apparatus. *J Urol* 1968; 99:585.
110. El Badawi A, Schenk EA: A new theory of the innervation of bladder musculature: III. Innervation of the vesicourethral junction and external urethral sphincter. *J Urol* 1974; 111:613.
111. Elliot TR: The innervation of the bladder and urethra. *J Physiol Lond* 1907; 35:367.
112. Elmer M: Action of drugs on the innervated and denervated urinary bladder of the rat. *Acta Physiol Scand* 1974; 91:289.
113. Elmer M: Atropine sensitivity of the rat urinary bladder during nerve degeneration. *Acta Physiol Scand* 1975; 93:202.
114. Enhorning G: Simultaneous recording of the intravesical and intraurethral pressures. *Acta Chir Scand* 1961; 276(suppl):1.
115. Erspamer GF, Negri L, Piccinelli D: The use of preparations of urinary bladder smooth muscle for bioassay of and discrimination between polypeptides. *Naunyn Schmiedebergs Arch Pharmacol* 1973; 276:61.
116. Fall M, Erlandson BE, Carlsson CA, et al: The effect of intravaginal stimulation on the feline urethra and urinary bladder neuronal mechanisms. *Scand J Urol Nephrol* 1977; 44(suppl):19.

117. Finkbeiner AE: In vitro effects of vasoactive intestinal polypeptide on guinea pig urinary bladder. *Urology* 1983; 22:275.
118. Finkbeiner AS, Bissada NK: In vitro effects of prostaglandins on the guinea pig detrusor and bladder outlet. *Urol Res* 1981; 9:281.
119. Fletcher TF, Bradley WE: Neuroanatomy of the bladder-urethra. *J Urol* 1978; 119:153.
120. Fredericks CM: Characterization of the rabbit detrusor response to histamine through pharmacologic antagonism. *Pharmacology* 1975; 13:5.
121. Gabella G: Structure of smooth muscles, in Bulbring F, Brading AF, Jones AW, et al (eds): *Smooth Muscle.* Austin, University of Texas Press, 1981, p 1–46.
122. Gajewski J, Downie J, Awad S: Experimental evidence for a central nervous system site of action in the effect of alpha adrenergic blockers on the external urethral sphincter. *J Urol* 1984; 133:403.
123. Ghonheim MA, Fretin JA, Gagnon DJ, et al: The influence of vesical distention on urethral resistance to flow: The collecting phase. *Br J Urol* 1975; 47:657.
124. Gilpin SA, Gosling JA: Smooth muscle in the wall of the developing human bladder and urethra. *J Anat* 1983; 137:503.
125. Gil Vernet S: *Morphology and Function of Vesico-Prostato-Urethral Musculature.* Treviso, Italy, Canora, 1968, pp 245–269.
126. Gjone R: A dual peripheral and supraspinal autonomic influence on the urinary bladder. *J Oslo City Hosp* 1965; 15:173.
127. Gjone R, Setekleiv J: Excitatory and inhibitory responses to stimulation of the cerebral cortex in the cat. *Acta Physiol Scand* 1963; 59:337.
128. Glazer E, Basbaum A: Leucine enkephalin: Localization in and axoplasmic transport by sacral parasympathetic preganglionic neurons. *Science* 1980; 208:1479.
129. Gosling J: The structure of the bladder and urethra in relation to function. *Urol Clin North Am* 1979; 6(Feb):31.
130. Gosling J: Anatomy, in Stanton SL (ed): *Clinical Gynecologic Urology.* St. Louis, CV Mosby Co, 1984, pp 3–12.
131. Gosling JA: Personal communication (letter), June 12, 1985.
132. Gosling JA, Chilton CP: The anatomy of the bladder, urethra and pelvic floor, in Mundy AR, Stephenson TP, Wein AJ (eds): *Urodynamics: Principles, Practice and Applications.* London, Churchill Livingstone, 1984, pp 3–13.
133. Gosling JA, Dixon JS, Critchley HOD, et al: A comparative study of the human external sphincter and periurethral levator ani muscles. *Br J Urol* 1981; 53:35.
133a. Gray TS, Morley JE: Neuropeptide Y: Anatomical distribution and possible function in mammalian nervous system. *Life Sci* 1986; 38:389.
134. Griffiths DJ: Hydrodynamics and mechanisms of the bladder and urethra, in Mundy AR, Stephenson TP, Wein AJ (eds): *Urodynamics: Principles, Practice and Applications.* London, Churchill Livingstone, 1984, pp 42–49.

135. Gruber CM: The autonomic innervation of the genitourinary system. *Physiol Rev* 1933; 13:497.
136. Gu J, Blank MA, Huang WM, et al: Peptide containing nerves in human urinary bladder. *Urology* 1984; 24:353.
137. Gu J, Restorich JM, Blank MA, et al: Vasoactive intestinal polypeptide in the normal and unstable bladder. *Br J Urol* 1983; 55:645.
138. Guth L: Axonal regeneration and functional plasticity in the central nervous system. *Exp Neurol* 1974; 45:606.
139. Guyton AC: *Textbook of Medical Physiology*. Philadelphia, WB Saunders Co, 1986, pp 120–135, 136–149, 686–696.
140. Gyermek L: Cholinergic stimulation and blockade on urinary bladder. *Am J Physiol* 1961; 201:325.
141. Gyermek L: Action of 5-hydroxytryptamine on the urinary bladder of the dog. *Arch Int Pharmacodyn Ther* 1962; 137:137.
142. Hald T, Bradley W: *The Urinary Bladder: Neurology and Dynamics*. Baltimore, Williams & Wilkins, 1982, pp 5–21, 22–36, 82–88.
143. Hammer R, Giachetti A: Muscarinic receptor subtypes: M1 and M2 biochemical and functional characterization. *Life Sci* 1982; 31:2991.
144. Hardman JG: Cyclic nucleotides and smooth muscle contraction: Some conceptual and experimental considerations, in Bulbring E, Brading AF, Jones AW (eds): *Smooth Muscle*. Austin, University of Texas Press, 1981, pp 249–262.
145. Hassouna M, Abdel-Hakim A, Abdel-Rahman M, et al: Response of the urethral smooth muscles to pharmacological agents: I. Cholinergic and adrenergic agonists and antagonists. *J Urol* 1983; 191:1262.
146. Haynes LW: Modulation of cholinergic transmission by VIP, a peptide co-transmitter. *Trends Pharmacol Sci* 1985; 6:427.
147. Hickey DS, Phillips JI, Hukins DWL: Arrangement of collagen fibers and muscle fibers in the female urethra and their implications for the control of micturition. *Br J Urol* 1982; 54:556.
148. Hindmarsh JR, Idowu OA, Yeates WK, et al: Pharmacology of electrically evoked contractions of human bladder. *Br J Pharmacol* 1977; 61:115P.
149. Hisamitsu T, deGroat WC: The effect of opioid peptides and morphine applied intrathecally and intracerebroventricularly on the micturition reflex in the cat. *Brain Res* 1984; 298:51.
150. Honda K, Osawa AM, Takenaka T: α_1-Adrenoceptor subtype mediating contraction of the smooth muscle in the lower urinary tract and prostate of rabbits. *Naunyn Schmiedebergs Arch Pharmacol* 1985; 330:16.
151. Hoyle CHV, Burnstock G: Atropine resistant excitatory junction potentials in rabbit bladder are blocked by α, β-methylene ATP. *Eur J Pharmacol* 1985; 114:239.
152. Hughes J, Kosterlitz HW: Introduction: Opioid peptides. *Br Med Bull* 1983; 39:1.
153. Husted S, Sjogren C, Andersson KE: Direct effects of adenosine and adenine nucleotides on isolated human urinary bladder and their influence on electrically induced contractions. *J Urol* 1983; 130:392.

154. Husted S, Sjogren C, Andersson KE: Substance P and somatostatin and excitatory neurotransmission in rabbit urinary bladder. *Arch Int Pharmacodyn* 1981; 252:72.
155. Hutch JA: A new theory of the anatomy of the internal urinary sphincter and the physiology of micturition: IV. The urinary sphincteric mechanism. *J Urol* 1967; 97:705.
156. Hutch JA, Rambo OA Jr: A new theory of the anatomy of the internal urinary sphincter and the physiology of micturition: III. Anatomy of the urethra. *J Urol* 1967; 97:696.
157. Ignarro LJ, Kadowitz PJ: The pharmacological and physiological role of cyclic GMP in vascular smooth muscle relaxation. *Ann Rev Pharmacol Toxicol* 1985; 25:171.
158. Ingersoll EH, Jones LL, Hegre ES: Effect on urinary bladder of unilateral stimulation of pelvic nerves in the dog. *Am J Physiol* 1957; 189:167.
159. Ito Y, Kimoto Y: The neural and non-neural mechanisms involved in urethral activity in rabbits. *J Physiol* 1985; 367:57.
160. Jacobowitz DM: The peripheral autonomic system, in Hubbard JI (ed): *The Peripheral Nervous System*, New York, Plenum, 1974, pp 87–110.
161. Jaffee JH, Martin WR: Opioid analgesics and antagonists, in Gilman AG, Goodman LS, Rall TW, et al (eds): *The Pharmacological Basis of Therapeutics.* New York, Macmillan Publishing Co, 1985, pp 491–531.
162. John A, Paton DM: Evidence for a role of prostaglandins in atropine-resistant transmission in the mammalian urinary bladder. *Prostaglandins* 1976; 11:595.
163. Jonas U, Tanagho E: Studies on vesicourethral reflexes. *Invest Urol* 1975; 12:357.
164. Jubelin B, Galeano C, Ladouceus D, et al: Effect of enkephalin on the micturition cycle of the cat. *Life Sci* 1984; 34:2015.
165. Kalsner S (chairman): The noradrenergic presynaptic receptor controversy (symposium). *Fed Proc* 1984; 43:1351.
166. Kaneko S, Minami K, Yachiku S, et al: Bladder neck dysfunction: The effect of the adrenergic agent phentolamine on bladder neck dysfunction and a fluorescent histochemical study of bladder neck smooth muscle. *Invest Urol* 1980; 18:212.
167. Kasakov L, Burnstock G: The use of the slowly degradable analog, α, β-methylene ATP to produce desensitization of the P-2 purinoceptor effect on nonadrenergic noncholinergic responses of guinea pig urinary bladder. *Eur J Pharmacol* 1983; 86:292.
168. Kawatani M, Lowe IP, Booth AM, et al: The presence of leucine-enkephalin in the sacral preganglionic pathway to the urinary bladder of the cat. *Neurosci Lett* 1983; 39:143.
169. Khalaf I, Elshawarby LA, Lehoux JG, et al: Release of prostaglandins into the pelvic venous blood of dogs in response to vesical distention and pelvic nerve stimulation. *Invest Urol* 1979; 17:244.
170. Khalaf IM, Ghonheim MA, Elhilali MM: The effect of exogenous prosta-

glandins F2 and E2 and indomethacin on micturition. *Br J Urol* 1981; 43:21.

171. Khalaf I, Toppercer A, Elhilali M: Urethral pressure changes on reflex micturition. *Invest Urol* 1979; 17:141.
172. Khanna OP: Effect of nonautonomic drugs on the vesical neck, in Hinman F Jr (ed): *Benign Prostatic Hypertrophy*. Berlin, Springer-Verlag, 1983, pp 384–404.
173. Khanna OP, Barbieri EJ, McMichael R: Effects of prostaglandins on vesicourethral smooth muscle of rabbit. *Urology* 1978; 12:674.
174. Khanna OP, Barbieri EJ, Altamura M, et al: Vesicourethral smooth muscle: Function and relation to structure. *Urology* 1981; 18:211.
175. Khanna OP, DeGregorio GJ, Sample RG, et al: Histamine receptors in urethrovesical smooth muscle. *Urology* 1977; 10:375.
176. Khanna OP, Heber D, Gonick P: Cholinergic and adrenergic neuroreceptors in urinary tract of female dogs: Evaluation of function with pharmacodynamics. *Urology* 1975; 5:616.
177. Kinder RB, Mundy AR: Atropine blockade of nerve mediated stimulation of the human detrusor. *Br J Urol* 1985a; 57:418.
178. Kinder RB, Mundy AR: Inhibition of spontaneous contractile activity in isolated human detrusor muscle strips by vasoactive intestinal polypeptide. *Br J Urol* 1985b; 57:20.
179. Kirchberger MA, Schwartz IL: Excitation and contraction of skeletal muscle, in West JB (ed): *Best and Taylor's Physiological Basis of Medical Practice*. Baltimore, Williams & Wilkins Co, 1985, pp 58–107.
180. Klarskov P, Gerstenberg T: Vasoactive intestinal polypeptide influence on lower urinary tract smooth muscle from human and pig. *J Urol* 1984; 131:1000.
181. Klarskov P, Gerstenberg TC, Ramirez D, et al: Non-cholinergic, non-adrenergic nerve mediated relaxation of trigone, bladder neck and urethral smooth muscle in vitro. *J Urol* 1983; 129:848.
182. Kleeman FJ: The physiology of the internal urinary sphincter. *J Urol* 1970; 104:549.
183. Klevmark B: Motility of the urinary bladder in cats during filling at physiologic rates: I. Intravesical pressure patterns studied by a new method of cystometry. *Acta Physiol Scand* 1974; 90:565.
184. Klevmark B: Motility of the urinary bladder in cats during filling at physiological rates: II. Effects of extrinsic bladder denervation on intramural tension and on intravesical pressure patterns. *Acta Physiol Scand* 1977; 101:176.
185. Klevmark B: Motility of the urinary bladder in cats during filling at physiological rates: III. Spontaneous rhythmic contractions in the conscious and anesthetized animal: Influence of distention and innervation. *Scand J Urol Nephrol* 1980; 14:219.

185a. Kluck P: The autonomic innervation of the human urinary bladder, bladder neck, and urethra: A histochemical study. *Anat Rec* 1980; 198:439.

186. Kock N, Pompeius R: Inhibition of vesical motor activity induced by anal stimulation. *Acta Clin Scand* 1963; 126:244.
187. Koff SA: Striated muscle determinants of intraurethral resistance. *Invest Urol* 1977; 15:147.
188. Koley B, Koley J, Saka JK: The effect of nicotine on spontaneous contractions of cat urinary bladder in situ. *Br J Pharmacol* 1984; 83:347.
189. Kondo A, Susset JG, Lefaivre J: Viscoelastic properties of bladder: I. Mechanical model and its mathematical analysis. *Invest Urol* 1972; 10:154.
190. Krane RJ, Olsson CA: Phenoxybenzamine in neurogenic bladder dysfunction: I. A theory of micturition. *J Urol* 1973a; 110:650.
191. Krane RJ, Olsson CA: Phenoxybenzamine in neurogenic bladder dysfunction: II. Clinical considerations. *J Urol* 1973b; 110:653.
192. Krell RD, McCoy JL, Ridley PT: Pharmacological characterization of the excitatory innervation to the guinea pig urinary bladder in vitro: Evidence for both cholinergic and non-adrenergic non-cholinergic neurotransmission. *Br J Pharmacol* 1981; 74:15.
193. Kunisawa Y, Kawabe K, Nijima T, et al: A pharmacological study of alpha adrenergic receptor subtypes in smooth muscle of human urinary bladder base and prostatic urethra. *J Urol* 1985; 134:296.
194. Kuo DC, Hisamitsu T, deGroat WC: A sympathetic projection from sacral paravertebral ganglia to the pelvic nerve and to post-ganglionic nerves on the surface of the urinary bladder and large intestine of the cat. *J Compr Neurol* 1984; 226:76.
195. Kuriyama H: Excitation-contraction coupling in various visceral smooth muscles, in Bulbring E, Brading AF, Jones AW, et al (eds): *Smooth Muscle.* Austin, University of Texas Press, 1981, pp 171–197.
196. Kuru M: Nervous control of micturition. *Physiol Rev* 1965; 45:425.
197. Langer SZ, Shepperson NB: Recent developments in vascular smooth muscle pharmacology: the postsynaptic 2 adrenoceptor. *Trends Pharmacol Sci* 1982; 11:440.
198. Langley JN, Anderson HK: The innervation of the pelvic and adjoining viscera: II. The bladder. *J Physiol* 1895; 19:71.
199. Langley JN, Anderson HK: The innervation of the pelvic and adjoining viscera: VII. Anatomical observations. *J Physiol* 1896; 20:372.
200. Lapides J: Neuromuscular vesical and ureteral dysfunction, in Campbell MF, Harrison JH (eds): *Campbell's Urology.* Philadelphia, WB Saunders Co, 1970, p 1343.
201. Lapides J: Structure and function of the internal vesical sphincter. *J Urol* 1958; 80:341.
202. Lapides J, Ajemian EP, Stewart BH, et al: Further observations on the kinetics of the urethrovesical sphincter. *J Urol* 1960; 84:86.
203. Lapides J, Sweet RB, Lewis LW: Role of striated muscle in urination. *J Urol* 1957; 77:247.
204. Larsen JJ: α and β Adrenoceptors in the detrusor muscle and bladder base of the pig and β adrenoceptors in the detrusor muscle of man. *Br J Pharmacol* 1979; 65:215.

205. Larsen JJ, Ottesen B, Fahrenkrug J, et al: Vasoactive intestinal polypeptide in the male genitourinary tract: Concentration and motor effect. *Invest Urol* 1981; 19:211.
206. Larsson B, Sjogren C, Andersson KE: Regional distribution of α-adrenoceptor subtypes in the female rabbit urethra. *Acta Physiol Scand* 1986; 126:39.
207. Lavin TN, Hoffman BB, Lefkowitz RJ: Determination of subtype selectivity of alpha adrenergic antagonists. *Mol Pharmacol* 1981; 20:28.
208. Learmoth JR: A contribution to the neurophysiology of the urinary bladder in man. *Brain* 1931; 54:147.
209. Lefkowitz RJ, Caron MG, Stiles GL: Mechanisms of membrane receptor regulation. *N Engl J Med* 1984; 24:1570.
210. Leger L, Charmay Y, Chayvialle JA, et al: Localization of substance P and enkephalin like immunoreactivity in relation to catecholamine containing cell bodies in the cat dorsolateral pontine tegmentum: Immunofluorescence study. *Neuroscience* 1983; 8:525.
211. Leoni JV, Wein AJ, Raezer DM, et al: The effect of β-adrenergic stimulation on the contractile response of canine detrusor muscle. *Invest Urol* 1973; 10:419.
212. Lepor H, Kuhar M: Characterization of muscarinic cholinergic receptor binding in the vas deferens, bladder, prostate and penis of the rabbit. *J Urol* 1984; 132:392.
213. Levin RM, Goldman M, Wein AJ: Effect of isoproterenol and EGTA on the volume-pressure relationship of the in-vitro whole bladder preparation. *Neurourol Urodynamics* 1984; 3:133.
214. Levin RM, High J, Wein AJ: Evidence against the presence of spare muscarinic receptors in the rabbit urinary bladder. *Neurourol Urodynamics* 1983c; 2:317.
215. Levin RM, Jacoby R, Wein AJ: Effect of adenosine triphosphate on contractility and adenosine triphosphatase activity of the rabbit urinary bladder. *Mol Pharmacol* 1981; 19:525.
216. Levin RM, Jacoby R, Wein AJ: High affinity divalent ion specific binding of ^{3}H-ATP to homogenates derived from rabbit urinary bladder: Comparison with divalent ion ATP-ase activity. *Mol Pharmacol* 1983b; 23:1.
217. Levin R, Ruggieri M, Velagapudi S, et al: Relevance of spontaneous activity in urinary bladder function: An in-vitro and in-vivo study. *J Urol* 1986; 136:517.
218. Levin RM, Ruggieri MR, Wein AJ: Functional effects of the purinergic innervation of the rabbit urinary bladder. *J Pharmacol Exp Ther* 1986; 236:452.
219. Levin RM, Shofer F, Wein AJ: Cholinergic, adrenergic and purinergic response of sequential strips of rabbit urinary bladder. *J Pharmacol Exp Ther* 1980; 212:536.
220. Levin RM, Staskin DR, Wein AJ: The muscarinic cholinergic kinetics of the human urinary bladder. *Neurourol Urodynamics* 1983a; 2:221.
221. Levin RM, Wein AJ: Direct measurement of the anticholinergic activity of

a series of pharmacologic compounds on the canine and rabbit urinary bladder. *J Urol* 1982; 128:396.
222. Levin RM, Wein AJ: Distribution and function of adrenergic receptors in the urinary bladder of the rabbit. *Mol Pharmacol* 1979a; 16:441.
223. Levin RM, Wein AJ: Effect of vasoactive intestinal peptide on the contractility of the rabbit urinary bladder. *Urol Res* 1981; 9:217.
224. Levin RM, Wein AJ: Quantitative analysis of alpha and beta adrenergic receptor densities in the lower urinary tract of the dog and the rabbit. *Invest Urol* 1979b; 17:75.
225. Liu CN, Chambers WW: Intraspinal sprouting of dorsal root axons: Development of new collaterals and preterminals following partial denervation of the spinal cord in the cat. *Arch Neurol Psychiatry* 1958; 79:46.
226. Lundberg JM, Hökfelt T: Coexistence of peptides and clasical neurotransmitters. *Trends Neurol Sci* 1983; 6:325.
227. Lundberg JM, Hua XY, FrancoCereceda A: Effects of neuropeptide Y on mechanical activity and neurotransmission in the heart, vas deferens, and urinary bladder of the guinea pig. *Acta Physiol Scand* 1984; 121:325.
228. Mahoney DT, Laferte RO, Blais DJ: Integral storage and voiding reflexes: Neurophysiologic concept of continence and micturition. *Urology* 1977; 9:95.
229. Maggi C, Evangelista S, Grimaldi G, et al: Evidence for the involvement of arachidonic and metabolites on spontaneous and drug induced contractions of rat urinary bladder. *J Pharmacol Exp Ther* 1984a; 230:500.
230. Maggi CA, Meli A: Modulation by β-adrenoceptors of spontaneous contractions of rat urinary bladder. *J Auton Pharmacol* 1982; 2:255.
231. Maggi CA, Santicioli P, Meli A: The effects of topical capsaicin on rat urinary bladder motility in vivo. *Eur J Pharmacol* 1984b; 103:41.
232. Maggi CA, Santicioli P, Meli A: $GABA_A$ and $GABA_B$ receptors in detrusor strips from guinea pig bladder dome. *J Auton Pharmacol* 1985a; 5:55.
233. Maggi CA, Santicioli P, Meli A: Dual effect of GABA on the contractile activity of the guinea pig isolated urinary bladder. *J Auton Pharmacol* 1985b; 5:131.
234. Maggi CA, Santicioli P, Meli A: Pharmacological evidence for the existence of two components in the twitch response to field stimulation of detrusor strips from the rat urinary bladder. *J Auton Pharmacol* 1985c; 5:221.
235. Mattiasson A: *On the Peripheral Nervous Control of the Lower Urinary Tract,* thesis. University of Lund, Sweden, 1984.
236. Mattiasson A, Andersson KE, Sjogren C: Adrenergic and non-adrenergic contraction of isolated urethral muscle from rabbit and man. *J Urol* 1985; 133:298.
237. McGuire EJ: Experimental observations on the integration of bladder and urethral function. *Trans Am Assoc Genitourinary Surgeons* 1977; 68:38.
238. McGuire EJ: Experimental observations on the integration of bladder and urethral function. *Invest Urol* 1978; 15:303.

239. McGuire EJ: Physiology of the lower urinary tract. *Am J Kidney Dis* 1983; 2:402.
240. McGuire EJ: Clinical evaluation and treatment of neurogenic vesical dysfunction, in Libertino J (ed): *International Perspectives in Urology.* Baltimore, Williams & Wilkins, 1984a, vol 2, pp 1–15.
241. McGuire EJ: Mechanisms of urethral continence and their clinical application. *World J Urol* 1984b; 2:272.
242. McGuire EJ, Herlihy E: Bladder and urethral responses to isolated sacral motor root stimulation. *Invest Urol* 1978; 16:219.
243. McGuire EJ, Herlihy E: Bladder and urethral responses to sympathetic stimulation. *Invest Urol* 1979; 17:9.
244. McLellan FC: *The Neurogenic Bladder.* Springfield, Ill, Charles C Thomas, 1939, pp 57, 116.
245. McNeal JE: The prostate and prostatic urethra: A morphologic synthesis. *J Urol* 1972; 107:1008.
246. Minneman KP, Molinoff PB: Classification and quantitation of beta adrenergic receptor subtypes. *Biochem Pharmacol* 1980; 29:1317.
247. Mobley TL, El Badawi A, McDonald DF, et al: Innervation of the human urinary bladder. *Surg Forum* 1966; 17:505.
248. Morita T, Nishizawa O, Noto H, et al: Pelvic nerve innervation of the external sphincter of urethra as suggested by urodynamic and horseradish studies. *J Urol* 1984; 131:591.
249. Morley JS: Chemistry of opioid peptides. *Br Med Bull* 1983; 39:5.
250. Movsesian AM: Calcium physiology in smooth muscle. *Prog Cardiovasc Dis* 1982; 25:211.
251. Mundy AR: Clinical physiology of the bladder, urethra and pelvic floor, in Mundy AR, Stephenson TP, Wein AJ (eds): *Urodynamics: Principles, Practice and Application.* New York, Churchill Livingstone, 1984a, pp 14–25.
252. Mundy AR: Neuropeptides in lower urinary tract function. *World J Urol* 1984b; 2:211.
253. Murray KHA, Geneley RCL: Endorphins—a role in urinary tract function? The effect of opioid blockade on the detrusor and urethral sphincter mechanisms. *Br J Urol* 1982; 54:638.
254. Nanninga J, Kaplan P, Lal S: Effect of phentolamine on peripheral muscle EMG activity in paraplegia. *Br J Urol* 1977; 49:537.
255. Nathan PW: The central nervous connections of the bladder, in Williams DJ, Chisholm GD (eds): *Scientific Foundations of Urology.* Chicago, Year Book Medical Publishers, 1976, vol 2, pp 51–58.
256. Nergardh A: Autonomic receptor functions in lower urinary tract: A survey of recent experimental results. *J Urol* 1975; 113:180.
257. Nergardh A: Neuromuscular transmission in the corpus fundus of the urinary bladder. *Scand J Urol Nephrol* 1981; 15:103.
258. Nergardh A, Boreus LD: Autonomic receptor function in the lower urinary tract of man and cat. *Scand J Urol Nephrol* 1972; 6:32.

259. Nergardh A, Boreus LO: The functional role of cholinergic receptors in the outlet region of the urinary bladder: An in vitro study in the cat. *Acta Pharmacol Toxicol* 1973; 32:467.
260. Nergardh A, Boreus LO, Haglo AS: Characterization of the adrenergic beta receptor in the urinary bladder of man and cat. *Acta Pharmacol Toxicol* 1977; 40:14.
261. Nesbit R, Lapides J: Tonus of the bladder during spinal shock. *Arch Surg* 1948; 56:138.
262. Nesbit R, Lapides J, Volk W, et al: The effects of blockade of the autonomic ganglia on the urinary bladder in man. *J Urol* 1947; 57:242.
263. Nilvebrant L, Andersson KE, Mattiasson A: Characterization of the muscarinic cholinoceptors in the human detrusor. *J Urol* 1985; 134:418.
264. Nilvebrant L, Sparf B: Muscarinic receptor binding in the guinea pig urinary bladder. *Acta Pharmacol Toxicol* 1983; 52:30.
264a. Nilvebrant L: On the muscarinic receptors in the urinary bladder and the putative subclassification of muscarinic receptors. *Acta Pharmacol Toxicol* 1986; 59(suppl 1):1.
265. Nishizawa O, Fukada T, Matsuzaki A, et al: Role of the sympathetic nerve in bladder and urethral sphincter function during the micturition cycle in the dog evaluated by pressure flow EMG study. *J Urol* 1985; 134:1259.
266. Nordling J: Influence of the sympathetic nervous system on lower urinary tract in man. *Neurourol Urodynamics* 1983; 2:3.
267. Nordling J, Meyhoff H, Hald T: Sympatholytic effect on striated urethral sphincter. A peripheral or central nervous system effect? *Scand J Urol Nephrol* 1981; 15:173.
268. Norlen L: Influence of the sympathetic nervous system on the lower urinary tract and its clinical implications. *Neurourol Urodynamics* 1982; 1:129.
269. Norlen LJ, Blaivas JG, Groden W, et al: Contractile effect of substance P on the canine urinary bladder in vivo. *Neurourol Urodynamics* 1983; 2:323.
270. Oelrich TM: The urethral sphincter muscle in the male. *Am J Anat* 1980; 158:229.
271. Oelrich TM: The striated urogenital sphincter muscle in the female. *Anat Rec* 1983; 205:223.
272. Ohtsuka M, Mori J, Tsujioka K, et al: Pharmacological study on sympathetic inhibition of the urinary bladder in dogs. *Jpn J Pharmacol* 1980; 30:181.
273. Owman C, Owman T, Sjoberg NO: Short adrenergic neurons innervating the female urethra of the cat. *Experientia* 1971; 27:313.
274. Pedersen E, Torring J, Kleman B: Effect of the alpha adrenergic blocking agent thymoxamine on the neurogenic bladder and urethra. *Acta Neurol Scand* 1980; 61:107.
275. Perry SV, Grand RJA: Mechanisms of contraction and the specialized protein components of smooth muscle. *Br Med Bull* 1979; 35:219.
276. Persson CGA, Anderson KE: Adrenoceptor and cholinoceptor mediated

effects in the isolated urethra of the cat and guinea pig. *Clin Exp Pharmacol Physiol* 1976; 3:415.

277. Plum F: Autonomous urinary bladder activity in normal man. *AMA Arch Neurol* 1960; 2:497.
278. Plum F, Colfelt R: The genesis of vesical rhythmicity. *AMA Arch Neurol* 1960; 2:487.
279. Polak JM, Bloom SR: Localization and measurement of VIP in the genitourinary system of man and animals. *Peptides* 1984; 5:225.
280. Raezer DM, Greenberg SH, Jacobowitz DM, et al: The innervation of the trigonal area of canine urinary bladder. *Urology* 1976; 7:369.
281. Raezer DM, Wein AJ, Jacobowitz D, et al: Autonomic innervation of canine urinary bladder: Cholinergic and adrenergic contributions and interaction of sympathetic and parasympathetic systems in bladder function. *Urology* 1973; 2:211.
282. Raz S, Caine M, Zeigler M: The vascular component in the production of intraurethral pressure. *J Urol* 1972b; 108:93.
283. Raz S, Zeigler M, Caine M: Isometric studies on canine urethral musculature. *Invest Urol* 1972a; 9:443.
284. Rockswold GI, Bradley WE, Chou SN: Innervation of the urinary bladder in higher primates. *J Compr Neurol* 1980a; 193:509.
285. Rockswold GI, Bradley WE, Chou SN: Innervation of the external urethral and external anal sphincters in higher primates. *J Compr Neurol* 1980b; 193:521.
286. Rohner TJ, Hannigan J: Effect of norepinephrine and isoproterenol on in vitro detrusor muscle contractility and cyclic AMP content. *Invest Urol* 1980; 17:324.
287. Rohner TJ, Raezer DM, Wein AJ, et al: Contractile responses of dog bladder neck muscle to adrenergic drugs. *J Urol* 1971; 105:657.
288. Roppolo JR, Booth AM, deGroat WC: The effects of naloxone on the neural control of the urinary bladder of the cat. *Brain Res* 1983; 264:335.
289. Rossier A, Fam B, Lee I, et al: Role of striated and smooth muscle components in the urethral pressure profile in traumatic neurogenic bladders: A neuropharmacologic and urodynamic study. Preliminary report. *J Urol* 1982; 128:529.
290. Ruch TC: The urinary bladder, in Ruch TC, Patton HD (eds): *Circulation, Respiration, and Fluid Balance.* Philadelphia, WB Saunders, 1974, pp 525–546.
291. Rud T, Andersson KE, Asmussen M, et al: Factors maintaining the urethral pressure in women. *Invest Urol* 1980; 17:343.
292. Ruffolo RR: Interactions of agonists with peripheral alpha adrenergic receptors. *Fed Proc* 1984; 43:2910.
293. Ruggieri M, Levin RM, Wein AJ: Muscarinic receptor subtypes in rabbit and human bladder smooth muscle. *Neurourol Urodynamics,* in press.
294. Sant GR: The anatomy of the external striated urethral sphincter. *Paraplegia* 1972; 10:153.

295. Santicioli P, Maggi CA, Meli A: The postganglionic excitatory innervation of the mouse urinary bladder and its modulation by prejunctional $GABA_B$ receptors. *J Auton Pharmacol* 1986; 6:53.
296. Saum WR, deGroat WC: The actions of 5-hydroxytryptamine on the urinary bladder and on vesical autonomic ganglia in the cat. *J Pharmacol Exp Ther* 1973; 185:70.
297. Saxena PR, Herligers J, Mylecharane EJ, et al: Excitatory 5-hydroxytryptamine receptors in the cat urinary bladder are the M and 5 HT_2 type. *J Auton Pharmacol* 1985; 5:101.
298. Schmidt RA: Urethrovesical reflexes and their inhibition, in Hinman F Jr (ed): *Benign Prostatic Hypertrophy*. Berlin, Springer-Verlag, 1983, pp 361–372.
299. Schulman CC, Duarte-Escalante O, Boyarsky S: The ureterovesical innervation: A new concept based on a histochemical study. *Br J Urol* 1972; 44:698.
300. Sibley GNA: A comparison of spontaneous and nerve mediated activity in bladder muscle from man, pig, and rabbit. *J Physiol* 1984; 354:431.
301. Sillen U: Central neurotransmitter mechanisms involved in the control of urinary bladder function. *Scand J Urol Nephrol*, suppl 58, 1980, pp 1–45.
302. Sillen U, Rubenson A: Central and peripheral motor effects of morphine on the rat urinary bladder. *Acta Physiol Scand* 1986; 126:181.
302a. Simonds WF, Booth AM, Thor KB, et al: Parasympathetic ganglia: Naloxone antagonizes inhibition by leucine-enkephalin and GABA. *Brain Res* 1983; 271:365.
303. Sjogren C, Andersson KE, Husted S, et al: Atropine resistance of transmurally stimulated isolated human bladder muscle. *J Urol* 1982; 128:1368.
304. Sjogren C, Andersson KE, Mattiasson A: Effects of vasoactive intestinal polypeptide on isolated urethral and urinary bladder smooth muscle from rabbit and man. *J Urol* 1985; 133:136.
305. Somlyo AP: The messenger across the gap. *Nature* 1985; 316:298.
306. Stanton SL: Urethral sphincter incompetence (stress incontinence), in Mundy AR, Stephenson TD, Wein AJ (eds): *Urodynamics: Principles, Practice, Application*. New York, Churchill Livingstone, 1984, pp 230–241.
307. Sundin T, Carlsson CA, Kock NA: Detrusor inhibition induced from mechanical stimulation of the anal region and from electrical stimulation of pudendal nerve afferents: An experimental study in cat. *Invest Urol* 1974; 11:374.
308. Sundin T, Dahlstrom A, Norlen L, et al: The sympathetic innervation and adrenoreceptor function of the human lower urinary tract in the normal state and after parasympathetic denervation. *Invest Urol* 1977; 14:322.
309. Taira N: The autonomic pharmacology of the bladder. *Annu Rev Pharmacol* 1972; 12:197.
310. Tanagho EA: The anatomy and physiology of micturition. *Clin Obstet Gynecol* 1978; 5 (April):3.
311. Tanagho EA: The ureterovesical junction: Anatomy and physiology, in

Chisholm GD, Williams D (eds): *Scientific Foundations of Urology*. Chicago, Year Book Medical Publishers, 1982, pp 295–404.
312. Tanagho EA: Anatomy of the lower urinary tract, in Walsh PC, Gillen RF, Perlmutter AD, et al (eds): *Campbell's Urology*. Philadelphia, WB Saunders, 1986, pp 46–74.
313. Tanagho EA, Meyers FH: The 'internal sphincter': Is it under sympathetic control? *Invest Urol* 1969; 7:79.
314. Tanagho EA, Meyers FH, Smith DR: Urethral resistance: Its components and implications: I. Smooth muscle component. *Invest Urol* 1969a; 7:136.
315. Tanagho EA, Meyers FH, Smith DR: Urethral resistance: Its components and implications: II. Striated muscle component. *Invest Urol* 1969b; 7:195.
316. Tanagho EA, Miller ER: Initiation of voiding. *Br J Urol* 1970; 42:175.
317. Tanagho EA, Pugh RCB: The anatomy of the ureterovesical junction. *Br J Urol* 1963; 35:151.
318. Tanagho EA, Smith DR: The anatomy and function of the bladder neck. *Br J Urol* 1966; 38:54.
319. Tanagho EA, Smith DR: Mechanism of urinary continence: I. Embryologic, anatomic, and pathologic considerations. *J Urol* 1968; 100:640.
320. Tanagho EA, Schmidt RA, Gomes deAranjo C: Urinary striated sphincter: What is its nerve supply? *Urology* 1982; 20:415.
321. Tang PC: Levels of brain stem and diencephalon controlling micturition reflex. *J Neurophysiol* 1955; 18:583.
322. Tang P, Ruch T: Non-neurogenic basis of bladder tonus. *Am J Physiol* 1955; 181:249.
323. Tang PC, Ruch TC: Localization of brain stem and diencephalic areas controlling the micturition reflex. *J Compr Neurol* 1956; 106:213.
324. Theobald RJ: The effect of arylazido aminoproprionyl ATP on atropine resistant contractions of the cat urinary bladder. *Life Sci* 1983; 32:2479.
325. Theobald RJ: The effect of $ANAPP_3$ on inhibition of pelvic nerve induced contractions of the cat urinary bladder. *Eur J Pharmacol* 1986; 120:351.
326. Thor KB, Roppolo JR, deGroat WC: Naloxone induced micturition in unanesthetized paraplegic cats. *J Urol* 1983; 129:202.
327. Todd JK, Mack AJ: A study of human bladder detrusor muscle. *Br J Urol* 1969; 41:448.
328. Tokunaka S, Murakami U, Hashi K, et al: Electrophoretic and ultrastructural analysis of the rabbit's striated external urethral sphincter. *J Urol* 1984; 132:1040.
329. Tsujimoto G, Timmins PV, Hoffman BB: Alpha adrenergic receptors in the rabbit bladder base smooth muscle: Alpha-1 adrenergic receptors mediate contractile responses. *J Pharmacol Exp Ther* 1986; 236:384.
330. Ursillo RC, Clark BB: The action of atropine on the urinary bladder of the dog and on the isolated nerve-bladder strip preparation of the rabbit. *J Pharmacol Exp Ther* 1956; 118:338.
331. Vaidyanathan S, Rao MS, Chary KSN, et al: Clinical impact of serotonin activity in the bladder and urethra. *J Urol* 1981a; 125:42.
332. Vaidyanathan S, Rao M, Chary K, et al: Enhancement of detrusor reflex

activity by naloxone in patients with chronic neurogenic bladder dysfunction: Preliminary report. *J Urol* 1981b; 126:500.
333. Van Buren GA, Anderson GF: Comparison of the urinary bladder base and detrusor to cholinergic and histaminergic receptor activation in the rabbit. *Pharmacology* 1979; 18:136.
334. Van Duyl WA: A model for both the passive and active properties of urinary bladder tissue related to bladder function. *Neurourol Urodynamics* 1985; 4:275.
335. Van Mastrigt R, Coolsaet BLRA, Van Duyl WA: The passive properties of the urinary bladder in the collection phase. *Urol Int* 1978; 33:14.
336. Vodusek DB, Light JK: The motor nerve supply of the external urethral sphincter muscles: An electrophysiologic study. *Neurourol Urodynamics* 1983; 2:193.
337. Wein AJ: Pharmacology of the bladder and urethra, in Stanton SL, Tanagho EA (eds): *Surgery of Female Incontinence.* Berlin, Springer-Verlag, 1986, pp 229–250.
338. Wein AJ, Benson GS, Jacobowitz DM: Lack of evidence of adrenergic innervation of the external urethral sphincter. *J Urol* 1979; 121:324.
339. Wein AJ, Gregory JG, Cromie WJ, et al: Sympathetic innervation and chemical sympathectomy of canine bladder. *Urology* 1974; 4:27.
340. Wein AJ, Levin RM: Comparison of adrenergic receptor density in the urinary bladder in man, dog, and rabbit. *Surg Forum* 1979; 30:576.
341. Wein AJ, Raezer DM: Physiology of micturition, in Krane RJ, Siroky MB (eds): *Clinical Neurourology.* Boston, Little Brown & Co, 1979, pp 1–33.
342. Westfall DP: Supersensitivity of smooth muscle, in Bulbring E, Brading AF, Jones AM, et al (eds): *Smooth Muscle.* Austin, University of Texas Press, 1981, pp 285–309.
343. Woodburne RT: Anatomy of the bladder, in Boyarsky S (ed): *The Neurogenic Bladder.* Baltimore, Williams & Wilkins, 1967, pp 3–17.
344. Woodburne RT: Anatomy of the bladder and bladder outlet. *J Urol* 1968; 100:474.
345. Woodside JR, McGuire EJ: Urethral hypotonicity after suprasacral spinal cord injury. *J Urol* 1979; 121:783.
346. Yablonsky F, Riffaud JP, Lacolle JY, et al: β-1 and β-2 adrenoceptors in the smooth muscle of male and female rabbit urethra. *Eur J Pharmacol* 1986; 121:1.
347. Zinner NR, Sterling AR, Ritter RC: Role of inner urethral softness in urinary continence. *Urology* 1980; 16:115.
348. Zinner NR, Sterling AM, Ritter RC: Structure and forces of continence, in Raz S (ed): Female Urology. Philadelphia, WB Saunders Co, 1983, pp 33–41.

SECTION II

Voiding Dysfunction: Diagnosis, Classification, and Management

Overview

Abnormalities of the micturition cycle are responsible for a large number of patient visits to the urologist. The symptoms and problems that result from these disorders can range from simply annoying and not serious to completely disabling and hazardous. These abnormalities may occur as a result of neurologic injury or disease, inflammatory or infectious disease, bladder outlet obstruction, structural changes in the bladder and urethra or loss of their supporting structures because of surgical or nonsurgical trauma or aging, or strictly psychogenic factors. For the purposes of description and teaching, micturition is best divided into two relatively discrete phases, one of bladder filling and urine storage, and one of bladder emptying. The previous chapter has considered in great detail the anatomic, neuromorphologic, neurophysiologic, neuropharmacologic, and mechanical details involved in both the storage and expulsion of urine by the lower urinary tract. It was emphasized and will be re-emphasized that, despite disagreements by "experts" on various details, one can succinctly summarize these processes from a conceptual point of view. Bladder filling and urine storage require:

1. Accommodation of increasing volumes of urine at a low intravesical pressure and with appropriate sensation.
2. A closed bladder outlet at rest that remains so during increases in intra-abdominal pressure.
3. Absence of involuntary bladder contractions.

Bladder emptying requires:

1. A coordinated contraction by the bladder smooth musculature of adequate magnitude.
2. Concomitant lowering of resistance at the level of the smooth sphincter and of the striated sphincter.
3. Absence of anatomic obstruction.

Any type of voiding dysfunction must by definition result from an abnormality of one or more of the factors involved in the two phases of the micturition cycle. This type of division, with its implied subdivisions under each category into causes related to the bladder and causes related to the outlet, seems to provide a reasonable rationale for consideration of all types of voiding dysfunction as disorders either related primarily to (1) bladder filling or urine storage or (2) bladder emptying. There are, indeed, some types of dysfunction that represent a combination of filling/storage and emptying disorders. However, within this type of scheme, these combined disorders become readily understandable and a clear rationale for treatment—or choices of treatments—is generally evident. In our description of various types of lower urinary tract dysfunction, we will try to emphasize this type of view of the clinical pathophysiology involved, because we believe that this provides the best rationale for the explanation of symptoms, urodynamic findings, and choices for therapy.

This chapter will begin with a very brief consideration of the pathophysiology, symptomatology, and general outline of treatment for disorders that fall primarily under the category of "failure to empty" and of "failure of filling/storage." We will then consider all aspects of the neurourologic evaluation, and the integration of the data so obtained within various classification systems for both neurogenic and nonneurogenic voiding dysfunction. We will then consider the treatment of all types of voiding dysfunction, again using primarily a simple-minded functional division of specific modes of therapy as to whether they primarily facilitate lower urinary tract emptying by increasing intravesical pressure or decreasing outlet resistance, or facilitate bladder filling and urine storage by inhibiting bladder contractility or increasing outlet resistance. Specific voiding dysfunctions associated with neurologic disease will be considered next, as will other types of voiding dysfunction, some of which are relatively clear-cut and some of which defy the usual type of pathophysiologic explanation.

FAILURE TO EMPTY

Absolute or relative failure to empty results from decreased bladder contractility, increased outlet resistance, or both. Absolute or relative failure of adequate bladder contractility may result from temporary or permanent alteration in any one of the neuromuscular mechanisms necessary for initiating and maintaining a normal detrusor contraction. Inhibition of the micturition reflex in a neurologically normal individual may occur via a reflex mechanism secondary to painful stimuli, especially from the pelvic and perineal areas, or may be psychogenic. Nonneurogenic causes include impairment of bladder smooth muscle function, which may result from overdistention, severe infection, or fibrosis. Increased outlet resistance is generally secondary to anatomic obstruction, but may be secondary to a failure of coordination of the smooth or striated sphincter during bladder contraction. Drug therapy may either decrease bladder contractility and/or increase outlet resistance. Treatment for failure to empty generally consists of attempts to increase intravesical pressure or facilitate the micturition reflex, to decrease outlet resistance, or both.

FAILURE TO STORE

The pathophysiology of failure of the lower urinary tract to fill with or store urine adequately may be secondary to reasons related to the bladder, the outlet, or both. Hyperactivity of the bladder during filling can be expressed as discrete involuntary contractions or as low compliance (Δ volume/Δ pressure) without a discrete and separable contraction. Involuntary contractions are most commonly seen in association with neurological disease or following neurological injury, but may also be associated with inflammatory or irritative processes in the bladder wall, with bladder outlet obstruction, or they may be idiopathic. Decreased compliance during filling may be secondary to the sequelae of neurological injury or disease, but may also result from any process that destroys the viscoelastic properties of the bladder wall. Decreased outlet resistance may result from damage to the innervation or the structural elements of the smooth or striated sphincter, neurologic disease or injury, or surgical or other mechanical trauma; aging may also be responsible for such pathology. Classical stress urinary incontinence in the female seems primarily to be a sphincter dysfunction caused by a failure of the normal transmission of increases in intra-abdominal pressure to the area of the bladder neck and proximal urethra. This is felt to be due mainly to a change in the anatomic position of the vesicourethral junction and proximal urethra during increases in intra-abdominal pressure, and is felt to accompany pelvic floor weakness or relaxation, which can be due to a number of causes. The treatment of abnormalities related to the filling/storage phase of micturition is directed toward inhibiting bladder contractility or decreasing sensory input during filling, or toward increasing outlet resistance, either continuously or just during abdominal straining.

The Neurourologic Evaluation

An orderly approach to the workup of the patient with voiding dysfunction includes the modalities as outlined in Table 9. As with all clinical problems, the degree of disease complexity, patient cooperation, time and equipment available, and economic resources will modify the progression through these diagnostic stages. In general, one should proceed using the simplest, least-invasive, least-expensive methods first, as these will often yield adequate information to support a reasonable therapeutic trial. When unsatisfactory results are achieved or a definite answer is elusive, then the more complex tests are introduced.

HISTORY

Assessment of the clinical history of individuals with voiding dysfunction should be designed to exclude previous neurologic disease, trauma, and surgery. A list of medications should be compiled, as these are frequently the sole cause for a change in voiding habits. Symptoms related to other organ systems that are compositely innervated by the somatic and autonomic nerves in the pelvis are to be included; this would include bowel and sexual function. Fecal incontinence, constipation, lower abdominal distention, and cramping may suggest neuropathy affecting intestinal or rectal sphincteric function. Changes in sexual function such as the frequency, duration, and rigidity of erections or a decrease in the volume of semen and force of ejaculation similarly would imply altered innervation of the pelvic organs.

TABLE 9.
Neurourologic Workup

History
Physical examination
Neurologic examination
Urine bacteriologic studies
Renal function studies
Intravenous urogram
Voiding cystourethrogram
Endoscopic examination
Videourodynamic studies

The functional classification of voiding dysfunction, i.e., failure to empty and failure to store, can provide a basis for collecting historical data from the patient. A "wet" patient with an empty bladder is most characteristic of a storage failure abnormality, while a "dry" patient with a bladder that cannot be emptied is typical of evacuation failure. Primary symptoms such as these are a useful guide to an ultimate diagnosis. However, the development of secondary symptoms or the combination of symptoms confuses the picture and makes the implementation of therapeutic measures based on historical factors alone fraught with error. Table 10 attempts to categorize the common presenting symptoms of a patient with the voiding dysfunction.

Incontinence (failure to store) may result from ureteral ectopy, congenital or acquired fistulae, or neuromuscular defects of the detrusor or urethral sphincter. Patients with wetness and ureteral ectopy or con-

TABLE 10.
Symptoms of Voiding Dysfunction

	Failure to Fill or Store	Failure to Empty
Incontinence	P*	S*
Urgency	P	S
Frequency	P	S
Nocturia	P	S
Enuresis	P	S
Pressure	P	P
Dysuria	?	?
Hesitancy	. . .	P
Straining to void	. . .	P

*P indicates primary symptom; S, secondary symptom (may develop consequent to the primary abnormality).

genital fistulae are almost all female and generally present as a consequence of failed toilet training. Not infrequently, these defects are associated with other abnormalities of the ureteral bud and/or urogenital sinus, and further examination should be undertaken. Deficiencies in the smooth or striated muscle or fibroelastic tissue that make up the bladder neck and proximal urethra and the surrounding structures can give rise to varying degrees of urinary incontinence. The characteristics of incontinence may be further divided into the following categories: stress, dripping, precipitous, or total. Varying in severity, leakage may occur only with associated increases in intra-abdominal pressure as occurs with stress urinary incontinence. A scarred, fibrotic, or noncompliant urethra and bladder neck, which may be seen after trauma, multiple surgical procedures, or radiation therapy, may also be associated with incontinence; this, however, generally results in a constant dripping type of leakage. Incontinence may also occur as a result of involuntary detrusor contractions or detrusor hyperreflexia. This type of incontinence is generally associated with some type of neurologic disease and is characterized by precipitous voiding with a more sustained type of leakage than is seen with pure sphincteric insufficiency. Total incontinence implies that little if any voiding occurs, and that urine essentially passes through the bladder and out, the continence mechanism being completely incompetent.

Incontinence is not always a symptom of primary failure to store urine adequately. Overflow or paradoxic incontinence may develop in a patient with insidious detrusor decompensation who has a failure-to-empty defect. The leakage in this case is generally associated with sudden increases in intra-abdominal pressure. Detrusor hyperreflexia can be seen as a result of outlet obstruction and failure to empty. The exact changes that result in increased detrusor contractility are unknown, but incontinence is the resultant symptom.

Urgency is defined as the extreme desire to void, either because of pain or because of a fear of leaking. The urgency that is associated only with pain is generally secondary to inflammatory disease of the lower urinary tract. Urodynamic studies may be normal except for hypersensitivity. The urgency that is associated with a fear of leaking, or a history of doing so, is usually associated with detrusor instability or hyperreflexia. Thus, urgency may either be a symptom of a primary failure to fill or store normally, or a manifestation of the detrusor hyperreflexia that develops secondary to bladder outlet obstruction. When using the term "urgency," it is important to at least try to distinguish between the impending sensation of micturition and the simple fear of leaking urine. The former is usually associated with detrusor hyperreflexia, while the latter may be associated with leakage from simple sphincteric incontinence.

An increase in daytime urinary frequency may simply be psychogenic in origin. However, such an increase may represent a genuine need to void, and in this case it may result from either pain on low-volume bladder distention (usually indicative of inflammatory disease of the lower urinary tract) or primary detrusor hyperreflexia. Increased frequency of urination may result secondarily from a failure to empty adequately, either because of a decreased functional bladder capacity (due to a substantial residual urine volume) or in association with outlet obstruction–induced hyperreflexia. Nocturia usually accompanies nonpsychogenic urinary frequency and may be associated, on the same basis, with either a failure of adequate urine storage or a failure of adequate urine emptying. Patients with true nocturnal enuresis often have detrusor hyperreflexia; therefore, this symptom may be seen in patients who exhibit a primary failure of storage or in patients who have developed hyperreflexia because of a failure to empty secondary to outlet obstruction.

The symptom of "pressure" defies exact definition. It is not quite the urge to void; rather, in many persons there is a feeling that the bladder is full or that the urge to void will occur shortly. Often no discernible voiding dysfunction is discovered in patients who complain of this symptom. However, it can be due to an intravesical pressure during filling that is pathologically elevated but below the level necessary to elicit the sensation of distention or urgency. This symptom also may be representative of the patient's accurate perception of the fact that the bladder does not in fact empty completely, and that a modest or large residual urine volume is present.

Hesitancy and straining to void, when associated with true voiding dysfunction, generally reflect a failure to empty adequately.

Finally, in considering the symptoms of voiding dysfunction, it must be remembered that combination abnormalities can occur. Outlet obstruction may exist in combination with detrusor hyperreflexia, and this combination may give rise to hesitancy, straining to void, frequency, nocturia, and urgency with urge incontinence. Likewise, elements of both sphincteric and detrusor incontinence can exist in the woman who complains of stress incontinence that is accompanied by frequency, nocturia, and—especially—urgency incontinence. An orderly review of these symptoms with the patient, noting the temporal aspects of each, will enhance the clinician's ability to tailor subsequent tests that will be needed to confirm any presumptive diagnoses.

The preceding section clearly describes the value of a symptomatic history in suggesting a voiding dysfunction that represents an abnormality of storage, of emptying, or of both. *Physical examination* may provide visual confirmation of the presence and degree of urinary incontinence in the form of cutaneous excoriation of the genitalia. A distended bladder suggests a failure to empty. Cutaneous scars may provide evidence of previous neurosurgical, orthopedic, or pelvic surgical procedures that may be related to the problem under evaluation, either because they were performed to correct a similar problem or because the problem under evaluation developed subsequent to a surgical procedure.

A careful neurologic examination is especially important as it may provide evidence of a neurologic lesion or disease that is presenting initially with symptoms of voiding dysfunction. Review should include inspection of the skull and vertebral column, assessment of mentation, sensory examination, motor function, and coordination evaluation. Concentrating on the pelvis, evaluation of rectal sphincter tone and the bulbocavernous reflex is essential to help establish the integrity of sacral reflex arcs. Acknowledgement of the presence of one or another type of neurologic disease may considerably alter the philosophy of treatment for a given patient.

Abnormal *renal function studies* may reflect an unsuspected failure of emptying or may reflect intrinsic renal or prerenal disease, thereby changing some of the considerations for treatment. *Urine bacteriologic studies* are needed as urinary tract infection can cause or worsen all of the symptoms of a failure to store and may coexist with other causes of storage failure. Persistent or recurrent infection may be a reflection of inadequate emptying with persistent residual urine.

Many urologists feel that *intravenous urography* is not necessary in patients with lower tract dysfunction. They point out that a significant abnormality is detected only in a small percentage of the patients studied. There is no argument, however, that upper tract deterioration can suggest emptying failure that has occurred on the basis of either bladder distention, pathologically elevated voiding pressures, or both. In addition, urography is useful in assessing the upper urinary tracts prior to the institution of any treatments designed to alter voiding function. Silent deterioration of the upper tracts can occur after surgical or pharmacologic therapy designed to decrease bladder contractility or increase outlet resistance, and it is therefore useful to have some sort of a baseline for later comparison.

Voiding cystourethrography as an isolated study may provide direct confirmation of leakage with stress and important details of bladder and urethral configuration and position. An alert uroradiologist can detect, in some cases, leakage secondary to an involuntary detrusor contraction without the aid of differential bladder and abdominal pressures. An abnormality of emptying might be suggested by secondary signs of outlet obstruction, such as trabeculation, cellules, diverticula, or vesicoureteral reflux. If obstruction has been documented, a VCUG carefully done during bladder contraction can generally pinpoint the site. *Endoscopic evaluation* may be helpful in detecting or suggesting previously unsuspected inflammatory or neoplastic disease or outlet obstruction.

Urodynamics

With the Assistance of Benad Goldwasser, M.D.

Urodynamics is a neurourologic diagnostic tool concerned with the identification and measurement of physiologic and pathologic factors involved in the storage, transportation, and evacuation of urine. The purpose of urodynamic testing is to identify and quantitate the etiologic factors that contribute to voiding dysfunction, whether it is a problem of storage or emptying. Since the bladder is a notoriously poor witness and will respond to a variety of pathologies with the same symptoms, the need for urodynamic testing becomes important before directing therapy. A number of studies have documented the poor correlation between the patient's symptoms and the findings of urodynamic testing. This is true both for patients without (Farrar et al., 1975; Powell et al., 1981) and those with (Blaivas et al., 1979; Blaivas, 1980) neurourologic disorders. In a study done in patients with multiple sclerosis, it was found that when treatment was instituted based on symptoms and signs, it was effective in 27% of patients. When treatment was based on urodynamic testing, it was effective in 83% of patients (Blaivas et al., 1979; Blaivas, 1980).

Urodynamic tests are not without their limitations and potential for misinterpretation. Ideally, the clinical symptom should be reproduced during the urodynamic testing sequence. If the symptom is not reproduced during routine testing, then the study must be repeated in as close an approximation as possible to the situation in which the patient's symptoms actually occur, be it rising, standing, coughing,

*Special Fellow in Neurourology and Prosthetics, Mayo Clinic, 1985–1986.

laughing, or jogging. Patients should be asked to evaluate the similarity of their usual voiding to the voiding sequence evaluated urodynamically. This helps establish the credibility of the urodynamic data. On the other hand, there may be certain symptoms produced during the testing sequence that have urodynamic correlates, but that do not constitute a part of the patient's original complaints. These findings may represent artifact or be early subclinical abnormalities not generally manifested during normal voiding, but brought to light by the challenge of urodynamic testing.

Interpreting sensory data during urodynamic testing is subjective at best. This is unfortunate as many patients with voiding dysfunction have only sensation abnormalities and have no demonstrable urodynamic abnormalities. It is relatively easy to assess whether the sensation of bladder filling is normal, decreased, or absent. However, there are a number of sensations that may occur during filling that are difficult to classify. The most troublesome of these is the symptom of urgency or the dire need to void. Although this can correlate with involuntary bladder contractions or detrusor hyperreflexia, it is not uncommon to reproduce this symptom during urodynamic testing and not be able to demonstrate a urodynamic abnormality. The explanation for this rests within the limitations of the test to be sensitive enough to record the subtle changes that occur in the bladder or outlet or the inhibitory factors that come into play in the laboratory setting.

Operator expertise is essential for successful completion of most studies and physician participation is recommended in the more complex tests.

There are four basic urodynamic modalities: (1) cystometry, (2) uroflowmetry (with residual volume determination), (3) urethral pressure profilometry, and (4) combined studies (with or without fluoroscopy). The exact sequence in which these tests are administered to the patient is entirely dependent on the presenting symptoms and the presumptive diagnosis based on other neurourologic tests. Table 11 lists the urodynamic modalities as they relate to evaluation of the bladder or the bladder outlet, and, in general, the simplest, least invasive test should be used first.

General urologic practices will derive most benefit from simple uroflowmetry and cystometry. Sphincter electromyography is important should neurogenic bladder dysfunction make up a significant proportion of the study population. In urogynecologic practices, cystometry, uroflowmetry, and urethral pressure studies will be of most value. Complex cases that cannot be evaluated adequately in this manner are best referred to a urodynamic center capable of performing multifunc-

TABLE 11.
Urodynamics Made Easy

	Bladder	Outlet
Filling/storage	$P_{det(FCMG)}$[1]	P_{ureth}[2] FLUORO[3]
Emptying	$P_{det(VCMG)}$[4]	P_{ureth}[2] FLUORO[3] EMG[5]
	FLOW[6] RU[7]	

1. Filling cystometrogram (recording of detrusor pressure during filling).
2. Urethral pressure(s).
3. Fluoroscopy.
4. Voiding cystometry (recording of detrusor pressure during voluntary or involuntary emptying).
5. EMG of periurethral striated muscle.
6. Flowmetry.
7. Residual urine determination.

tion studies—with the option of combined videocystourethrography—which is staffed by a urodynamic technician with knowledge and expertise in this specialty.

It is important to keep in mind constantly that urodynamic testing is but one part of the overall evaluation. It is imperative that all portions of the neurourologic evaluation and the conclusions drawn from them be carefully reviewed and, when discrepancy exists between the symptoms and the urodynamic findings, these studies should be questioned and repeated, especially before irreversible therapy is undertaken.

CYSTOMETRY

Cystometry is the method by which changes in bladder pressure are measured with progressive increase in bladder volume. The test is basically designed to evaluate the filling/storage phase of detrusor function. The presence or absence of a detrusor contraction, although an important observation, is not necessary to glean important information from this test.

The normal adult bladder capacity averages 400–750 ml. Within this capacity, bladder pressure should not rise above 15 cm H_2O, the mean rise in normal bladders being 6 cm H_2O. Schematically, the normal cystometrogram may be divided into four phases (Fig 40). There is

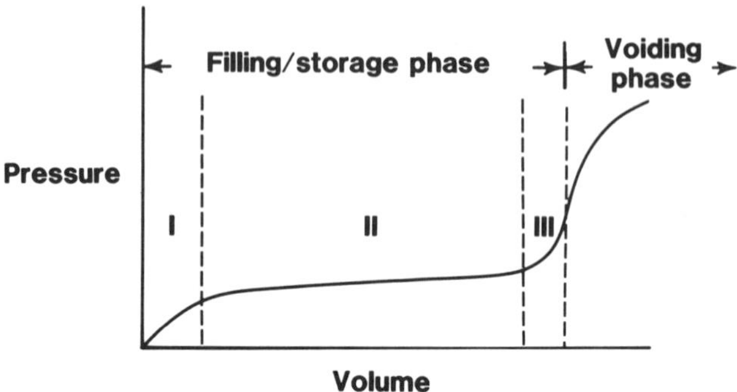

FIG 40.
Characteristics of the normal cystometrogram.

an initial rise in pressure to achieve resting bladder pressure. The second phase—the tonus limb—reflects the vesicoelastic properties of the smooth muscle, collagen, and mucopolysaccharides of the bladder wall. During this filling/storage phase, bladder pressure should increase by very little as the normal bladder is able to accommodate to increasing urine volumes. Rapid filling rates may generate a steeper tonus limb. Bladder wall fibrosis of various etiologies (infection, radiation, etc.) and detrusor hypertrophy may also cause compromised accommodation with a steeper tonus limb. At peak capacity, the detrusor muscle and other elastic tissue have stretched to their limit and any additional increase in volume will be accompanied by a rise in intravesical pressure. During this third stage, the patient is still able to suppress voluntary voiding contractions. Ruch and Tang (1969) have demonstrated that the characteristic shape of the cystometry curve is independent of neural control and is an inherent property of the structural elements of the bladder wall. The fourth phase of the normal cystometrogram is the generation of a voluntary voiding reflex that is dependent on intact neural pathways to the micturition center located in the brain stem. The normal patient should be able to suppress voiding even at capacity. It is not uncommon during a study to find that the patient is unable to generate a micturition reflex at command. This is more common in females and is related to psychological inhibition resulting from the unnatural circumstances of the study. Performance of this phase of the cystometrogram with the male patient in an erect posture and the female on a commode may facilitate generating a micturition reflex. Alternatively, voiding may be stimulated by administering 2.5 mg of bethanechol subcutaneously. If voiding does not occur in response to bethanechol administration, the bladder should be emptied and filled again while measuring bladder pressures to test for evidence of denervation supersensitivity (see below).

Both water and gas (carbon dioxide) are used for cystometry. Controversy exists as to the relative merits of each. From a practical point of view, there seems not to be a statistically significant difference between the two. The advantage of gas (carbon dioxide) is that it is clean and efficient, allowing rapid rate of bladder filling, and thereby takes little time to perform. On the other hand, when the bladder is filled at a rapid rate, accommodation is impaired, with resultant low values of total capacity. Carbon dioxide is irritating to the urothelium and some patients complain of discomfort and dysuria. Because gas is compressible, phasic bladder contractions of small amplitude may escape recording and significant high-pressured contractions may appear as of low amplitude. Gas may also leak unobtrusively at instrument connections and also from the bladder around the catheter, particularly if outflow resistance is low.

The cystometric variables that may be observed during the study are those of compliance, contractility, sensation, and capacity. Although the stable bladder should remain so even at an unphysiologic rate of filling of 100 ml/min, certain patients require a slower rate of bladder filling. These include patients with a known neurological condition suspected of having a hyperreflexic bladder, those with bladders with decreased compliance, and children. In these situations the bladder should be filled at a rate of 25–50 ml/min. During filling, a record is made of the bladder volumes at which first sensation of filling, sensation of urgency to void, and the sensation of maximal capacity occur. During the filling phase, provocative measures such as coughing and the Valsalva maneuver should be utilized to observe for increased detrusor contractility. The pressure measured within the bladder is composed of pressure induced by the detrusor itself and also by intra-abdominal pressure. Therefore, pressure increments recorded on a simple cystometrogram may at least partially reflect intra-abdominal pressure rises. To eliminate such artifactual interferences, it may be necessary to measure simultaneously intra-abdominal pressure by means of a rectal catheter. Cystometers are available that will electronically subtract the rectal pressure from the total bladder pressure, thus giving the subtracted bladder pressure or detrusor pressure. This measurement is important both for provocative cystometry and for voiding studies to determine the efficiency of the voiding contraction.

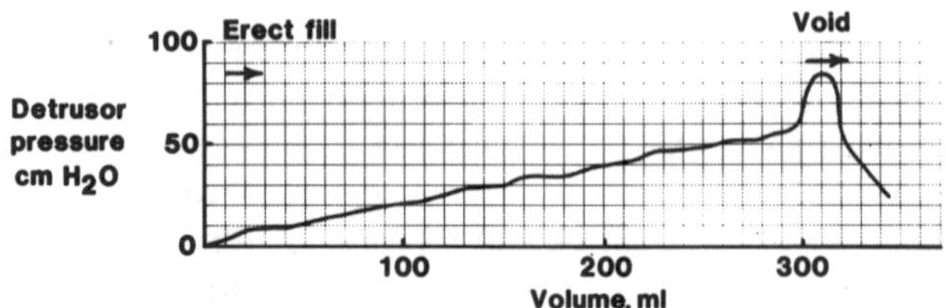

FIG 41.
Cystometrogram depicting decreased detrusor compliance.

Abnormal Cystometric Patterns

Abnormalities of bladder function that may be detected by cystometry include decreased detrusor compliance, increased detrusor contractility or detrusor hyperreflexia, involuntary detrusor contraction, increased bladder compliance, and decreased detrusor contractility or detrusor areflexia.

Bladder compliance refers to the change in detrusor pressure that accompanies an increase in bladder volume during filling. Normally, this should not exceed 15 cm H_2O. A bladder with decreased compliance is one in which the pressure rises steeply with filling (Fig 41). Reduced compliance may result from detrusor hypertrophy, fibrotic changes in the bladder wall, bladder wall inflammation, and possibly neurologic lesions.

Involuntary detrusor contraction refers to a phasic rise in bladder pressure. This may occur in response to provocation such as a cough, stress, or posture change, or may occur spontaneously (Fig 42). States of increased detrusor contractility have been referred to as "detrusor instability" or "detrusor hyperreflexia." In general, the term detrusor hyperreflexia refers to detrusor function that is a direct result of associated neurologic disease, while detrusor instability is seen in the absence of neurologic disease (Hald, 1984). Detrusor hyperreflexia com-

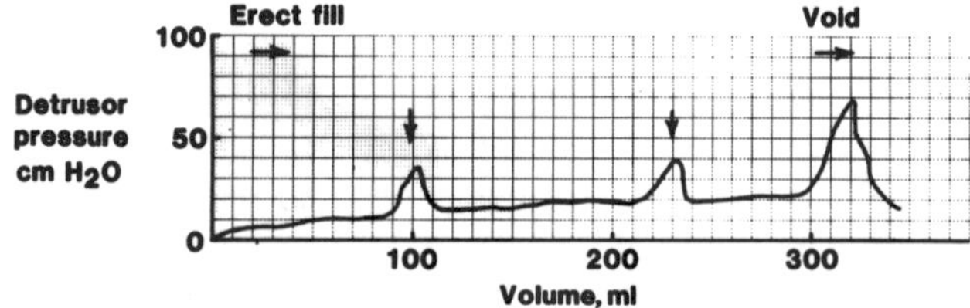

FIG 42.
Cystometrogram depicting increased detrusor contractility.

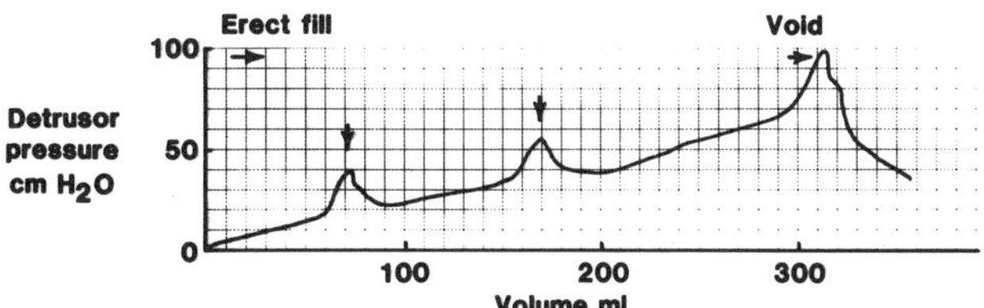

FIG 43.
Cystometrogram showing decreased compliance and increased detrusor contractility.

monly occurs due to suprapontine cerebral disorders, such as cerebrovascular accidents or parkinsonism. This may also occur in patients with suprasacral spinal cord disease processes, such as multiple sclerosis or trauma with or without concomitant detrusor-sphincter dyssynergia.

With marked detrusor instability (or hyperreflexia), the compliance may also be reduced, probably secondary to detrusor muscle hypertrophy (Fig 43). At the most severe end of the spectrum of increased detrusor contractility is the bladder with reduced capacity, in which detrusor hyperreflexia occurs at a low volume (Fig 44). Steepness of the curve is due to muscle contraction as well as to reduced compliance. This may be due to a neurogenic etiology, though it may be seen in patients with severe outlet obstruction. Since both decreased compliance and detrusor hyperreflexia result in a precipitous bladder pressure elevation, differentiation of the two can be difficult.

A large-capacity bladder of normal or increased compliance (Fig 45) may result from decreased sensation as commonly seen in the diabetic patient or from chronic outlet obstruction. It may also be a behavioral

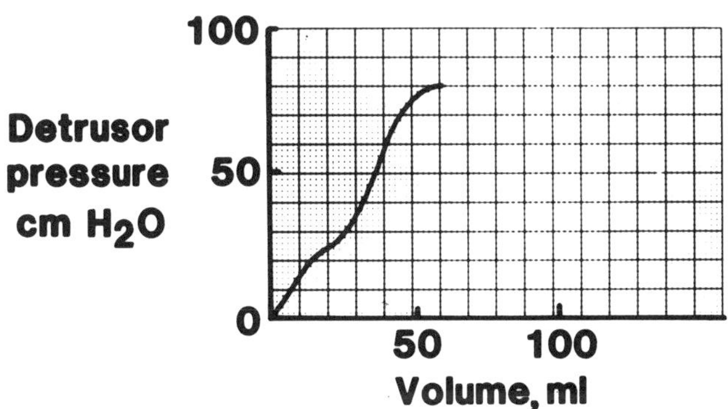

FIG 44.
Cystometrogram showing detrusor hyperreflexia.

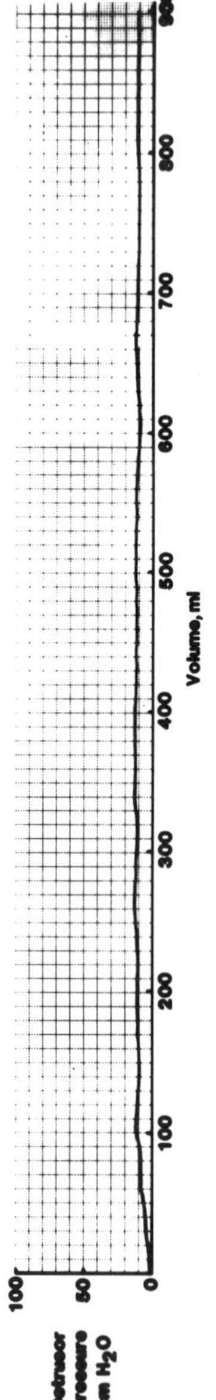

FIG 45.
Cystometrogram demonstrating increased detrusor compliance.

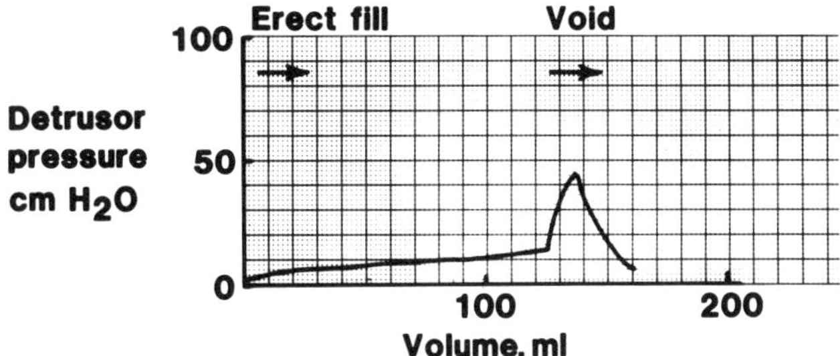

FIG 46.
Cystometrogram depicting normal compliance and contractility but small capacity.

phenomenon in patients who learned to voluntarily inhibit voiding for long periods. Weir and Jaques (1974) found that 30% of patients with bladder capacities in excess of 800 ml were urodynamically normal, so that increased bladder capacity in itself is not necessarily an indication of pathology, especially in patients who can generate a normal detrusor contraction and void to completeness.

Decreased bladder capacity may be purely sensory in origin (normal compliance and stability) and is commonly seen in females with the idiopathic frequency syndrome and in those with an inflamed bladder. These patients are usually able to produce a voluntary detrusor contraction (Fig 46).

BETHANECHOL SUPERSENSITIVITY TEST

Bethanechol chloride is an acetylcholine-like parasympathomimetic agent that exhibits a relatively selective action on the urinary bladder and gut with little or no action at therapeutic dosages on ganglia or on the cardiovascular system (Koelle, 1975; Ursillo, 1967). It is cholinesterase-resistant and causes a contraction in vitro of smooth muscle from all areas of the bladder (Raezer et al., 1973). It has minimal effect on the normal bladder, decreasing the capacity slightly, increasing detrusor tone, and increasing the maximum voluntary micturition pressure. It will not cause the normal bladder to become unstable.

The bethanechol supersensitivity test is based on Cannon's law of denervation, which states that when an organ is deprived of its nerve supply it will develop hypersensitivity to its own neurotransmitter substance. Lapides reported this to be quite accurate in patients with de-

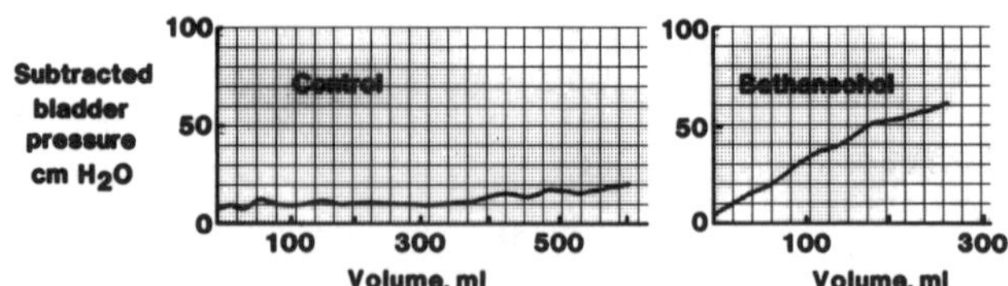

FIG 47.
Cystometrogram with positive bethanechol stimulation test.

nervated bladder (Lapides et al., 1962). However, others (Blaivas et al., 1980) have found significant rates of false negative and false positive responses.

The test requires the subcutaneous injection of 2.5 mg of bethanechol chloride followed in 15–30 minutes by repeated cystometric examination. In patients with areflexic bladders of neurogenic etiology, a rise in pressure of at least 15 cm H_2O at 100 ml filling, in excess of the pretreated cystometric pressure, will result (Fig 47). This does not occur in normal patients and in those with myogenically decompensated bladders. A positive test should not imply a potential benefit from the therapeutic use of oral bethanechol chloride (Barrett, 1981).

The use of bethanechol chloride is contraindicated in patients with bronchial asthma, peptic ulcer, hyperthyroidism, enteritis, bowel obstruction, bladder outlet obstruction, cardiac disease, or a history of recent gastrointestinal surgery (Wein, 1979, 1980).

PROPANTHELINE (PRO-BANTHINE) STIMULATION TEST

Propantheline blocks acetylcholine at muscarinic receptor sites. The test, which is of limited clinical value, is based on the ability of propantheline bromide (as well as of other antimuscarinic agents, such as glycopyrrolate, isopropamide, hyoscyamine, and anisotropine methylbromide) to abolish or cause a decrease in amplitude and frequency of involuntary bladder contractions and to increase the bladder capacity in patients with hyperreflexia of neurologic etiology (Fig 48).

The production of propantheline bromide has been discontinued and glycopyrrolate, 0.1 mg, is currently being used for this test. It is of particular value in the evaluation of the unstable bladder in the man with suspected bladder outlet obstruction where it is important to know whether the instability is of neurologic etiology or secondary to obstruction. This of course has an implication on the therapy that will

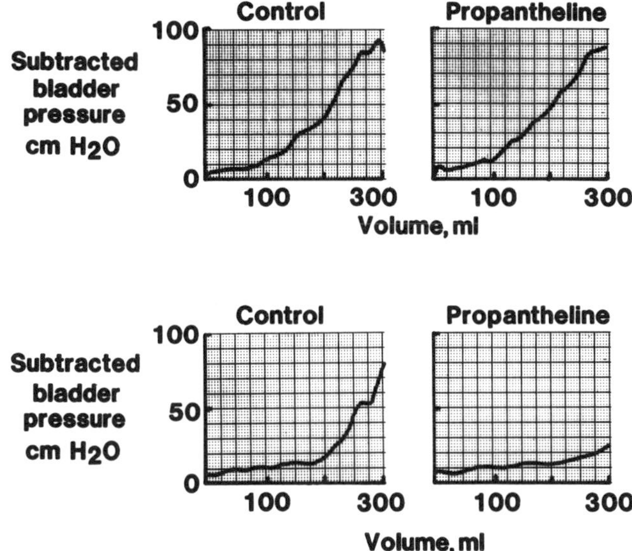

FIG 48.
Cystometrogram before and after administration of 15 mg parenteral propantheline. A positive response is indicated by flattening of tonus limb *(bottom panels)*. No change indicates positive study *(top panels)*.

be recommended to the patient. Whereas in the patient with obstructive unstable bladder, the instability may resolve following relief of obstruction, the patient with a neurologic etiology will most likely become incontinent if surgical treatment is instituted to reduce outlet obstruction. Contraindications to glycopyrrolate include patients with glaucoma and those with obstructive gastrointestinal disease.

UROFLOWMETRY

Flow rate is defined as the volume of fluid expelled from the urethra per unit time and is expressed in milliliters per second. Modern instruments allow us to record not only the overall rate but also a flow pattern (Fig 49). The urine flow rate is an expression of the combined activity of the detrusor and urethra. A normal flow rate will usually indicate a good function of both.

An obstruction in the urethra (benign prostatic hyperplasia, urethral stricture, etc.) may be overcome by a more forceful detrusor contraction, which would bring higher bladder pressures during the stage

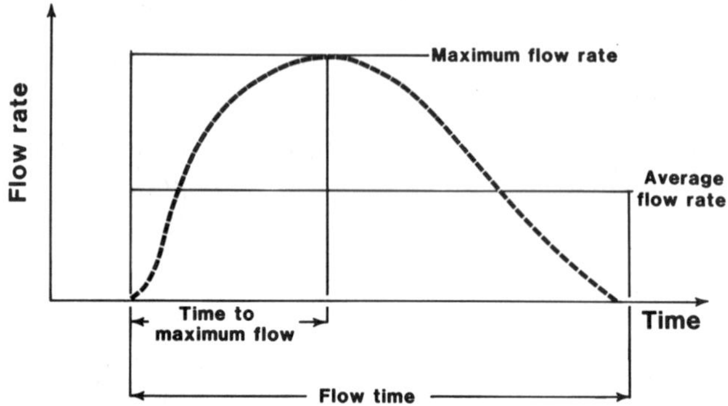

FIG 49.
Characteristics of normal uroflow.

of micturition. This may result in a normal peak flow rate—at least during the early stages of the obstruction—but a reduced average flow rate. Therefore, for a full definition of lower tract function, simultaneous pressure (cystometry) and flow studies during voiding may be indicated. However, a urine flow study even by itself has value as a screening test for lower urinary tract dysfunction, for preoperative and postoperative assessment of lower urinary tract surgery, and to study the effects of pharmacologic agents on urethral resistance and voiding efficiency.

Urine Flow Rate Parameters

To the clinician, the urine flow rate parameters (Table 12) of most importance are the maximum flow rate, voided volume, and flow pattern. Our measurement of urine flow rate is dependent mostly on the patient's comfort with the environment in which the test is conducted and lack of feelings of intimidation in the urodynamics laboratory. Ad-

TABLE 12.
Urine Flow Rate Parameters

1. *Flow time.*—Time over which measurable flow occurs
2. *Time to maximum flow.*—Time elapsed from the onset of flow to maximum rate
3. *Maximum flow rate.*—The maximal rate of flow
4. *Voided volume.*—The total volume expelled by way of the urethra
5. *Average flow rate.*—The voided volume divided by flow time
6. *Voiding time.*—The total duration of micturition, including interruptions
7. *Flow pattern.*—May be continuous, interrupted, or specifically described

ditionally, the patient must have an adequately full bladder, as urine flow rate is dependent on voided volume. Ideally, urine flow interpretation should be for volumes of at least 150 ml. Interpretation of flow rates with smaller voided volumes should be done with caution. Volumes of over 500 ml are also accompanied by reduced flow rates, perhaps due to overstretching of the detrusor fibers. However, flow rates are also related to the sex and age of the patient. Most data in the literature relate to measurements of flow in men younger than 55 years and cite norms of 15 and 25 ml/second for mean and maximum rates. Abrams (1984) states correctly that normality should be defined in terms of age, and that the use of nomograms relating to young men when assessing the older male patient is a doubtful practice. Females have significantly higher flow rates than males matched for age and voided volumes. The values presented in Table 13 are quoted from Abrams (1984) and represent the minimal flow rate for a given sex, age, and voided volume.

The normal flow pattern exhibits a rapid rise to maximum flow rate, attaining this level within one third of the ultimate voiding time, and in addition at least 45% of the total volume voided should be evacuated within this same period and before maximum flow is achieved. After achieving maximum rate, flow decreases more slowly; hence, a true bell-shaped curve is not achieved. In normal patients, average flow rate should be approximately 50% of the maximum urine flow rate.

If abdominal straining is used to augment voiding, the stream is interrupted (Fig 50). Other causes of an interrupted stream may be voluntary sphincter contraction during voiding by the patient with detrusor sphincter dyssynergia or, more commonly, by an anxious patient,

TABLE 13.
Minimum Acceptable Urine Flow Rates*

Age, yr	Minimum Voided Volume, ml	Flow Rates, ml/sec	
		Males	Females
54–7	100	10	10
8–13	100	12	15
14–45	200	21	18
46–55	200	22	15
56–80	200	9	10

*From Abrams P: The urethral pressure profile measurement, in Mundy AR, et al (eds): *Urodynamics: Principles, Practice, and Application.* Edinburgh, Churchill-Livingstone, 1984.

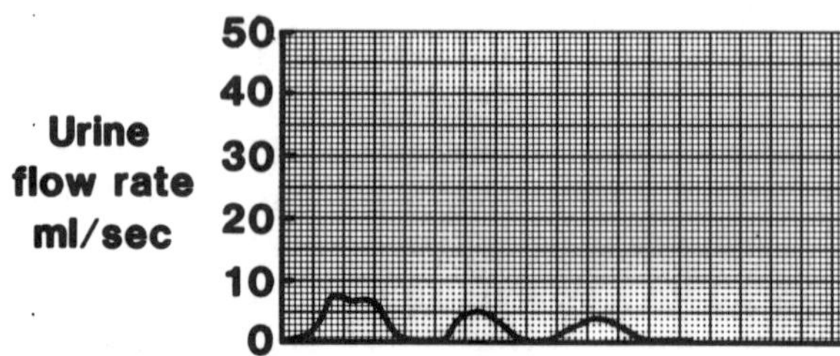

FIG 50.
Uroflow with interrupted stream during straining to void.

and artifactual recording, which most commonly occurs when a male patient directs the urinary stream across the collecting funnel (Fig 51).

In outlet obstruction, a flat, elongated curve with a low maximum flow rate is seen characteristically, which is reached in the initial part of the trace (Fig 52). In the patient with detrusor underactivity, the flow pattern will be intermittent, as abdominal muscles are used to augment voiding. The urine flow rate is reduced and the maximum flow rate is seen in the middle part of the tracing.

Considerable care must be taken not to overinterpret flow study results, and considerable clinical judgment is necessary in their interpretation. Abnormal findings should be confirmed by the use of more elaborate urodynamic studies.

RESIDUAL URINE VOLUME

Residual urine volume is another parameter that integrates the activity of the bladder and outlet during the emptying phase of micturition. A consistently increased residual urine volume generally indicates

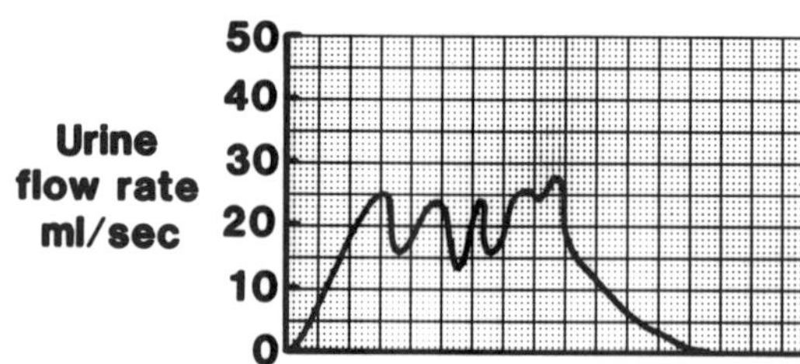

FIG 51.
Uroflow with interrupted pattern due to intermittent sphincter activity.

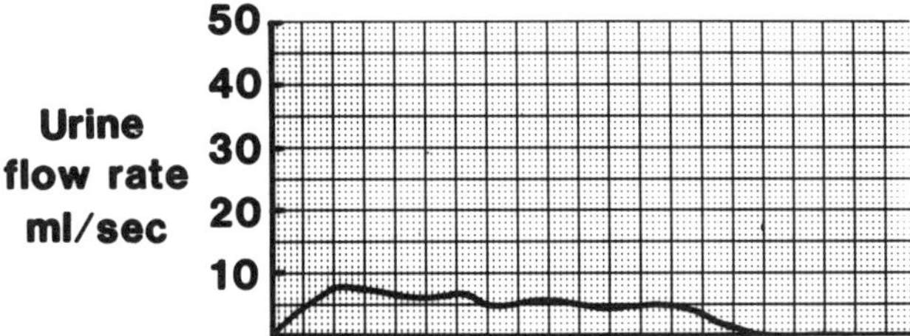

FIG 52.
Uroflow with abnormal flow rate characteristic of detrusor outlet obstruction.

increased outlet resistance, decreased bladder contractility, or both. Absent residual urine is compatible with normal lower urinary tract function during emptying but may also exist in the presence of significant disorders of filling/storage (incontinence) and disorders of emptying in which the intravesical pressure is sufficient to overcome increases in outlet resistance up to a certain point. Typical of this is the patient with outlet obstruction due to benign prostatic obstruction. Initially, despite significant obstruction, the detrusor is capable of emptying the bladder by contracting with a greater force, leading to hypertrophy and increased intravesical pressure. However, with time, the detrusor will fail, leading to increased residual volumes and decrease in intravesical pressures produced during voiding. This is an important example of the fact that it is extremely rare to be able to make an adequate diagnosis on the basis of any single urodynamic study. All of the study results must fit together and these must ultimately be compatible with the symptoms and with the results of the rest of the neurourologic evaluation.

ELECTROMYOGRAPHY

Electromyography (EMG) is the study of the bioelectric potentials generated by depolarization of skeletal muscle. Skeletal muscle is innervated by neurons whose cell bodies lie in the anterior horn of the spinal cord. The anterior horn cell in the grey matter of the spinal cord, its axon, and all of the muscle fibers (their number may vary) that it innervates is called a "motor unit." An excitatory impulse from an anterior horn cell causes contraction of all the muscle fibers in that motor unit, which is brought about by membrane depolarization. The electrical discharge produced on contraction of the muscle fibers of the motor unit by their depolarization is termed "motor unit action potential." This may be detected by electrodes and displayed on an oscilloscopic screen or strip chart, or it may be converted to an audible sound. Individually recorded on an oscilloscope, the motor unit action potentials may take a variety of configurations, being biphasic, triphasic, or, rarely, polyphasic. In the relaxed state, the normal striated muscle is almost electrically quiescent, and only infrequent action potentials are recorded. However, with progressive muscle contraction, increasing numbers of motor units are recruited and each motor unit fires at a more rapid rate. These firings can be individually recorded electromyographically, and the configuration of the action potentials is of significance in diagnosis. At the point of maximal contraction, motor unit action potentials are so frequent that total overlap occurs and EMG separation cannot be achieved, resulting in an interference pattern. It takes considerable EMG experience to interpret the various parameters recorded on an oscilloscope during sphincter EMG. Identification of these variations is important in making an accurate neurologic diagnosis. Individual motor unit action potentials may be detected by needle electrodes placed directly into or near the muscle to be studied. When surface electrodes are used, individual motor unit action potentials are not visualized; rather, an overall gross recording of the activity of the muscle is detected (Barrett, 1980). If one is not interested in motor unit action potentials, surface electrodes are adequate. They will detect whether the pelvic floor muscles are contracting or relaxing at any given instant. However, being unable to detect individual motor unit action potential, surface electrodes cannot help in assessing the integrity of these muscles and their nerve supply.

During cystometric bladder filling there should be incremental increase in EMG activity as more motor units are recruited. This activity will reach a maximum when peak bladder capacity is reached and at the command to void there should be sudden cessation of sphincter activity, which should persist throughout voiding (Blaivas et al., 1977). On completion of bladder emptying, resumption of baseline sphincter activity occurs. In assessing external sphincter activity, the patient is asked to interrupt voiding in the middle of the stream, at which point there should be an abrupt increase in sphincter activity that should be sufficient to stop the flow. Resumption of voiding should occur thereafter; however, if the holding pattern is maintained, the detrusor reflex should ideally be lost in approximately 10 seconds (Webster, 1982).

Abnormal EMG patterns may be detected in a number of situations. Detrusor sphincter dyssynergia describes sphincter activity that

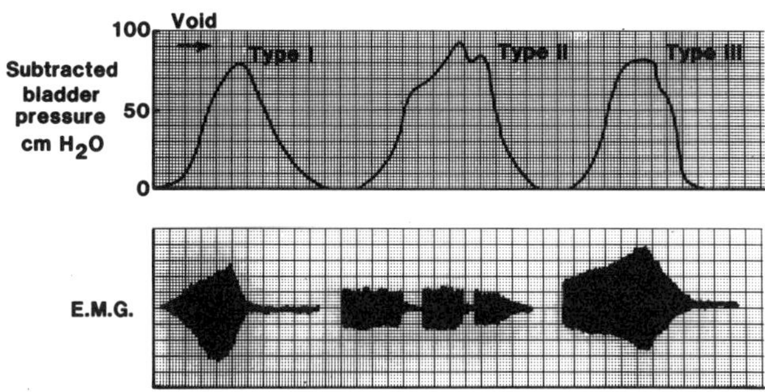

FIG 53.
Varieties of external sphincter discoordination. (Adapted from McGuire EJ: Electromyographic evaluation of sphincter function and dysfunction. *Urol Clin North Am* 1979; 6:121.)

is inappropriate to the activity of the detrusor. Three varieties of such discoordination (Fig 53) were described (McGuire, 1979). One pattern involves an appropriate increase in EMG activity with bladder filling, which is followed by inappropriate involuntary increase in activity at the onset of detrusor contraction. Thus, the detrusor contracts against a closed sphincter.

A second type of discoordination involves failure to develop a proper reflex detrusor contraction because of increased EMG activity during voiding, which causes inhibition of the detrusor motor nucleus in the sacral spinal cord with resultant inhibition of detrusor contraction. This type of discoordination may be seen in patients with suprasacral spinal cord injury.

The third type involves contraction and relaxation of the sphincter during bladder filling. This amounts to periods of uninhibited sphincter relaxation, which is associated with reflex detrusor contraction leading to urgency and urge incontinence.

Simultaneous EMG activity with an increase in intravesical pressure is not always sphincter dyssynergia. Detrusor striated sphincter dyssynergia is undoubtedly the most overdiagnosed entity in the field of voiding dysfunction. Patients suspected of having this diagnosis should always be further investigated with urodynamic and/or radiologic evaluation to study the activity of the bladder and the outlet during the emptying phase of micturition. It must be remembered that true detrusor striated sphincter dyssynergia is extremely uncommon (or does not exist) in patients without neurologic disease. Such a diagnosis in such a patient deserves exhaustive study before it is in fact confirmed.

Sphincter electromyographic studies have gained popularity for the investigation of children with voiding dysfunction (Maizels and Firlit, 1979). It is suggested that learned dysfunctional sphincter habits may be responsible for voiding abnormalities, with resultant recurrent urinary infections, reflux, and upper tract deterioration. An attempt has been made to retrain these patients by the use of biofeedback techniques utilizing sphincter electromyography during voiding (Maizels et al., 1979). The patient can appreciate from an EMG audio monitor whether or not sphincter relaxation is being accomplished; hence, positive reinforcement may correct the problem.

EVOKED RESPONSES

Evoked responses are potential changes in neural tissue, recorded using averaging techniques, resulting from distant stimulation, usually electrical (*Sixth Report on the Standardization of Terminology of Lower Urinary Tract Function,* 1985). Evoked responses may be used to test the integrity of peripheral, spinal, and central nervous pathways. As with nerve conduction studies, the conduction time (latency) may be measured. In addition, information may be gained from the amplitude and configuration of these responses. An example of such procedures is the sacral evoked response, which is measured by the latency of the bulbocavernosus reflex (Nordling and Meyhoff, 1979; Blaivas et al., 1981; Blaivas, 1984). The bulbocavernosus reflex arc is mediated by afferent and efferent pudendal nerve fibers. The reflex is seemingly polysynaptic, traversing at least several spinal cord segments. Clinically the bulbocavernosus reflex is elicited by briskly squeezing the glans penis or clitoris and observing or feeling a reflex contractility response of the external anal sphincter or bulbocavernosus muscle. Alternatively, the reflex may be stimulated by pulling the balloon of a Foley catheter against the bladder neck. The bulbocavernosus reflex is present in almost all normal men and in approximately 70% of normal women. Absence of this reflex in a man is strongly suggestive of a sacral neurological lesion, but it is present in approximately 50% of patients with an incomplete lower motor neuron lesion. Since it is difficult to grade the reflex clinically, measurement of the bulbocavernosus reflex latency offers a more quantitative means of evaluating the sacral reflex arcs.

When one side of the penis is stimulated electrically, as by a surface stimulating electrode, there is a bilateral contractile response in the bulbocavernosus muscle that may be detected by needle electrodes placed bilaterally into this muscle (Blaivas et al., 1981; Krane and Siroky, 1980). Considerable EMG expertise is required to determine the onset of the evoked response because of the possibility of interference from units that are firing either randomly or as a result of the patient's anxiety. Although some authors have therefore recommended that evoked responses of 20 to 30 stimulations be electronically averaged to determine the latency, Blaivas (1984) claims that the shortest latency, rather than the average, is a more specific means of evaluating the sacral segments, since the bulbocavernosus reflex is polysynaptic.

The bulbocavernosus reflex is a crossed response and it is therefore possible to stimulate on one side and record from both the ipsilateral and contralateral bulbocavernosus muscles. This is useful in detecting subtle abnormalities that affect only a single afferent or efferent pathway. Thus, when stimulating one side of the penis, recordings may be made from both sides of the bulbocavernosus muscle. The other side of the penis is then stimulated and the latencies from the bulbocavernosus muscle again determined. In this fashion, it is possible to evaluate the right and left afferent and efferent pathways individually. The normal bulbocavernosus reflex latency varies from approximately 30–40 msec, but the exact values vary slightly from one laboratory to another. Any neurological process that interferes with the integrity of the reflex arc will result in a prolonged latency. Common disorders that result in prolonged latencies include diabetes mellitus, alcoholic neuropathy, and prolapsed disks. Less commonly, a prolonged latency may be a very early manifestation of a spinal cord tumor or multiple sclerosis. Bulbocavernosus reflex latencies may also be obtained by stimulating the proximal urethra or bladder and neck instead of the penis. However, limited experience has been gained with these techniques. A word of caution is warranted in the interpretation of the result of sacral evoked responses. This test quantitates the integrity of innervation of the striated pelvic floor and perineal muscles and the supraspinal neurological pathways involved in lower urinary tract function. It does not give information concerning the status of the smooth muscle of the detrusor, bladder neck, and proximal urethra. Although in general it is reasonable to assume that when a neurological lesion is found to affect the striated perineal floor muscles, it is likely that the same process also involves the detrusor, since the pudendal and parasympathetic nuclei in the sacral spinal cord are practically adjacent to one another. Nevertheless, certain neurological disorders may involve one portion of the nervous system and spare another.

URETHRAL PRESSURE PROFILE

The urethral pressure profile (UPP) is a graphic recording of the pressure within the urethra at each point along its length. In 1969, Brown and Wickham described a technique that is the basis for modern perfusion urethral profilometry. They utilized a specially designed catheter with multiple side holes and an occluded tip. Fluid infused along the catheter escaped through the side holes and the UPP measured the resistance of the urethral walls to distention by this escaping fluid. This resistance is expressed in terms of the pressure necessary to maintain a steady flow of fluid through the catheter system. The UPP recording commences in the bladder and constant withdrawal of the catheter is accomplished through the entire length of the urethra. Being a measure of the urethra's response to distention, various factors affecting urethral compliance will alter the appearance of the profile curve. Contributing to the normal urethral compliance are smooth muscle activity, striated muscle activity, fibroelastic component of the urethral wall, vascular tension due to the rich spongy network around the urethra, and an extrinsic compression component of varying degrees. Obviously, alteration in any of these variables may significantly alter the appearance of the curve. However, the diagnostic value of the static UPP is limited because it is a study that is carried out neither during filling/storage nor during emptying. In other words, it is a study done at rest and it is difficult to prove that the events recorded bear any relationship to what goes on in the bladder or in the outlet during filling/storage or emptying.

Despite these shortcomings, static infusion profilometry does have a certain value in evaluating artificial sphincter function, gel prosthesis function, and the success of medical or surgical therapy for sphincteric incontinence. Alterations in the static profile certainly correlate with some disease entities, such as stress incontinence, an enlarged prostate, and striated sphincter dyssynergia. However, the overlap is invariably large and, because of this, the utility of infusion profilometry as a specific diagnostic study is limited. More recently, other methods of UPP measurement have been developed. These methods include dynamic UPP and stress UPP. Before we elaborate on these more sophisticated techniques, let us review some aspects of static UPP.

STATIC URETHRAL PRESSURE PROFILE

Although this technique may be modified by altering the position of the patient and the degree of bladder filling, the static UPP measures urethral pressure with the patient lying down, the bladder at rest, and the urethra closed. Although perfusion profilometry may be the method most commonly used, the other two techniques used to measure static UPP are the balloon catheter technique and the catheter tip transducers.

PERFUSION URETHRAL PRESSURE PROFILE

This technique uses a catheter with side holes through which saline or gas is perfused with a motorized syringe pump. The pressure is measured via a side arm from the catheter. The pressure registered by the transducer represents the resistance to flow from the catheter side hole, as previously mentioned. Consequently, when the catheter is in the bladder, only bladder pressure opposes the outflow of saline and the measured pressure is low. The catheter is then withdrawn at a constant rate through the entire length of the urethra. The initial pressure recorded on the chart strip recording is the intravesical pressure, followed by a positive deflection at the bladder neck and progressive increase in urethral pressure to the midportion of the urethra in the female (Fig 54) and the membranous urethra in the male (Fig 55).

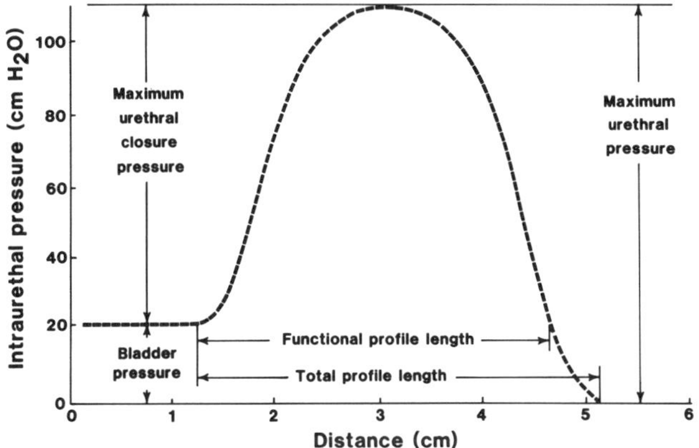

FIG 54.
Normal perfusion urethral pressure profile in a woman.

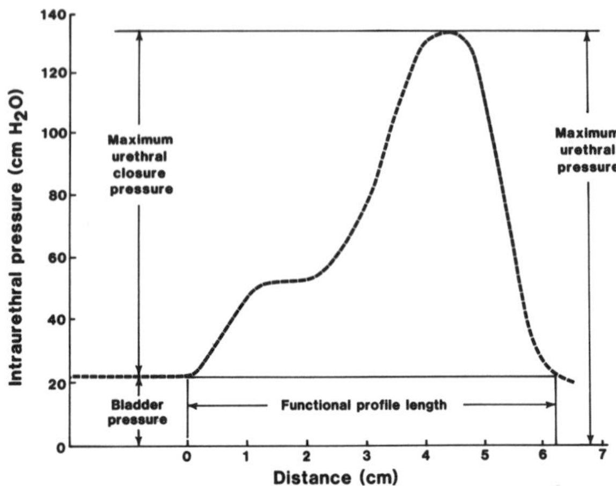

FIG 55.
Normal perfusion urethral pressure profile in a man.

Beyond this point, pressure progressively decreases again until the external meatus is reached. Recommended nomenclature for UPP has been proposed by the International Continence Society. The most frequently measured parameters are: (1) maximum urethral pressure, which is the maximum pressure of the profile; (2) maximum urethral closing pressure, which is the difference between the maximum urethral pressure and bladder pressure; and (3) functional profile length, which is the length of the urethra along which the pressure exceeds bladder pressure. Perfusion profilometry may be performed using gas instead of saline. However, it has been demonstrated that carbon dioxide perfusion rate of 120 ml/min is needed to achieve a satisfactory reading of urethral pressure. The use of such high flow rates makes the practical recording of urethral pressure very difficult in that the bladder is rapidly filled and the investigator is measuring urethral pressure whilst the bladder is being distended swiftly. In addition, the speed of gas flow may theoretically lead to the recording of artificially high pressures due to the gas pushing the urethral walls apart. In this instance, the gas profile may be measuring urethral elasticity rather than urethral pressure.

BALLOON CATHETER SYSTEM

With this system, the eye holes of the catheter are covered by a fine plastic balloon. This technique relies on a closed system that must be free of all bubbles or leaks. Although accurate, frequent calibration and frequent replacement of balloon catheters is required due to a gradual change in compliance of the thin-walled balloons.

CATHETER TIP TRANSDUCER

This technique utilizes a catheter on which one or two transducers are mounted. The transducer is at the site of recording and obviates the problems inherent in recording at a distance from the organ being monitored. It allows for urethral pressure measurement during voiding and double transducer tip catheters allow for the simultaneous measurement of intravesical and urethral pressure. The disadvantages of the Mickel transducer catheter are its fragility and expense.

Whatever technique is used to measure UPP, it is probably essential to simultaneously record external sphincter activity. This will ensure that unintentional external sphincter contraction does not cause artifactual increase in maximum closing pressure. Many patients find it impossible to inhibit the external sphincter during the perfusion withdrawal process, and this is even more true of those with hypersensitive urethras and neurogenic bladder dysfunction. Simultaneous measurement of rectal pressure is advocated as a means to identify unintentional abdominal straining, which might also alter the normal profile curve.

In the normal female patient, there is a gradual tendency for the maximum urethral pressure to decrease with age. This occurs mainly after the menopause. The shape of the UPP curve is symmetrical. In male patients, there is no decrease in maximum urethral pressure with age. However, there is a tendency for the length of the prostatic urethra to increase, particularly over the age of 45 years. The shape of the UPP curve in the male is asymmetrical. In the proximal part of the profile, there is a variable plateau due to the bladder neck and prostatic tissues. In the distal part of the profile, the pressure recorded is higher than from the distal female urethra due to the length and configuration of the male urethra. However, the distal urethra is rarely of clinical significance except on the rare occasion when the profile is recorded in a patient with a urethral stricture.

STRESS URETHRAL PRESSURE PROFILE

The stress UPP is best performed using a dual-sensor catheter tip transducer. The sensors should be separated by a 5–10 cm interval. The catheter is introduced into the bladder and then slowly withdrawn through the urethra while the patient is asked to cough at regular intervals. In order that coughs may be recorded for each 0.2 cm of urethral length, a slow withdrawal speed of 0.1 cm/sec is used (Abrams, 1984).

In normal patients, the increased pressure seen during coughing on the intravesical pressure trace is also seen superimposed on the urethral pressure trace. In normal patients, the raised intra-abdominal pressure is transmitted to the proximal two-thirds of the female urethra. In patients with genuine stress incontinence, there is a failure of pressure transmission. The findings on stress UPP have a far better correlation with the presence of genuine stress incontinence than does the static UPP. Stress urinary incontinence in women is the main indication for stress UPP.

DYNAMIC PRESSURE PROFILE

Static infusion profilometry is criticized mainly because it provides limited information as to the pressure in the outlet at rest. It supplies no information as to the outlet's behavior during filling, storage, and voiding.

The dynamic pressure profile is intended to show variation in sphincteric closure pressure under various physiological events, as well as under various stresses and commands. This dynamic pressure profile is obtained easily by the membrane catheter or microtransducer technique, but is practically impossible to obtain by perfusion techniques (Tanagho, 1984). The pressure profile will rise normally when the bladder is filled. In addition, postural change will affect the urethral pressure. The lowest pressure will be recorded when the patient is in the supine position. Sitting up will cause an increase in pressure, and further increase in functional length and magnitude of closing pressure will occur when the upright position is assumed. Sharp increase in intra-abdominal pressure, as by coughing, and low sustained increase in intra-abdominal pressure, as from bearing down, should result in simultaneous increase of pressure in the urethra, which is normally much higher than the increase in intra-abdominal pressure.

A drop in urethral pressure just before normal voiding occurs has been reported (Tanagho, 1979). Whether meaningful information can be gleaned from urethral measurement during voiding is debatable and the technique is unlikely to replace the conventional ways of assessing dynamic urethral function by fluoroscopy. However, where fluoroscopic evaluation is unavailable, dynamic profilometry may be applied to diagnose such uncommon causes of obstruction as proximal sphincter dyssynergia. The establishment of a pressure gradient in an area of the urethra that is normally wide open with a detrusor contraction establishes the diagnosis of obstruction. An elevated bladder pressure that falls off sharply at some point between the bladder neck and the bulbomembranous urethral junction is sufficient to diagnose proximal sphincter dyssynergia (McGuire, 1984b).

Dynamic UPP measurement may prove to be useful in the assessment of pharmacotherapy, but this field has been little explored as yet.

MULTIFUNCTION STUDIES

As mentioned earlier in this chapter, the clinical applicability of urodynamics depends to a large extent on the reenactment of the patient's symptom complex during the urodynamic assessment. Which urodynamic study to perform will depend on the nature of the clinical problem, the available electronic equipment, the ease with which the studies can be performed, and the interest and expertise of the urodynamic technician. In most clinical settings, it is usually practical and cost-effective to screen patients by performing uroflowmetry, measurement of postvoid residual volume, and cystometry (Blaivas, 1984). These three simple tests will help understand the patient's symptoms in the vast majority of cases. However, occasionally a more sophisticated study is called for, the indications for which include (Blaivas et al., 1981): (1) when simple diagnostic procedures have proved inconclusive, (2) when the patient has persistent symptoms despite what appears to be appropriate treatment, (3) when the patient has a preexisting condition known to be associated with complex urodynamic abnormalities, and (4) when history and physical examination suggest neurologic pathology that requires more elaborate investigation for diagnosis.

Despite what has previously been stated, the patient with an overt neurological disease (such as spinal cord injury or multiple sclerosis) in whom a urodynamic evaluation is required should probably routinely undergo a multifunction study, preferably with simultaneous cystourethrography. This is because such conditions are often accompanied by unpredictable pathophysiology.

Ideally, abdominal pressure should be measured so that subtracted bladder pressure can be monitored during voiding studies, as it is this entity that will alter in obstruction or detrusor dysfunction. This is par-

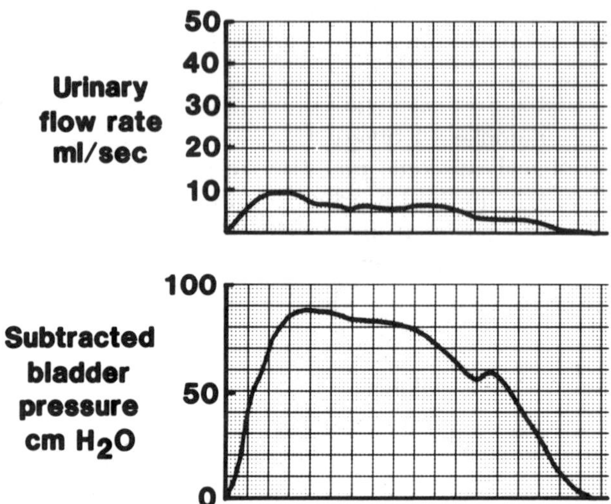

FIG 56.
Abnormal uroflow consistent with outlet obstruction.

ticularly important when the detrusor contractions are of small magnitude and when voiding is accompanied by abdominal straining.

A poor urinary flow rate may be caused by outflow obstruction (Fig 56), impaired detrusor contractility (Fig 57), or a combination of both. From a practical standpoint, bladder outlet obstruction may be defined as a poor urinary flow rate in the presence of an "adequate" detrusor contraction (Blaivas, 1984). For an individual patient, however, it may be difficult to determine whether or not the detrusor pressure is "adequate" with respect to the flow rate, and for this reason many investigators have attempted to formulate a mathematical definition of bladder outlet obstruction by constructing a "resistance coefficient." The hydrodynamic principles from which these resistance coefficients are derived assume that the bladder behaves as a geometric sphere and that the urethra behaves as a rigid tube. This is clearly not the case, and this limits the usefulness of these formulas. If a bladder has normal contractility, the pressure generated during contraction is high, and a low flow rate is produced (see Fig 56), then a formula is not needed to verify that an obstruction exists. On the other hand, if the bladder is decompensated and incapable of producing an adequate rise in intravesical pressure, then there is no way that obstruction (or resistance) can be quantitated by these formulas. These formulas assume that if obstruction exists the bladder is capable of monitoring a propor-

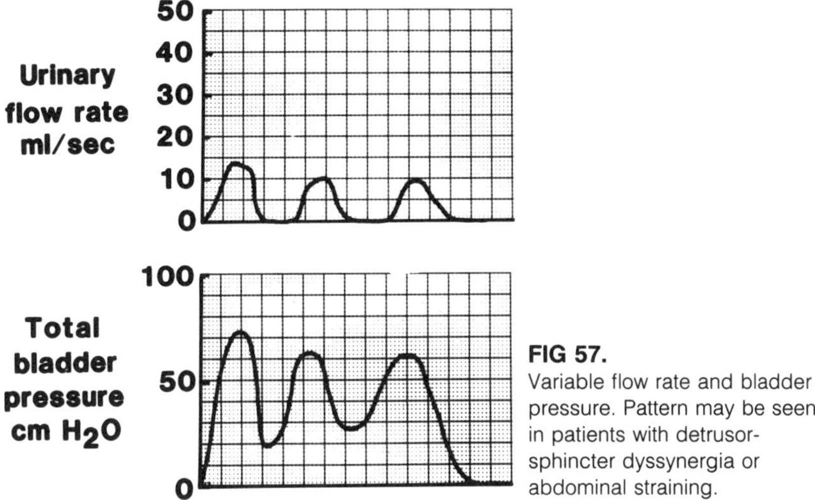

FIG 57.
Variable flow rate and bladder pressure. Pattern may be seen in patients with detrusor-sphincter dyssynergia or abdominal straining.

tionate contraction in response to the obstruction. This is not always the case. If the bladder cannot contract, or contracts poorly, then obstruction cannot be defined. Thus, it appears that when these formulas are most necessary they are least accurate, and are therefore of little clinical use at present.

Synchronous cystometry and sphincter EMG is a most useful urodynamic technique for assessing neurologic function (Blaivas, 1977, 1984). This examination helps define the interrelationship between the striated external urethral sphincter and the detrusor during the storage and voiding phases of micturition.

The most important information to be gained from simultaneous cystometry and EMG relates to the presence or absence of detrusor external sphincter dyssynergia (DSD). In normal patients or those with detrusor instability or detrusor hyperreflexia due to neurologic lesions above the brain stem, the external urethral sphincter relaxes completely immediately prior to the onset of the rise in detrusor pressure. The relaxation continues throughout the detrusor contractions unless the patient voluntarily attempts to interrupt micturition. Detrusor external sphincter dyssynergia is characterized by an involuntary contraction of the external sphincter coincident with or immediately preceding the rise in detrusor pressure. Blaivas (1981a) has classified DSD into three types (see Fig 53). Type 1 is characterized by an abrupt increase in EMG activity whose onset is approximately coincident with the onset of the measurable detrusor contraction. At the peak of the detrusor contraction there is a sudden complete relaxation of the external sphincter, and widening ensues as the detrusor pressures fall. In type 2 there are sporadic sphincter contractions throughout the detrusor contraction. Type 3 is characterized by a crescendo-decrescendo pattern of external sphincter contraction, which parallels the detrusor contraction. Detrusor sphincter dyssynergia is an abnormal reflex that occurs only when the neurologic pathways between the pons and sacral micturition center are interrupted. In the absence of such a neurologic lesion, extreme caution should be exercised in diagnosing DSD.

Pseudodyssynergia is believed to be an abnormality of learned behavior in which the patient subconsciously or consciously attempts to inhibit micturition as it progresses (Wein and Barrett, 1982). This results in "voluntary" contraction of the external sphincter throughout micturition. These pseudodyssynergic syndromes are encountered most frequently in children with persistent voiding symptoms, in men with prostatitis, and in women with the urethral syndrome.

It is not possible to distinguish between true dyssynergia and pseudodyssynergia by simultaneous cystometry and EMG unless intra-abdominal pressure is measured concurrently. In pseudodyssynergia there is usually some elevation of intra-abdominal pressure as the patient tightens the abdominal and pelvic floor musculature.

Another, possibly more simple, way to screen for detrusor-sphincter dyssynergia is by performing the combined test of uroflow and EMG (Barrett and Wein, 1981). When uroflow is accompanied by no external sphincter activity, dyssynergia may be excluded.

STOP FLOW TEST

This is a combined measurement of uroflow and intravesical pressure, which is performed to evaluate the isometric detrusor pressure. The patient is asked to void. After the stream is well initiated and intravesical pressure is being recorded, the stream is abruptly stopped. In normal detrusor function the detrusor pressure usually increases to a level well above voiding pressure. Theoretically, this test reflects on the integrity of detrusor tone and contractility.

VIDEOURODYNAMICS

Videourodynamics is a technique utilizing synchronously recorded urodynamic studies and cystourethrography for the evaluation of complex lower urinary tract problems. It comprises the performance of pressure/flow/external-sphincter EMG studies during filling, storage, and voiding phases of the micturition cycle, together with the periodic screening of the synchronous cystourethrographic appearance of the bladder and outflow tract.

Radiographic contrast material is used as the infusant for cystometry, permitting radiographic visualization of the lower urinary tract. Urodynamic parameters are transduced and displayed on a storage oscilloscope. A television camera scans the oscilloscope screen and the resulting image is displayed on a television monitor. The fluoroscopic image of the bladder and urethra is electronically mixed with that of the urodynamic data and displayed on the same monitor. The advantage of these studies is that they combine the objectivity of urodynamics with the visual radiographic image of the part being studied, making for far more logical interpretation of results. The financial investment required to establish such a study center limits its use to the medical center setting where a large enough patient population in whom such a study is indicated is seen, making this investment justified.

Videourodynamics has proved particularly valuable in the identifi-

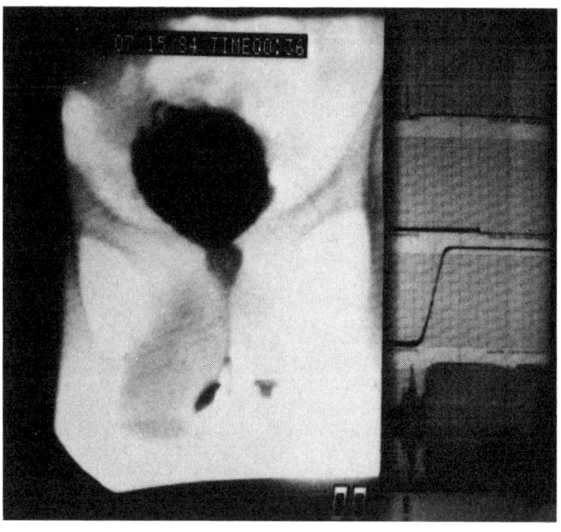

FIG 58.
Videourodynamic study in a 15-year-old paraplegic (T5) boy who had high residual urine volumes and recurrent urinary infection. Intravesical pressure exceeded 100 cm H_2O (scale, 0–100 cm H_2O) and EMG activity was excessive during the detrusor contraction. Although the bladder neck opened, the prostatic urethra was dilated to a level of the external sphincter. There was no urinary flow *(top strip recording)* or increase in abdominal pressure *(second strip recording from top)*. This is classic detrusor-external sphincter dyssynergia.

cation of complex bladder outlet obstruction problems. If bladder outlet obstruction has been diagnosed or is suspected, but the site of obstruction is not clear, a micturitional static urethral pressure profile determination will usually provide definitive diagnostic criteria (Blaivas, 1981). The demonstration of a drop in pressure between the bladder and the membranous urethra during voiding, at which time the bladder and proximal urethra are normally isobaric, establishes the diagnosis of an obstruction between the bladder and the site of the decreased pressure. Fluoroscopy will also allow visualization of the site of obstruction (Yalla et al., 1980).

Detrusor external sphincter dyssynergia is characterized by involuntary contraction of the external urethral sphincter during involuntary detrusor contractions (Fig 58). This may be readily identified by fluoroscopy during voiding. If a patient was treated by external sphincterotomy and a question arises as to the efficacy of surgery, this may be best evaluated by a videourodynamic study.

Videourodynamics is also valuable in the evaluation of some women with stress incontinence. The symptoms of stress incontinence may be caused not only by urethral and bladder hypermobility, but also by denervation of the smooth muscle of the proximal urethra, as following radical pelvic surgery or in myelodysplasia. The latter condition maybe diagnosed by demonstrating an open bladder neck during bladder filling and a proximal urethra that is isobaric with the bladder. The practical implication of this is the choice of surgical repair, which is quite different for the two.

Classification of Voiding Dysfunction

The purpose of any classification system is to facilitate understanding and management and to avoid confusion among those who are concerned with the problem for which the system was designed. A classification system should be able to serve as a sort of an intellectual shorthand and to convey, in a few key words or phrases, the essence of a clinical situation. An ideal classification system for voiding dysfunction should include or imply a number of factors. Foremost among these should be the conclusions reached from urodynamic testing during the filling/storage and the emptying phases of micturition. Expected clinical symptoms should be able to be inferred from a given category within an ideal system, as should the knowledge of whether the individual has normal sensory appreciation. The approximate site and type of a neurologic lesion or a lack of one may also be implied. If the various categories in the classification system accurately portray pathophysiology, treatment options should then be obvious, and a treatment "menu" evident. Most current systems of classification for voiding dysfunction were formulated primarily to describe those types of dysfunction secondary to neurologic disease or injury. The ideal classification system should be applicable to all types of voiding dysfunction. Besides the primarily neurologic systems, urodynamic and functional classification schemes also exist. We will review the major systems or types of systems currently used for the classification of neurogenic and nonneurogenic voiding dysfunction and comment about the advantages, disadvantages, and applicability of each. In so doing, we will describe many of the common forms of micturitional abnormalities.

THE BORS-COMARR CLASSIFICATION

Bors and Comarr (Bors, 1957; Comarr, 1967; Bors and Comarr, 1971) made a remarkable contribution with their classification system, one which was deduced by pure logic from clinical observation of patients with traumatic spinal cord injury (Table 14). This system is applicable only to patients with neuropathic dysfunction and considers (1) the anatomic localization of the lesion, (2) the neurologic completeness or incompleteness of the lesion, and (3) a designation as to whether the lower urinary tract is "balanced" or "unbalanced." The latter terms are based simply on the percentage of residual urine relative to bladder capacity. Unbalanced refers to the presence of greater than 20% residual urine in a patient with an upper motor neuron lesion or 10% in a patient with a lower motor neuron lesion. This relative residual urine volume would ideally imply coordination (synergy) or lack of coordination (dyssynergy) between the smooth and striated sphincters of the outlet and the bladder during bladder contraction or attempted micturition by abdominal straining or the Credé maneuver.

The determination of whether a lesion is complete or incomplete is

TABLE 14.
The Bors-Comarr Classification

Sensory neuron lesion
Incomplete, balanced
Complete, imbalanced
Motor neuron lesion
Balanced
Imbalanced
Sensory motor neuron lesion
Upper motor neuron lesion
Complete, balanced
Complete, imbalanced
Incomplete, balanced
Incomplete, imbalanced
Lower motor neuron lesion
Complete, balanced
Complete, imbalanced
Incomplete, balanced
Incomplete, imbalanced
Mixed lesion
Upper somatomotor neuron, lower visceromotor neuron
Lower somatomotor neuron, upper visceromotor neuron
Normal somatomotor neuron, lower visceromotor neuron

made on the basis of a thorough neurologic examination. This system assumes that the sacral spinal cord is the primary reflex center for micturition. Lower motor neuron in this system is a term used to describe collectively the preganglionic and postganglionic parasympathetic autonomic fibers that innervate the bladder and outlet and originate as preganglionic fibers in the sacral spinal cord. This term is used in an analogy to efferent somatic nerve fibers, such as those of the pudendal nerve, which originate in the same sacral cord segment but terminate directly on pelvic floor striated musculature without the interposition of ganglia. Upper motor neuron is used in this classification system to refer to those descending autonomic pathways above the sacral spinal cord (the origin of the parasympathetic nerve supply to the bladder and outlet).

In the Bors-Comarr system, an upper motor neuron bladder refers to the pattern of micturition that results from an injury to the suprasacral spinal cord, after the period of spinal shock has passed, assuming that the sacral spinal cord and the sacral nerve roots are intact and that the pelvic and pudendal nerve reflexes are intact. A lower motor neuron bladder refers to the pattern that results if the sacral spinal cord or sacral roots are damaged and the reflex pattern through the autonomic and somatic nerves that emanate from these segments is absent. In essence, this classification system implies that if skeletal muscle spasticity exists below the level of the lesion, the lesion is above the sacral spinal cord and is by definition an upper motor neuron lesion. This type of lesion is characterized by detrusor hyperreflexia during the filling/storage phase of micturition. If there is flaccidity of the skeletal muscle below the level of a lesion, a lower motor neuron lesion is said to exist, implying associated detrusor areflexia. Exceptions do occur and are classified in the "mixed lesion" group, characterized either by detrusor hyperreflexia in association with a flaccid skeletal muscle paralysis below the level of the lesion or by detrusor areflexia with skeletal muscle spasticity or normal skeletal muscle tone below the level of the lesion.

The use of this classification system is best illustrated by example. An upper motor neuron lesion, complete, imbalanced, is a neurologically complete lesion above the level of the sacral spinal cord that results in skeletal muscle spasticity below the level of the injury. Detrusor hyperreflexia exists, but with a residual urine volume of greater than 20% of bladder capacity, which implies that there is obstruction in the area of the bladder outlet (generally striated sphincter dyssynergia) during the hyperreflexic detrusor contraction. This is typically seen in a complete T10 paraplegic. A lower motor neuron lesion, complete, imbalanced, is typified by a neurologically complete lesion at the level of the sacral spinal cord or of the sacral roots that results in skeletal muscle flaccidity below that level. Detrusor areflexia results, and whatever maneuvers the patient may use to increase intravesical pressure are not sufficient to decrease residual urine to less than 10% of bladder capacity.

The Bors-Comarr classification system applies best to post-spinal shock, spinal cord–injured patients with complete neurologic lesions. It is difficult to use in patients with multicentric neurologic diseases and cannot be used at all for voiding dysfunction from nonneurologic causes. Additionally, it should be recognized that the terms upper and lower motor neuron do not, strictly speaking, apply to bladder innervation. The autonomic nervous system pathways from the spinal cord to the bladder contain not just one neuron but both preganglionic and postganglionic fibers, and the neural circuit from the spinal cord to the bladder is not truly analogous to the lower motor neuron of the somatic nervous sytem. Additionally, a neurologic description does not always imply a certain clinical or urodynamic picture. The period of spinal shock that immediately follows severe cord injuries is associated with bladder areflexia, whatever the status of the sacral somatic reflexes.

Temporary or permanent changes in bladder and/or bladder outlet activity during filling/storage or emptying may occur secondary to a number of factors such as chronic overdistention, urinary infection, or reinnervation phenomenon, making it impossible to always predict correctly lower urinary tract activity solely on the basis of the level of a neurologic lesion. Although the terms balanced and imbalanced are helpful in that they describe the presence or absence of a certain relative percentage of residual urine, these do not necessarily imply the true functional significance of the lesion, which depends on the potential for damage to the lower or upper urinary tract and also on the social and vocational disability that results.

THE GIBBON AND HALD-BRADLEY CLASSIFICATION

Gibbon (1976) pointed out that the complexity of the Bors-Comarr system could be lessened considerably by eliminating reference to the completeness of the lesion and to its balanced or unbalanced nature (Table 15). He also suggested that a rearrangement into suprasacral, sacral, and mixed categories would preserve the neurologic basis of the scheme, while simplifying it even further for everyday use by urolo-

TABLE 15.
The Gibbon Classification

Suprasacral lesion
Sacral lesion
Motor
Sensory
Motor and sensory
Mixed lesion

gists. However, he noted that, for reasons similar to those just mentioned, the utility of such a system is limited. Hald and Bradley (1982) further modified the Gibbon system into what they described as a simple neurotopographical classification (Table 16). Within this classification system, a supraspinal lesion is characterized by synergy between detrusor contraction and the smooth and striated sphincters, but a defective inhibition of the voiding reflex exists. Detrusor hyperreflexia is the most constant finding. Sensation is usually preserved. However, depending on the site of the lesion, detrusor areflexia and defective sensation may be seen. A suprasacral spinal lesion is generally equivalent to what is described as an upper motor neuron lesion in the Bors-Comarr classification. An infrasacral lesion is equivalent to a lower motor neuron lesion. Peripheral autonomic neuropathy is most frequently encountered in the diabetic and is characterized by a deficient bladder sensation, gradually increasing residual urine, and ultimate decompensation, with loss of detrusor contractility. A muscular lesion is described as involving the detrusor itself, the smooth sphincter, or any portion or all of the striated sphincter. The resultant dysfunction is dependent on which structure is affected. Detrusor dysfunction is the most common, and generally results from decompensation following long-standing bladder outlet obstruction.

TABLE 16.
The Hald-Bradley Classification

Supraspinal lesion
Suprasacral spinal lesion
Infrasacral lesion
Peripheral autonomic neuropathy
Muscular lesion

THE BRADLEY CLASSIFICATION

Bradley's "loop system" of classification is another primarily neurologic system based on his concept of central nervous system control of the lower urinary tract as consisting of four neurologic loops (see Section I for full description).

Loop 1 consists of neuronal connections between the cerebral cortex and the micturition center in the pontine-mesencephalic reticular formation. Loop 1 coordinates voluntary control of the detrusor reflex. Interruption of this loop may be seen in conditions such as brain tumor, cerebrovascular accident or disease, and cerebral atrophy with dementia. The final result is usually detrusor hyperreflexia.

Loop 2 includes the intraspinal pathway of detrusor muscle afferents to the brain-stem micturition center and the motor impulses from this center to the sacral spinal cord. Strictly speaking, it does not include peripheral sensory or motor pathways and so is not a true "loop," but does include the long routed portion of the sensory afferent fibers that originate in the bladder musculature and synapse in the brain stem. Loop 2 is thought to coordinate and provide for a detrusor reflex of adequate temporal duration to allow total evacuation of intravesical contents. Partial interruption of this loop by spinal cord injury is felt to result in a detrusor reflex of low threshold and in poor emptying, as manifested by residual urine. Spinal cord transsection of this circuit acutely produces detrusor areflexia and urinary retention, the urinary tract correlates of spinal shock. After spinal shock has passed, detrusor hyperreflexia results. According to the loop theory, this reflex bladder activity occurs subsequent to a process similar to collateral sprouting from afferent to efferent pathways at the level of the transsection.

Loop 3 consists of the peripheral detrusor afferent axons and their pathway in the spinal cord, which terminates by synapsing on pudendal motor neurons that ultimately innervate the periurethral striated muscle. This loop provides the neurological substrate for coordinated reciprocal action of the bladder and striated sphincter. Dysfunction of this loop may be responsible for detrusor striated sphincter dyssynergia or for involuntary sphincter relaxation.

Loop 4 consists of two components. Loop 4A consists of the suprasacral afferent and efferent innervation of the pudendal motor neurons to the periurethral striated musculature. Loop 4B consists of afferent fibers from the periurethral striated musculature, which synapse on pudendal motor neurons, i.e., the segmental innervation of the periurethral striated muscle. In contrast to stimulation of detrusor afferent fibers, which produce inhibitory postsynaptic potentials in pudendal motor neurons through loop 3, pudendal nerve afferents produce excitatory postsynaptic potentials in these motor neurons through loop 4B. This provides for contraction of the periurethral striated muscle during bladder filling and urine storage. The sensory impulses concerned arise from muscle spindles and tendon organs in the pelvic floor musculature. Loop 4 provides for volitional control of the striated sphincter. Abnormalities of the suprasacral portion result in abnormal responses of the pudendal motor neurons to bladder filling and emptying, which may be manifested as detrusor striated sphincter dyssynergia or/and loss of voluntary contraction of the striated sphincter on command.

This classification system is very sophisticated and is a tribute to the ingenuity and neurophysiological expertise of its originator. For the neurologist this method of classification may be an excellent way to conceptualize the relevant neurophysiology, assuming that there is agreement on the existence and significance of all four loops, and the types and locations of the lesion produced in these loops by various injuries and disease processes. Many urologists, however, find this classification difficult to use for all types of neurogenic voiding dysfunction, and not at all applicable to voiding dysfunction of other etiology.

Cystometry and sphincter EMG are the primary tools for categorizing the different loop lesions; however, it may be extremely difficult to test the intactness of each loop system, even using extremely sophisticated neuromuscular testing. Multicentric and partial lesions are difficult to describe in this system and the type and functional significance of voiding dysfunction they produce are not necessarily implied by their anatomic localization.

THE LAPIDES CLASSIFICATION

Lapides (1967, 1970) contributed significantly to the classification and care of the patient with neuropathic voiding dysfunction by popularizing a modification of a scheme originally proposed by McLellan in 1939 (Table 17). The systems are virtually identical except that Lapides further divided McLellan's category of atonic bladder into motor neurogenic and sensory neurogenic bladder. The Lapides classification is the scheme most familiar to urologists and describes in recognizable shorthand the clinical and cystometric condition in most types of neu-

TABLE 17.
The Lapides Classification

Sensory neurogenic bladder
Motor paralytic bladder
Uninhibited neurogenic bladder
Reflex neurogenic bladder
Autonomous neurogenic bladder

rogenic voiding dysfunction. In the uninhibited neurogenic bladder and reflex neurogenic bladder groups, the exact categorization further implies whether the striated sphincter is dyssynergic (reflex neurogenic bladder) or synergic (uninhibited neurogenic bladder) during bladder contraction.

A sensory neurogenic bladder results from any disease that selectively interrupts the sensory fibers between the bladder and spinal cord or the afferent tracts to the brain. Most commonly, this is seen with diabetes mellitus, tabes dorsalis, and pernicious anemia. The first clinical changes consist only of impaired sensation of bladder distention. Unless voiding is initiated out of habit or on a timed basis, varying degrees of bladder overdistention often result, with resultant hypotonicity. With bladder decompensation significant amounts of residual urine usually are found and, at this time, the cystometric curve generally demonstrates a large bladder capacity with a flat low-pressure filling curve (high compliance). The bethanechol supersensitivity test is usually positive in the early stages, but may later become negative as decompensation of the bladder smooth muscle occurs.

A motor paralytic bladder results from disease processes that destroy the parasympathetic motor innervation of the bladder. Herpes zoster and extensive pelvic surgery or trauma can produce a motor paralytic bladder. The early symptoms may vary from painful urinary retention to a relative inability to initiate and maintain normal micturition. In the early stages the filling limb of the cystometrogram is normal with normal sensation, but without a voluntary bladder contraction at bladder capacity. Later, chronic overdistention and bladder decompensation may occur and a large-capacity bladder with a flat low-pressure filling limb and, generally, a large residual urine volume will result. The bethanechol test is positive and remains so unless severe decompensation occurs.

The uninhibited neurogenic bladder was described originally as resulting from injury or disease in the "corticoregulatory tract." The sacral spinal cord was presumed to be the reflex center for micturition and this corticoregulatory tract was believed normally to exert an inhibitory influence on the primary micturition reflex. A destructive lesion in this tract would then result in overfacilitation of the micturition reflex. Cerebrovascular accident, brain or spinal cord tumor, and demyelinating disease are the most common causes of this type of lesion. This generally results in a voiding dysfunction characterized clinically by frequency, urgency, and incontinence and cystometrically by normal sensation with detrusor hyperreflexia at low filling volumes. Residual urine is characteristically small or absent unless anatomic outlet obstruction or true involuntary smooth or striated sphincter dyssynergia occurs. The patient usually can initiate a bladder contraction voluntarily but is often unable to do so during cystometry because sufficient urine storage cannot occur before detrusor hyperreflexia is stimulated.

The term reflex neurogenic bladder is most commonly used to describe the post–spinal shock condition existing after complete interruption of the sensory and motor pathways between the sacral spinal cord and the brain stem. This occurs most commonly in traumatic spinal cord injury and transverse myelitis, but may occur with extensive demyelinating disease or tumor as well. Typically, the patient has no bladder sensation and is unable to initiate micturition voluntarily. Incontinence results because of low-volume detrusor hyperreflexia, which generally occurs with striated sphincter dyssynergia. This type of lesion is equivalent to a complete upper motor neuron lesion in the Bors-Comarr system.

An autonomous neurogenic bladder results from complete motor and sensory separation of the bladder from the sacral spinal cord. Any disease process that destroys the sacral spinal cord or causes extensive damage to the sacral roots or pelvic nerves may result in this state of affairs. The patient is unable to initiate micturition voluntarily, has no bladder reflex activity, and no specific bladder sensation. This type of bladder is equivalent to the complete lower motor neuron lesion in the Bors-Comarr system. This is also the type of dysfunction seen in patients with spinal shock. The characteristic cystometric pattern is initially similar to the late stages of the motor or sensory paralytic bladder with a marked shift to the right of the filling curve and a large bladder capacity at low intravesical pressure. However, secondary changes in the filling limb may occur that cause an increase in slope (decreased compliance). This may be secondary to chronic inflammatory change or to the effects of the denervation with secondary neuromorphologic and neuropharmacologic changes. Emptying capacity in an autonomous neurogenic bladder may vary from nil to a large percentage of bladder capacity, depending on the ability of the patient to increase intravesical pressure and on the resistance offered during this increase by the smooth and striated muscle of the bladder outlet.

These five classic cystometric categories and their usual clinical settings are easily understood and remembered, and this system therefore provides an excellent framework for teaching the fundamentals of neurogenic voiding dysfunction to students and nonurologists. Unfortunately, many patients do not exactly fit into one or another of these classic descriptions. Gradations of sensory, motor, and mixed lesions occur, and the patterns produced after different types of peripheral denervation may vary widely from those classically described. The detrusor hyperreflexia associated with the classic uninhibited neurogenic bladder may be associated with dyssynergic striated sphincter activity as well as synergic activity. Secondary changes caused by infection, chronic distention, and reinnervation can be superimposed on and alter any of these classic patterns.

THE URODYNAMIC CLASSIFICATION

With the development of more sophisticated urodynamic equipment and techniques to categorize the activity of the bladder and the outlet during the filling/storage and emptying phase of micturition, systems of classification have been formulated based solely on objective urodynamic data. Evolution of this type of classification system

TABLE 18.
The Krane-Siroky Urodynamic Classification

Detrusor hyperreflexia (or normoreflexia)
Coordinated sphincters
Striated sphincter dyssynergia
Smooth sphincter dyssynergia
Nonrelaxing smooth sphincter
Detrusor areflexia
Coordinated sphincters
Nonrelaxing striated sphincter
Denervated striated sphincter
Nonrelaxing smooth sphincter

has paralleled urodynamic expertise and, in the United States, was pioneered by Krane and Siroky (1979, 1984) whose initial urodynamic classification system is shown in Table 18. When exact urodynamic classification is possible, this system provides a truly exact description of the particular voiding dysfunction under consideration. If a normal or hyperreflexic detrusor exists with coordinated smooth and striated sphincters and without anatomic obstruction, total bladder emptying should be produced. Striated sphincter dyssynergia is most commonly seen in the patient with a complete suprasacral spinal cord injury after the period of spinal shock has passed. Smooth sphincter dyssynergia is seen most classically in autonomic dysreflexia, when it is characteristically associated with detrusor hyperreflexia and striated sphincter dyssynergia. Detrusor hyperreflexia is most commonly associated with neurologic lesions above the sacral spinal cord, but may be associated with inflammatory or infectious disease or may be idiopathic. Detrusor areflexia may be secondary to bladder muscle decompensation or to various other conditions that produce inhibition at either the level of the brain-stem micturition center, sacral spinal cord, bladder ganglia, or bladder smooth muscle. Patients with a voiding dysfunction that falls into this category generally attempt bladder emptying by abdominal straining or the Credé maneuver. Their continence status and the efficiency of their emptying efforts are determined by the status of the smooth and striated sphincters of the outlet.

This classification system is easiest to use when detrusor hyperreflexia or normoreflexia exists, since sufficiently sophisticated and reproducible urodynamic techniques exist to describe the activity of the smooth and striated sphincters during bladder contraction. Thus, a typical T10 paraplegic exhibits detrusor hyperreflexia, smooth sphincter synergia, and striated sphincter dyssynergia. When a voluntary or hyperreflexic bladder contraction cannot be elicited, this system is more difficult to use since it is not appropriate to speak of true dyssynergia in the absence of an opposing bladder contraction.

Urodynamic classification systems assume total urodynamic agreement among the classifiers. Often this is easy to obtain, but one has only to attend the case presentation sections of various neurourology symposia to realize that there are many voiding dysfunctions that do not fit neatly into such a classification system. This does not mean that such a system is not the ideal system, but simply that the "experts" sometimes do not agree about the significance of the data generated using a given urodynamic evaluation. As sophisticated urodynamic technology and understanding improve, this type of classification system of voiding dysfunction may supplant others in general use.

THE FUNCTIONAL SYSTEM

Classification of voiding dysfunction can also be formulated on a functional basis, describing the dysfunction simply in terms of whether the deficit produced is primarily one of the filling/storage phase of micturition or of the emptying phase (Wein, 1981, 1984; Quesada et al., 1968; Bors and Comarr, 1971; Wein et al., 1976) (Table 19). This type of classification system is an excellent alternative when a particular dysfunction does not lend itself to a generally agreed-on classification in one of the other systems. Our groups have adopted and promoted this system primarily because of dissatisfaction with attempts to exactly classify urodynamically some types of voiding dysfunction.

This simple-minded scheme assumes only that, whatever their differences, all "experts" would agree on certain general principles concerning the micturition cycle. Bladder filling and urine storage require: (1) accommodation of increasing volumes of urine at a low intravesical pressure and with normal and appropriate sensation, (2) absence of involuntary bladder contractions, and (3) a bladder outlet that is closed at rest and remains so with stress. Storage failure can then result because of problems related to bladder hyperreflexia or/and low compliance and because of a permanent or intermittent decrease in outlet resistance. Bladder emptying requires: (1) a coordinated bladder contraction of adequate magnitude, and (2) lack of anatomic obstruction and concomitant lowering of resistance at the level of the smooth and striated sphincter. Failure to empty can then result from inadequate bladder contractility or increased outlet resistance. Failure in either category generally is not absolute, but is more often relative.

Such a system can easily be "expanded" and made more complicated to include etiologic or urodynamic connotations (Table 20). However, the simplified system avoids argument in those complex situ-

TABLE 19.
The Functional Classification

Failure to store
Because of the bladder
Because of the outlet
Failure to empty
Because of the bladder
Because of the outlet

TABLE 20.
The Expanded Functional Classification

- Failure to store
  - Because of the bladder
    - Detrusor hyperactivity
      - Involuntary contractions
        - Suprasacral neurologic disease
        - Bladder outlet obstruction
        - Idiopathic
      - Decreased compliance
        - Fibrosis
        - Idiopathic
      - Sensory urgency
        - Inflammatory
        - Infectious
        - Neurologic
        - Psychologic
        - Idiopathic
  - Because of the outlet
    - Stress incontinence
    - Nonfunctional bladder neck/proximal urethra
- Failure to empty
  - Because of the bladder
    - Neurologic
    - Myogenic
    - Psychogenic
    - Idiopathic
  - Because of the outlet
    - Anatomic
      - Prostatic obstruction
      - Bladder neck contracture obstruction
      - Urethral stricture
    - Functional
      - Smooth sphincter dyssynergia
      - Striated sphincter dyssynergia

ations in which the exact etiology or urodynamic mechanism for a voiding dysfunction cannot be agreed on. A different type of logical extension of this system functions especially well as a "menu" for the treatment of voiding dysfunction (see Tables 22 through 26).

Proper use of this system for a given voiding dysfunction obviously requires a reasonably accurate notion of what the urodynamic data show. However, an exact diagnosis is not required for treatment. Some patients do not have just a discrete storage or emptying failure, and the existence of combination deficits must be recognized to properly utilize this system of classification. For example, the T10 paraplegic generally exhibits a relative failure to store because of detrusor hyperreflexia and a relative failure to empty because of striated sphincter dyssynergia. In such a combination deficit, to utilize this classification system one must assume that either one deficit is primary and that significant improvement will result from its treatment alone or that the voiding dysfunction can be converted primarily to a disorder either of storage or emptying by means of surgical or pharmacologic therapy. The resultant deficit can then be treated or circumvented. Using the same example, the combined deficit in a T10 paraplegic can be converted primarily to a failure to store by surgical procedures directed at the dyssynergic striated sphincter and the resultant incontinence (secondary to detrusor hyperreflexia) circumvented (in a male) with an external collecting device. Alternatively, the deficit can be converted to primarily a failure to empty by surgical or pharmacologic measures designed to abolish or reduce the detrusor hyperreflexia, and the resultant failure to empty can then be circumvented with clean intermittent catheterization. Other examples of combination deficits include impaired bladder contractility with sphincter dysfunction, bladder outlet obstruction with detrusor hyperactivity, and bladder outlet obstruction with sphincter malfunction.

The major problem with this classification system is that not every voiding dysfunction can in fact be reduced or converted primarily to a failure of storage or emptying. Additionally, although the functional classification of therapy that is a correlate of this scheme seems logical, there is a danger of accepting an easy therapeutic solution and of thereby overlooking an etiology for a voiding dysfunction that is reversible at the primary level of causation. Nonneurogenic voiding dysfunction can, however, be classified within this system, with the possible exception of those dysfunctions involving primarily the sensory aspect of micturition. Unfortunately, those disorders are virtually ignored by all classification systems, unless one broadly includes such disorders as the urgency-frequency syndrome without urodynamic abnormalities under the category of "failure to store."

THE INTERNATIONAL CONTINENCE SOCIETY CLASSIFICATION

Finally, the International Continence Society (ICS) has proposed a classification based on the functional state of the bladder and urethra, which operates with a "three by three" system (ICS Standardization Committee, 1981) (Table 21). Overactive detrusor function is indicated

TABLE 21.
The International Continence Society Classification

Detrusor
Normal
Overactive
Underactive
Urethra
Normal
Overactive
Incompetent
Sensation
Normal
Hypersensitive
Hyposensitive

when, during the filling phase, there are involuntary detrusor contractions that the patient cannot suppress. Involuntary bladder contractions that are associated with known neurologic disease fall under the category of detrusor hyperreflexia, while the term "unstable detrusor" or "bladder instability" is applied to such activities that occur in a patient without known neurologic disease. The term "compliance" refers to the volume-pressure relationship in a bladder, and the term "low compliance" represents another form of detrusor overactivity, consisting of a tonically high pressure rise in response to a given increment in bladder volume. The underactive detrusor may be described as noncontractile (no contraction under any circumstances), areflexic (the complete absence of centrally coordinated contractions secondary to neurologic disease); a patient with an underactive detrusor may be described as having a high-compliance bladder (a capacious bladder that shows little change in pressure in response to a given volume increment). An overactive urethral closure mechanism contracts involuntarily against the detrusor contraction (dyssynergia) or fails to relax during attempted micturition. An incompetent urethral closure mechanism allows urinary incontinence. This may occur only during a rise in intraabdominal pressure (stress incontinence) or it may be persistent, in which case continuous leakage will occur. It may also be due to an involuntary fall in urethral pressure in the absence of detrusor activity (the unstable urethra).

Within the ICS system, the condition of a classical T10 paraplegic would be classified as follows: overactive detrusor, overactive urethra, hyposensitive; the condition of a stroke patient with urgency incontinence would most likely be classified as follows: overactive detrusor, normal urethra, normal sensation; the condition of a patient with stress incontinence would be classified as follows: normal detrusor, incompetent urethra, normal sensation.

No type of classification system for voiding dysfunction is perfect. Some systems clearly apply only to neuropathic disorders. Others are more widely applicable, but each has its obvious shortcomings. Each offers something to every clinician, the amount being dependent on his level and type of training, interest, experience, and prejudices regarding the accuracy and interpretation of urodynamic data. The ideal approach for a given patient remains a thorough neurourologic evaluation and an attempt at categorization using each classification system described. If the clinician can classify a given patient's condition in each system, or understand why he cannot, he has a working knowledge of the situation sufficient to proceed with treatment. However, if the clinician is familiar with only one or two of these classification systems and a given patient does not fit these and the reason is uncertain, the patient should be studied further and the voiding dysfunction better characterized, certainly before irreversible therapy is undertaken.

Treatment of Voiding Dysfunction

This section will consider the various therapies available for the treatment of voiding dysfunction. There are only a discrete number of such therapies available, and these are easily categorized on a functional basis according to their effect on the bladder or on the outlet (Tables 22 and 23). This basic outline will be followed in discussing each therapy. Some of the surgical forms of therapy are well discussed elsewhere in this text; therefore, an attempt has been made to restrict detailed descriptions of surgical technique or illustrations of some of those procedures that are important but do not receive extensive coverage in other chapters.

The initial choice of a surgical vs. a nonsurgical mode of management for a given problem is based on a great many factors. Although many urologists who lecture and write about the management of voiding dysfunction are associated primarily with one approach or procedure or another, all would doubtless agree on certain goals of management satisfied by the ideal treatment for voiding dysfunction (Table 24). One of the most important concepts to be put forth in recent years is a urodynamic clarification of exactly what "adequate storage at low intravesical pressure" means. McGuire (1984) and co-workers (1981, 1983) have clearly shown that upper tract deterioration is apt to occur when storage, even though adequate in terms of continence, occurs at sustained intravesical pressures of greater than 40 cm H_2O. Application of this concept to patients with storage problems because of decreased bladder compliance has resulted in the concept of the "leak-point" as a very significant piece of urodynamic data. Patients with leakage pressures less than 40 cm H_2O, or those who can store (or whose bladders

TABLE 22.
Therapy to Facilitate Bladder Emptying

- Increasing intravesical pressure/bladder contractility
  - External compression, Valsalva
  - Promotion or initiation of reflex contractions
    - Trigger zones or maneuvers
    - Bladder training, tidal drainage
  - Pharmacologic therapy
    - Parasympathomimetic agents
    - Prostaglandins
    - Blockers of inhibition
      - α-Adrenergic antagonists
      - Opioid antagonists
  - Electrical stimulation
    - Directly to the bladder
    - To the spinal cord or nerve roots
  - Reduction cystoplasty
- Decreasing outlet resistance
  - At a site of anatomic obstruction
    - Prostatectomy
    - Urethral stricture repair/dilation
  - At the level of the smooth sphincter
    - Transurethral resection or incision of the bladder neck
    - Y-V plasty of the bladder neck
    - Pharmacologic therapy
      - α-Adrenergic antagonists
      - β-Adrenergic agonists
  - At the level of the striated sphincter
    - External sphincterotomy
    - Urethral overdilation
    - Pudendal nerve block or interruption
    - Pharmacologic therapy
      - Skeletal muscle relaxants
        - Centrally acting relaxants
        - Dantrolene
        - Baclofen
      - α-Adrenergic antagonists
    - Biofeedback, psychotherapy
- Circumventing problems
  - Intermittent catheterization
  - Continuous catheterization
  - Urinary diversion

can be pharmacologically or surgically manipulated to store) at a pressure less than that, will not experience upper tract deterioration in the absence of other complicating factors, such as significant vesicoureteral reflux with urinary tract infection.

In treating patients with voiding dysfunction, a perfect result is

TABLE 23.
Therapy to Facilitate Urine Storage

- Inhibiting bladder contractility/decreasing sensory input/increasing bladder capacity
  - Timed bladder emptying
  - Pharmacologic therapy
    - Anticholinergic agents
    - Musculotropic relaxants
    - Polysynaptic inhibitors
    - Calcium antagonists
    - β-Adrenergic agonists
    - α-Adrenergic antagonists
    - Prostaglandin inhibitors
    - Tricyclic antidepressants
    - Dimethyl sulfoxide
    - Bromocriptine
  - Biofeedback, bladder retraining
  - Bladder overdistention
  - Electrical stimulation (reflex inhibition)
  - Interruption of innervation
    - Central (subarachnoid block)
    - Peripheral (sacral rhizotomy, selective sacral rhizotomy)
    - Perivesical (peripheral bladder denervation)
  - Augmentation cystoplasty
- Increasing outlet resistance
  - Physiotherapy
  - Electrical stimulation of the pelvic floor
  - Pharmacologic therapy
    - α-Adrenergic agonists
    - Tricyclic antidepressants
    - β-Adrenergic antagonists
    - Estrogen
  - Vesicourethral suspension (SUI)
  - Bladder outlet reconstruction
  - Surgical mechanical compression
  - Nonsurgical mechanical compression
- Circumventing problem
  - Antidiuretic hormone–like agents
  - External collecting device
  - Intermittent catheterization
  - Continuous catheterization
  - Urinary diversion

rarely, if ever, achieved, and a very flexible approach must therefore be adopted in choosing therapy. This approach must take into account the individual wishes of each patient and the practicality of each proposed solution in each case, especially in those patients with neurologic disease (Table 25). The decision as to whether initial therapy is to be surgical or nonsurgical is best made with the patient and with his

TABLE 24.
Voiding Dysfunction: Goals of Management

Upper urinary tract preservation or improvement
Absence or control of infection
Adequate storage at low intravesical pressure
Adequate emptying at low intravesical pressure
Adequate control
No catheter or stoma
Social acceptability/adaptability
Vocational acceptability/adaptability

or her family. In every case, the patient and family must be informed of all possible methods of management, including reversibility and side effects that occur with some regularity, ultimate best and worst possible result, and frequency and extent of follow-up. It has always been our subjective bias that the simplest, least destructive, and most reversible form of therapy that has a chance of satisfying the goals of treatment should be tried first. It is important to remember that a combination of therapeutic maneuvers, drugs, and surgery can sometimes be used to achieve a particular end, especially if they act through different mechanisms and their side effects are not synergistic. There are circumstances and locales in which hospital resources and bed usage efficiency must also be considered, especially in this day and age when some health care systems and third-party payers have placed considerable financial restraints on health care.

Absolute or relative indications for changing or augmenting a particular regimen exist, and, likewise, these are generally agreed on, al-

TABLE 25.
Patient Factors to Consider in Choosing Therapy

Prognosis of underlying disease, especially if progressive or malignant disease
Limiting factors: inability to perform certain tasks (hand dexterity, ability to transfer)
Mental status
Motivation
Desire to remain catheter- or appliance-free
Desire to avoid surgery
Sexual activity status
Reliability
Educability
Psychosocial environment; interest, reliability, and cooperation of family
Economic resources
Age

TABLE 26.
Reasons to Change or Augment a Given Regimen

Upper urinary tract deterioration
Recurrent sepsis or fever of urinary tract origin
Lower urinary tract deterioration
Inadequate storage
Inadequate emptying
Inadequate control
Unacceptable side effects
Skin changes secondary to incontinence or collecting device

though the relative importance of the indication for change might be disputed (Table 26). Remember that here, too, the term "inadequate," when applied to storage or emptying, does not imply only completeness, but includes performance of the function at unacceptably high intravesical pressures.

THERAPY TO FACILITATE BLADDER EMPTYING

Increasing Intravesical Pressure/Bladder Contractility

External Compression: Valsalva

Manual compression of the bladder (Credé maneuver) is most effective in those patients with decreased bladder tonicity who can generate a pressure greater than 50 cm H_2O with this maneuver and whose outlet resistance is borderline or decreased (Glahn, 1974; Wein et al., 1976). The technique of voiding by the open-hand Credé method involves the placement of the thumb of each hand over the area of the left and right anterior superior iliac spine and of the digits over the suprapubic area, with slight overlap at the finger tips (Opitz, 1984). The slightly overlapped digits are then pressed into the abdomen and, when they have gotten behind the symphysis, downward, to compress the fundus of the bladder. Both hands are then pressed as deeply as possible downward into the real pelvic cavity. At times, the compression of the bladder can be accomplished more efficiently by the use of the fist of one hand (closed-hand method) or a rolled-up towel. A similar increase in intravesical pressure may be achieved by abdominal straining. The technique of straining (Valsalva) involves sitting and resting the abdomen forward on the thighs in both men and women. During straining in this position, hugging of the knees and legs may be advantageous to prevent any bulging of the abdomen. To increase intravesical pressure in this manner requires voluntary control of the abdominal wall and diaphragmatic muscles, or, in the case of the Credé maneuver, adequate hand control. Straining at the time the Credé maneuver is applied should be avoided because this increases the intra-abdominal pressure and causes bulging of the abdominal wall, which then tends to lift the compressing hands off the fundus of the bladder. The Credé maneuver is much easier in a patient with a lax, lean abdominal wall than with a taut or obese one, and is more readily performed in a child than in an adult.

Voiding by these maneuvers is unphysiologic and is resisted by the same forces that normally resist stress urinary incontinence. In our experience, adaptive change (funneling) of the bladder neck and proximal urethra does not generally occur with external compression maneuvers of any kind. In patients with intact pelvic floor striated muscle reflexes, increases in outlet resistance may actually occur. If adequate emptying does not occur, other types of therapy to decrease outlet resistance may be considered, but these may adversely affect continence. Vesicoureteral reflex is a relative contraindication to Credé or Valsalva maneuvers, especially in patients who are capable of generating a high intravesical pressure by so doing. The greatest likelihood of success with this mode of therapy is in the patient with an areflexic and hypotonic or atonic bladder, and some outlet denervation (striated or smooth sphincter or both). Such a patient not uncommonly has stress incontinence as well. The continued use of external compression or Valsalva maneuver implies that the intravesical pressure between attempted voidings is consistently below that necessary to cause upper tract deterioration. This may be an erroneous assumption, and close follow-up is necessary, especially in those patients with close to normal outlet resistance, to avoid this complication. The most flagrant misuse of this form of management is in the patient with a decentralized or denervated bladder in whom decreased compliance during filling has developed. Such a patient may silently develop intravesical pressures greater than those necessary to cause upper tract deterioration with minimal filling.

Promotion or Initiation of Reflex Contraction

In those types of spinal cord injury or disease characterized by detrusor hyperreflexia, manual stimulation of areas within the sacral and lumbar dermatomes may sometimes provoke a reflex bladder contraction (Bors, 1957; Comarr, 1959; Gibbon, 1974). Pulling the skin or hair of the pubis, scrotum, or thigh, squeezing the clitoris, or digital rectal stimulation are examples of the type of activity that sometimes induces "trigger voiding" in these patients. According to Glahn (1974), the most effective method of inducing such a contraction is rhythmic suprapubic manual pressure (seven or eight pushes every 3 seconds). This is thought to produce a summation effect on the tension receptors in the bladder wall, resulting in an afferent neural discharge, which activates the bladder reflex arc. Ideally, the contraction so produced will be sustained and of adequate magnitude. Patients who are potentially able to induce bladder contractions by such a maneuver should be encouraged to find their own optimal "trigger points" and position for urination. Manual dexterity and either the ability to transfer to a commode or an external collecting device are required. Unfortunately, this type of patient often has sphincter dyssynergia, and such maneuvers may have to be combined with measures to decrease outlet resistance at the level of the striated and/or smooth sphincter.

Occasionally, this form of induced bladder contraction is possible and desirable in patients with supraspinal disease and involuntary bladder contractions. If induced emptying can be carried out frequently enough in these patients so as to keep bladder volume below the threshold for activation of the micturition reflex, incontinence can be "controlled." This actually amounts to a form of timed voiding. If regular frequent attempts at voiding are unsuccessful, these maneuvers may be helpful as an initial sensory cue (Opitz, 1984).

Some clinicians still feel that the establishment of a rhythmic pattern of bladder filling and emptying by maintaining a copious fluid intake and by periodically clamping and unclamping an indwelling catheter or with intermittent catheterization can "condition" or "train" the micturition reflex. Others, with whom we would agree, feel that there is no cause-and-effect relationship between the attainment of balanced lower urinary tract function and such programs, and that such regimens benefit patients primarily by focusing their attention on the urinary tract and by ensuring an adequate fluid intake.

Pharmacologic Manipulation

Parasympathomimetic Agents

Since at least a major portion of the final common pathway in physiologic bladder contraction is stimulation of the muscarinic cholinergic receptor sites at the postganglionic parasympathetic neuromuscular junction, agents that imitate the actions of acetylcholine (ACh) might be expected to be useful in the management of patients who cannot empty because of inadequate bladder contractility. Acetylcholine itself cannot be used for therapeutic purposes because of actions at central and ganglionic levels and because of its rapid hydrolysis by acetylcholinesterase and by nonspecific cholinesterase (Taylor, 1980). Many acetylcholine-like drugs exist. However, only bethanechol chloride exhibits a relatively selective action on the urinary bladder and gut with little or no action at therapeutic dosages on ganglia or on the cardiovascular system (Ursillo, 1967; Taylor 1980). It is cholinesterase-resistant and causes a contraction in vitro of smooth muscle from all areas of the bladder (Raezer et al., 1973).

Bethanechol has been recommended for the treatment of postoperative or postpartum urinary retention in a subcutaneous dose of 5–10 mg. In this instance, it should be used only if the patient is awake and alert and if there is no outlet obstruction (Wein, 1986). For over 30 years it has been used in the treatment of the atonic or hypotonic bladder (Lee, 1949) and it has been reported to be effective in achieving "rehabilitation" of the chronically atonic or hypotonic detrusor (Lapides, 1964; Diokno and Koppenhoeffer, 1976; Sonda et al., 1979). When so used, it is recommended that the drug be initially administered subcutaneously in a dose of 5–10 mg (usually 7.5 mg) every 4–6 hours. This is done preferably with an intermittent bladder decompression regimen. The patient is asked to try to void 20–30 minutes after each dose. When the residual urine volume has decreased to an acceptable level, the dose is gradually decreased and ultimately changed to an oral dose of 50 mg four times daily.

In cases of partial bladder emptying, a therapeutic trial with an oral dose of 25–100 mg, four times daily, may be utilized in conjunction with attempted voiding every four hours. Bethanechol has also been used to stimulate or facilitate the development of reflex bladder contractions in patients with suprasacral spinal cord injury (Perkash, 1975). Twiddy et al. 1980) have, in fact, concluded that—in spinal cats at least—intact pelvic reflex pathways are required for bethanechol to produce what they described as a brisk and sustained increase in intravesical pressure during bladder filling.

Although anecdotal success in specific patients seems to occur occasionally, attempts to facilitate bladder emptying in series of patients where bethanechol was the only variable have been generally disappointing. A pharmacologically active subcutaneous dose (5 mg) did not demonstrate significant changes in flow parameters or residual urine volume in women with a residual urine volume equal to or greater than 20% of bladder capacity, but no evidence of neurologic disease or outlet obstruction, or in a group of 27 "normal" women of approximately the same age (Wein et al., 1980a). A similar dose likewise failed to produce urodynamic evidence of improved emptying in patients with a positive bethanechol supersensitivity test (Wein et al., 1980b). This dosage did increase the intravesical pressure at all points along the filling limb of the cystometrogram, and also decreased the bladder capacity threshold, findings previously described by others (Lapides et al., 1963; Sonda et al., 1979). In adequate doses, bethanechol is capable of eliciting an increase in tension in bladder smooth muscle such as would be expected from in vitro studies, but its ability to stimulate or facilitate a physiologic-like bladder contraction in the vast majority of patients with voiding dysfunction has been unimpressive. Similar sentiments, at least with respect to its use in neuropathic dysfunction, have been expressed by Gibbon (1975), Merrill and Rotta (1977), Yalla et al. (1977), and Light and Scott (1982). In fact, it is difficult to find reproducible urodynamic data that support recommendations for the usage of bethanechol in any specific category of patients. Most, if not all, long-term studies in such patients are neither prospective nor double-blind, and do not exclude the effects of other simultaneous regimens, such as treatment of urinary infection, bladder decompression by continuous or intermittent catheterization, timed voiding with the Credé maneuver and other types of treatment affecting the bladder or outlet, an important lesson when considering the design of drug protocols for treatment of voiding dysfunction. Short-term studies in which the drug was the only variable have generally failed to demonstrate significant efficacy in terms of flow and residual urine volume data. Whether repeated doses of any cholinergic agonist can achieve a clinical effect that a single dose cannot is speculative. If this is not the case, the long-term response to therapy could be predicted by a urodynamic assessment before and after a short trial. It is generally agreed that, at least in a denervated bladder, an oral dose of 200 mg is required to produce the same effect as a subcutaneous dose of 5 mg (Diokno et al., 1976; Philp et al., 1980).

Much of the emotion surrounding the question of whether bethanechol is efficacious can be dispelled by a brief urodynamically controlled trial in which institution of therapy is the only variable (Blaivas, 1984). In the laboratory, a functioning micturition reflex is an absolute requirement for the production of a sustained bladder contraction by a subcutaneous injection of drug (Downie, 1984). Clinically, there is little logic for its use in patients with detrusor hyperreflexia who already have bladder contractions, though the contractions are uncontrollable. Patients with incomplete lower motor neuron lesions seem to constitute the most reasonable group for a trial of bethanechol (Awad et al., 1984), though caution is advised in drawing conclusions regarding efficacy of a single modality when other modes of treatment (such as bladder decompression) are employed simultaneously.

No agreement exists as to whether cholinergic stimulation produces an increase in urethral resistance (Wein, 1980b). It would appear that pharmacologically active doses do in fact increase urethral closure pressure, at least in patients with neurogenic bladder dysfunction with detrusor hyperreflexia (Sporer et al., 1978). If so, a reasonable question would seem to be whether cholinergic agonists could be combined with agents to decrease outlet resistance to facilitate emptying. Khanna (1976) reported that a combination of a total daily oral dose of bethanechol of 50–100 mg with 20–30 mg of oral phenoxybenzamine produced satisfactory results in a group of patients with an atonic bladder and functional outlet obstruction. Our own experience with such therapy, utilizing even 200 mg of oral bethanechol daily, has been extremely disappointing. Certainly, most clinicians would agree that a daily dose of 50–100 mg rarely affects any urodynamic parameter at all.

The potential side effects of the cholinergic agonists and the anticholinesterase agents are similar and include flushing, nausea, vomiting, diarrhea, gastrointestinal cramps, bronchospasm, headache, salivation, sweating, and difficulty with visual accommodation (Taylor, 1980). Intramuscular or intravenous use is contraindicated, as such use can precipitate acute and severe side effects, resulting in acute circulatory failure and cardiac arrest. Contraindications to the use of this general category of drug include bronchial asthma, peptic ulcer, bowel obstruction, enteritis, history of recent gastrointestinal surgery, cardiac arrhythmia, hyperthyroidism, and any type of bladder outlet obstruction.

Prostaglandins

It has been hypothesized (see previous chapter) that prostaglandins are intimately involved in and necessary for bladder contractile activity. Using this rationale, Bultitude et al. (1976) reported that instillation of 0.5 mg of prostaglandin E_2 (PGE_2) into the bladders of females with varying degrees of urinary retention resulted in acute emptying and in improvement of long-term emptying in two thirds of the patients studied. Desmond et al. (1980) reported further results with intravesical use of this agent in patients whose bladders exhibited no contractile activity or in whom bladder contractility was relatively impaired. Twenty of 36 patients showed a strongly positive and six showed a weakly positive immediate response. Fourteen patients were reported to show prolonged beneficial effects, all but one of whom had shown a strongly positive immediate response. Stratification of the data revealed that an intact sacral reflex arc was a prerequisite for any type of positive response. The authors noted additionally that the effects of PGE_2 appeared to be additive or synergistic with cholinergic stimulation in some patients. Vaidyanathan et al. (1981) reported that intravesical instillation of 7.5 mg of 15(*S*)-15-methyl prostaglandin F_2 produced reflex voiding in some patients with incomplete suprasacral spinal cord lesions. The favorable response to a single dose of drug, when present, lasted from 1.0–2.5 months. Other investigators including Stanton (1978) and Delaere et al. (1981) have reported absolutely no success with this type of treatment. Prostaglandins have a relatively short half-life and it is difficult to understand how any effects after a single application can last up to even several months. If such does occur, it must be the result of a "triggering effect" on some as yet unknown physiologic or metabolic mechanism. Potential side effects of prostaglandin usage include bronchospasm, chills, hypotension, tachycardia, cardiac arrhythmia, convulsions, hypocalcemia, and diarrhea (Moncada et al., 1980).

Blockers of Inhibition

As discussed in the preceding chapter, a sympathetic reflex exists, at least in the cat, which promotes urine storage by exerting an inhibitory effect on pelvic parasympathetic ganglionic transmission. This effect, although inhibitory, is α-adrenergic in nature. Some have suggested on this basis that α-adrenergic blockade, in addition to decreasing outlet resistance, may in fact facilitate transmission through these ganglia and thereby enhance bladder contractility. Methyldopa (Raz et al., 1977) has been used with this rationale with at least some good initial results. Likewise, on this basis, Raz and Smith (1976) have advocated a trial of an α-adrenergic blocking agent for the treatment of nonobstructive urinary retention. Although we and others have had occasional anecdotal success using this or another exotic approach, we would caution against the assumption that improvement during administration of a drug occurs solely because of it.

The recent knowledge "explosion" in the field of neuropeptide physiology has also provided potentially new insights into lower urinary tract function and its pharmacologic alteration. Endogenous enkephalins are thought to exert a tonic inhibitory effect on the micturition reflex (see Section I), and agents such as narcotic antagonists offer a new possibility for stimulating reflex bladder activity (Vaidyanathan et al., 1981; Thor et al., 1981). Comprehensive clinical trials will doubtless be done in the future.

Electrical Stimulation

Clinical trials of direct electrical stimulation of the bladder originated in 1940 (Dees, 1965), but have met with only partial success and intermittent enthusiasm since that time. Merrill (1974, 1975), Merrill and Conway (1974), and Halverstadt and Parry (1975) reviewed the literature through the mid-1970s and reported the results of their clinical trials. Direct electrical stimulation was most effective in patients with hypotonic and areflexic bladders. Initial success, defined as a low postvoid residual with sterile urine, was achieved in only 50%–60% of patients, and secondary failure, usually related to equipment malfunction, often supervened. The spread of current to other pelvic structures whose stimulus thresholds were lower than that of the bladder often resulted in abdominal, pelvic, and perineal pain; a desire to defecate; contraction of the pelvic and leg muscles; and erection and ejaculation in males. It was also noted that the increase in intravesical pressure was not generally coordinated with bladder neck opening or with pelvic floor relaxation, and that other measures to accomplish these ends might be necessary. Grimes et al. (1973, 1975) applied electrical stimulation directly to the sacral spinal cord, attempting to take advantage of the remaining intact motor pathways to initiate micturition. Although some short-term success was noted, many of the side effects seen with direct bladder stimulation occurred, since the stimulus, so applied, was also unphysiologic. Enthusiasm for both of these approaches has waned considerably, and resurrection seems unlikely.

Tanagho (1986) and his associates have logically pursued neurostimulation for both emptying and storage problems, and have recently described the evolution of their work (Schmidt, 1983; Tanagho, 1986). They too tried direct spinal cord stimulation but found that a very high rise in outlet resistance resulted. Although some emptying occurred, it was with a high intravesical pressure, a high outlet pressure, and occurred only at the end of stimulation, when the outlet resistance decreased. They found that it was not possible, at the spinal cord level, to separate a bladder center from a striated sphincter center. However, they have pursued, with some success, stimulation of individual sacral nerve roots. In an ingenious series of experiments, they found that, to achieve maximal specific detrusor stimulation with minimal sphincter activation, it was necessary to separate the dorsal component from the ventral component of the sacral root involved and to isolate and selectively section the somatic fibers of the sacral root to be stimulated.

Reduction Cystoplasty

On the surface, a reduction cystoplasty seems an attractive alternative for patients with chronic urinary retention who have large decompensated bladders. Using techniques of reduction cystoplasty involving either fundus invagination or detrusor duplication (but not simple excision of bladder tissue only), symptomatic successes with lower bladder capacity and lower residual urine volumes have been achieved (Roberts et al., 1979; Hanna, 1982; Kinn, 1985). However, it is puzzling that, in spite of such improvement, at least Roberts et al. and Kinn report absolutely no change in bladder or sphincter activity. In patients with no bladder contractility, flow rates seemed to change only when outlet reduction is also performed. However, there may in fact be merit in Hanna's suggestion (1982) that such procedures are rational in selected patients with very large bladder capacities who exhibit poor emptying because of only a partial deficiency of detrusor contractility.

Decreasing Outlet Resistance at a Site of Anatomic Obstruction

Prostatic enlargement and urethral stricture are two of the more common causes of bladder outlet obstruction in males. The pathophysiology of their development and their surgical and nonsurgical correction are very well dealt with elsewhere in this volume.

Decreasing Outlet Resistance at a Level of the Smooth Sphincter

Transurethral Resection or Incision of the Bladder Neck

Emmett (1945) performed the first transurethral bladder neck resection in a patient with neurogenic bladder dysfunction in 1937, and for years this procedure represented the first line of surgical attack in cases of poorly balanced bladder function. Originally, the operation was performed primarily in two groups of patients: (1) those with weak or absent detrusor contractions, and (2) those with anatomic or functional obstruction at the level of the bladder neck and proximal urethra, which prevents emptying even with a sustained detrusor contraction (Gibbon et al., 1965; Bunce, 1967; Wein et al., 1976). Some urologists still prefer to resect the bladder neck whenever signs of outlet obstruction are associated with a neuropathic bladder, and treat other areas of outlet resistance later, if this proves necessary (Glahn, 1974; Gibbon, 1974a, 1974b).

More refined urodynamic techniques have resulted in the realization that dyssynergia at the level of the bladder neck or proximal urethra is uncommon, both in patients with neurologic disease and in patients with obstruction but without neurologic disease. We think that the prime indication for this procedure is the demonstration of true obstruction at the bladder neck or proximal urethra level by combined detrusor pressure-flow studies with either fluoroscopic demonstration of a failure of opening of the smooth sphincter area or a micturitional urethral profile showing that the bladder pressure falls off sharply at some point between the bladder neck and the area of the striated sphincter (McGuire, 1984). In the past, it was felt that another category of patient for whom this procedure would be useful was one with a sacral spinal cord lesion and an areflexic bladder who could achieve a measurable increase in intravesical pressure by straining and/or use of the Credé maneuver, but who could not empty the bladder adequately by these methods (Wein et al., 1976). Currently, we feel that the procedure simply creates a form of "graded" stress incontinence in these patients, and that other alternatives for adequate emptying should be sought first. Although documented instances of bladder neck obstruction in women have been reported (Diokno et al., 1984), extreme caution must be exercised in surgically treating this entity in females because of the risk of incontinence.

Techniques of resection include: (1) a thorough circumferential resection of all tissue between the internal orifice and the verumontanum (in males); (2) a limited resection of dorsal tissue from the 3 o'clock through the 9 o'clock position; (3) a resection further limited to the posterior lip; and (4) transurethral incision of the bladder neck at the 5 o'clock and/or 7 o'clock position. Turner-Warwick (1984) recommends a single full-thickness incision in one position in the male, extending from the bladder base down to the level of the verumontanum. He recommends deepening the incision until pinpoints of reflected light reveal minute interstitial fat globules between the latticework of the residual prostatic capsule fibers. Hemostasis is achieved by electrocoagulation with the flat surface of the knife electrode. Turner-Warwick (1984) reports the incidence of diminished volume of ejaculate to be only 10%, and in fewer than 5% of his patients has it been absent altogether. Our experience in this regard falls somewhere between the reported incidences of Moisey et al. (1982) (16%) and of Blaivas and Norlen (1984) (50%).

Y-V Plasty of the Bladder Neck

A simple Y-V plasty of the bladder neck can accomplish the same effect as a transurethral resection or incision. However, especially in females, an "overcorrection" can result, and it would seem logical to recommend this only when an open surgical procedure is already required to correct a concomitant disorder. When outlet reduction is required to render a refractory, poorly emptying bladder totally incontinent prior to inserting an artificial sphincter, an open Y-V plasty—though originally mentioned as a possibility (Scott et al., 1974)—certainly makes subsequent placement of a bladder neck cuff extremely difficult.

Pharmacologic Therapy

Krane and Olsson (1973a, 1973b) endorsed the concept of a physiologic internal sphincter partially controlled by tonic sympathetic stimulation of contractile α-adrenergic receptors in the smooth musculature of the bladder neck and proximal urethra. Further, they hypothesized that some obstructions that occur at this level during detrusor contraction are a result of inadequate opening of the bladder neck and/or of inadequate decrease in resistance in the area of the proximal urethra. They also theorized and presented evidence that α-adrenergic blockade could be useful in promoting bladder emptying in such a patient with an adequate detrusor contraction but without anatomic obstruction or detrusor–striated sphincter dyssynergia. Abel et al. (1974) called attention to the fact that such a functional obstruction, which they, too, presumed to be mediated by the sympathetic nervous system, could be maximal in the urethra rather than at the bladder neck, and coined the term "neuropathic urethra." The implication that α-adrenergic blockade could be useful in certain patients with a failure to empty despite an adequate increase in intravesical pressure was first made by Kleeman in 1970 and was subsequently supported by others (Johnston and Farkas, 1975; Stockamp, 1975; Whitfield et al., 1976). Successful results, usually defined as an increase in flow rate, decrease in residual urine, and improvement in upper tract appearance (where pathological), could often be correlated with an objective decrease in urethral profile closure pressures. Although one would expect success with such therapy to be most evident in patients without detrusor–striated sphincter dyssynergia as reported by Hachen (1980), Mobley (1976) reported a startling 86% success rate in 21 patients with a reflex neurogenic bladder, with a corresponding success rate of 66% in what was termed "flaccid" and 57% in what was termed "autonomous" neurogenic bladder dysfunction, success being defined as postvoid residual urine volume consistently less than 100 ml. Such effects could be explained by a decrease in perineal striated muscle activity induced by α-adrenergic blockade (Nanninga et al., 1976), an effect that is probably mediated by a central mechanism, as evidence of adrenergic innervation of the human striated sphincter is lacking (Wein et al., 1979; Rossier et al., 1982). Scott and Morrow (1978), on the other hand, noted excellent results with phenoxybenzamine therapy in 9 of 10 patients with a flaccid bladder and a flaccid external sphincter, a single patient with an upper motor neuron bladder with intact sympathetic innervation, but only 8 of 21 patients with hyperreflexia and autonomic dysreflexia, and 0 of 6 patients with an upper motor neuron bladder and sympathetic denervation (lesion between T10 and L2).

There is also a rationale for the addition of α-adrenolytic therapy in the patient with inadequate emptying secondary to neuropathic voiding dysfunction after conventional pharmacologic treatment has failed. Parasympathetic decentralization has been reported to lead to a marked increase in adrenergic innervation of the bladder, with a resultant conversion of the usual β (relaxant) response of the bladder body in response to sympathetic stimulation to an α (contractile) effect (Norlen et al., 1976; Sundin et al., 1977). Although the alterations in innervation have been disputed (Nordling et al., 1980), the alteration in receptor function has not. Koyanagi (1979) showed supersensitivity of the urethra to α-adrenergic stimulation in a group of patients with autonomous neurogenic bladders. This implies a similar change in adrenergic receptor function in the urethra following parasympathetic decentralization. Parsons and Turton (1980) observed a similar phenomenon but provided a different pharmacologic explanation. They ascribed the cause to adrenergic supersensitivity of the urethral smooth muscle caused by sympathetic decentralization, resulting in an inappropriately high sensitivity to alterations in circulating catecholamine levels brought about as a part of normal cardiovascular homeostasis. Nordling et al. (1981) described a similar phenomenon in females after radical hysterectomy and ascribed this change to damage to the sympathetic innervation of the lower urinary tract.

The pentolamine stimulation test (Olsson et al., 1977) can usually predict the effectiveness of α-adrenolytic therapy in a given situation. Flow rates are measured before and after an intravenous dose of 5 mg, and the values are plotted on a nomogram that relates flow rate to volume voided. An increase of 0.8 units on the nomogram predicts improved voiding with oral α-adrenergic blocker therapy.

Phenoxybenzamine is the α-adrenolytic agent that was most commonly used in the treatment of voiding dysfunction (Wein, 1986). The initial adult dosage of this agent is 10 mg/day. The dose may be increased by 10 mg every 4–5 days to a recommended maximum of 60 mg/day. Daily doses larger than 10 mg are generally divided and given every 8–12 hours. The maximum effect of a particular dose usually becomes apparent only after a week following the initiation of or a change in therapy. After discontinuation, the effects of daily administration persist for about the same period of time. In our experience, patients who responded favorably to this agent generally did so at doses less than 30 mg and did not respond to dose increases with incremental improvement. Some patients who responded to 10 mg daily could be maintained on an even lower dose. Potential side effects include orthostatic hypotension, reflex tachycardia, nasal congestion, diarrhea, miosis, sedation, nausea, and vomiting (secondary to local irritation). Ejaculatory failure, due to lack of seminal emission and not to retrograde ejaculation, frequently occurs, but without any adverse effect on erection. Those who still use phenoxybenzamine for long-term therapy should be aware of the recently reported adverse in vitro and in vivo mutagenicity studies with this agent (see latest *Physicians' Desk Reference*). Further, the manufacturer has indicated a dose-related incidence of gastrointestinal tumors in rats. Although this agent has been in use for some 30 years in humans without any adverse epidemiologic associations, it is obvious that one must now carefully consider the potential medical-legal ramifications of long-term phenoxybenzamine therapy, especially in younger persons.

Prazosin hydrochloride is one of a class of new antihypertensive agents with an affinity for postsynaptic α_1 receptors, at least in vascular smooth muscle (Weiner, 1980), in contrast to classical α-adrenergic blocking agents such as phentolamine and phenoxybenzamine, which have blocking properties at both α_1 and α_2 receptor sites. Prazosin has been shown to cause α_1 blockade in the smooth muscle of the canine and human urethra (MacGregor and Diokno, 1981) and, in addition, it has been safely used clinically to lower outlet resistance in some patients (Andersson et al., 1981). Therapy with prazosin is generally begun in daily divided doses of 2–3 mg. The dose may be very gradually increased to a maximum of 20 mg daily, although we seldom use more than 9–12 mg daily in three divided doses. The potential side effects of prazosin are consequent to its α_1 blockade. Additionally, there occasionally occurs the "first-dose phenomenon," a symptom complex of faintness, dizziness, palpitation, and, infrequently, syncope, thought to be due to acute postural hypotension. The incidence of this phenomenon can be minimized by restricting the initial dose of the drug to 1 mg and by administering this at bedtime. Other side effects associated with chronic prazosin therapy are generally mild and rarely necessitate withdrawal of the drug. Thus far, reports of adverse effects on seminal emission have been sparse.

Other agents with some α-adrenergic blocking properties at various levels of neural organization have urologic side effects that may be therapeutically useful in certain circumstances. Methyldopa is an antihypertensive agent that is converted to α-methyl norepinephrine, and that functions as a false neurotransmitter at a central and perhaps peripheral level, with the end result being a decreased peripheral sympathetic effect. Raz et al. (1977) have reported improved emptying in patients with neurogenic bladder dysfunction with this agent. Clonidine is another antihypertensive agent whose net action results in a decreased peripheral sympathetic effect, reflected in the urinary tract by a decrease in the urethral closure pressure profile (Nordling and Meyhoff, 1979). Other commonly used pharmacologic agents with significant α-adrenergic blocking properties include chlorpromazine and haloperidol (Weiner, 1980).

These and other agents with α-adrenergic blocking properties at various levels of neural organization have been utilized in patients with various types of voiding dysfunction. Our own experience would suggest that a trial of such an agent in such patients may certainly be worthwhile, as the effect or noneffect will become obvious in a matter of days, and the pharmacologic side effects are of course reversible. However, our results with such therapy in these patients have been considerably less spectacular than those of at least some other investigators.

β-Adrenergic stimulation has been shown experimentally to decrease the urethral pressure profile and by inference urethral resistance (Raz and Caine, 1971). Vaidyanathan et al. (1980) reported a decrease in urethral closure pressure after administration of terbutaline, a relatively specific β_2 agonist. Whether this drug or other pharmacologically similar agents will prove useful to facilitate bladder emptying by decreasing outlet resistance remains to be investigated.

Decreasing Outlet Resistance at the Level of the Striated Sphincter

External Sphincterotomy

Therapeutic destruction of the external urethral sphincter was first performed in 1936 (Watkins) in a patient with nonspastic obstruction. Although this procedure was mentioned again by Baumrucker in 1943, the first large clinical series was reported in 1958 by Ross et al. The primary indication for this procedure is the failure of the bladder to empty in a male patient with a suprasacral lesion, and good but involuntary detrusor contractions when prostatic obstruction and obstructive inflammatory lesions at the bladder neck have been ruled out and when other types of management have been unsuccessful or are not possible.

A substantial improvement in bladder emptying occurs in 70%–90% of cases (Wein et al., 1976). Upper tract deterioration is rare after successful sphincterotomy, and vesicoureteral reflux—if present previously—often disappears because of lower bladder pressures and the reduced incidence of infection in a catheterless patient with a low residual urine volume. Although an external collecting device is generally worn postoperatively, total dripping incontinence or severe stress incontinence should be unusual unless the proximal sphincter mechanism (bladder neck and proximal urethra) has been compromised, either by prior surgical therapy or as a secondary effect of the striated sphincter dyssynergia.

Different techniques have historically been used for external sphincterotomy, including incisions at the 5 and 7 o'clock positions, the 3 and 9 o'clock positions, the 2, 4, 8, and 10 o'clock positions, and the 11 and 1 o'clock positions (Wein et al, 1976). The 12 o'clock sphincterotomy, originally proposed by Madersbacher and Scott (1975), is our method of choice for a number of reasons, which have been confirmed and commented on by others (Madersbacher and Scott, 1975; Yalla et al., 1977; Hachen, 1977; Madersbacher, 1986). First of all, the anatomy of the striated sphincter is such that its main bulk is anteromedial. The blood supply, on the other hand, is primarily lateral; thus there is less of a chance of significant hemorrhage with an incision at the 12 o'clock position. There is disagreement about the rate of postoperative erectile impotence in those individuals who have erections in series that have utilized the 3 and 9 o'clock technique. Estimates vary from 5%–30%, and whatever the true figure is, it is clear that most would agree that this complication is far less common (approximately 5%) with incision in the anteromedial position (Madersbacher, 1986). Other complications of external sphincterotomy may include significant hemorrhage and urinary extravasation. Urethral stricture rarely occurs at the site of sphincterotomy.

External sphincterotomy can be performed using a knife electrode or by resection with a loop electrode. The incision must extend from the level of the verumontanum at least to the bulbomembranous junction. A gradually deepening incision allows good visual control and minimizes the chances of significant hemorrhage and extravasation.

Sphincterotomy failure generally indicates an inadequate incision or resection of tissue. Failure may also be due to the presence of another unsuspected obstruction (e.g., at the bladder neck), or to inadequate bladder contractions, either those of insufficient magnitude or those that are poorly sustained. Residual urine does not always indicate "failure," as low pressure but incomplete emptying in an individual may be quite acceptable.

Urethral Overdilation

Urethral overdilation to 40–50 F usually achieves the same objective as external sphincterotomy in females (Gibbon, 1974a). External sphincterotomy is rarely carried out, however, in females because of the lack of a suitable external collecting device. In young boys, when sphincterotomy is contemplated, a similar stretching of the posterior urethra can be accomplished through a perineal urethrostomy, obviating or postponing the need for formal sphincterotomy (Johnston and Farkas, 1975).

Pudendal Nerve Block or Interruption

Relief of obstruction at the level of the striated sphincter can also be achieved by a pudendal neurectomy, which was first described in 1899 by Rocket (Stark, 1969). Historically, this method enjoyed the same popularity in patients with fixed neurologic lesions and striated sphincter dyssynergia, but is seldom used today (Wein et al., 1976). In the rare instance of usage, therapeutic assessment of the results of a pudendal block should precede the formal procedure, which should be carried out only unilaterally. Bilateral nerve section results in an unacceptably high rate of impotence in the male, and may result in fecal and severe stress urinary incontinence.

Pharmacologic Therapy

There is no class of pharmacologic agents that will selectively relax the striated musculature of the pelvic floor. Chlordiazepoxide, methocarbamol, orphenadrine, and diazepam belong to a group of agents classified as centrally acting muscle relaxants (Bianchine, 1980). The primary side effect of all members of this group is sedation, which many feel is primarily responsible for their muscle-relaxing effect when administered orally. In general, we have not found the recommended oral doses to be effective in controlling the classical types of striated sphincter dyssynergia seen secondary to neurological disease. If the etiology of incomplete emptying in a neurologically normal patient is obscure, and the patient has what appears to be inadequate relaxation of the pelvic floor striated musculature, a trial of an agent such as diazepam may be worthwhile. The theoretical rationale in such circumstances is either that of relaxation of the pelvic floor striated musculature during bladder contraction or of such relaxation removing a stimulus that is inhibitory to bladder activity. Improvement under such circumstances may simply be due, however, to the drug's antianxiety effect or to the intensive explanation, encouragement, and modified biofeedback therapy that usually accompanies this type of treatment in such patients.

Dantrolene sodium is a skeletal muscle relaxant that has been shown to dissociate excitation-contraction coupling at a site distal to the neuromuscular end-plate—in the sarcoplasmic reticulum (Bianchine, 1980). It has been shown to have therapeutic benefits for chronic spasticity associated with CNS disorders. The drug has been used in patients with classical detrusor striated sphincter dyssynergia, and was initially reported as being very successful in improving voiding function in these patients (Murdock et al., 1976). Therapy in adults is begun at a dose of 25 mg twice daily, increasing the dose weekly by 50- to 100-mg increments up to a recommended daily maximum of 400 mg given in divided doses. Hackler et al. (1980) achieved improvement in voiding function in approximately half of their patients treated with dantrolene, but found that such improvement required doses of 600 mg/day. Although the drug has no autonomic side effects, it may induce a generalized weakness severe enough to compromise its therapeutic benefits, especially at higher doses. Other potential side effects include euphoria, dizziness, diarrhea, and hepatotoxicity. The toxicity to liver is seemingly related to high-dose long-term usage, and has apparently resulted in some fatalities.

Baclofen is an agent that is thought to hyperpolarize primary afferent fiber terminals in the spinal cord (Bianchine, 1980) and to inhibit monosynaptic and polysynaptic spinal reflex activity (Duncan et al., 1976). It has been found useful in the treatment of skeletal spasticity due to a variety of causes. Treatment is started at an initial dose of 5 mg, three times daily, and the dose is doubled every three days until a daily total dose level of 60 mg is reached. The manufacturer recommends that the total daily dose not exceed 20 mg, four times daily. Florante et al. (1980) reported that 73% of their patients with voiding dysfunction secondary to acute and chronic spinal cord injury showed lower striated sphincter responses and decreased residual urine volume following treatment, but only with an average daily oral dose of

120 mg. Hachen and Krucker (1977) found a 75 mg daily oral dose to be ineffective in patients with striated sphincter dyssynergia and traumatic paraplegia, whereas they found a daily intravenous dose of 20 mg to be highly effective. Potential side effects of baclofen include drowsiness, insomnia, rash, pruritus, dizziness, and weakness. Hallucinations may sometimes occur after abrupt withdrawal.

Biofeedback, Psychotherapy

Biofeedback is a useful adjunct in the improvement of voluntary control of neural, visceral, and skeletal responses (Miller, 1975; Miller and Dworkin, 1977; Schwartz, 1979). Understanding the concept of biofeedback is much easier than formulating an all-inclusive unequivocal definition of the term. Literally, the feedback is information (data) about biologic processes that is used in a training program whose goal is the acquisition of some voluntary control over these processes. The data utilized in biofeedback may be as sophisticated as visual or auditory information produced by modern electronic equipment that is monitoring a physiologic process, or it may be as simple as a self-kept record of symptoms and biologic events (such as a chart for recording the time and volume of voiding and the presence of urgency and incontinence). The list of physiologic processes subject to some self-control includes blood pressure, heart rate, blood flow, sweat gland activity, skin temperature, body temperature, respiratory function, genital responses, bowel and bladder motility, and skeletal muscle control.

Schwartz (1979) points out that the clearest evidence for the efficacy of biofeedback is in the regulation of skeletal muscle activity. As he further states, this should not be surprising since, of all bodily systems, the skeletal muscles are under the most voluntary control. Hinman (1974, 1980) and Allen (1972, 1980) were perhaps the first to recognize that nonneurogenic striated sphincter dyssynergia (or a disorder qualitatively similar to it) can occur on a psychogenic basis and cause gross upper tract damage. Each used a combination of psychologic retraining, suggestion, medication, and parent cooperation in a treatment program. Wear and colleagues (1979) described the use of a urodynamic display of external sphincter EMG activity to facilitate this type of treatment. They reported significant clinical improvement in four of eight patients so treated. Maizels and co-workers (1979) further simplified this technique by using anal skin electrodes for the repeated display of striated sphincter activity without pain or significant inconvenience to the patient. Successful therapy in this type of situation obviously requires a strongly motivated patient who is capable of understanding the instruction for biofeedback training.

Circumventing Problems

Intermittent Catheterization

Intermittent catheterization (IC) has proved to be the most effective means of attaining a catheter-free state in the majority of patients with acute spinal cord lesions (Frankel, 1974). It is also an extremely effective method of treating the adult or child whose bladder fails to empty, especially when efforts to increase intravesical pressure and/or decrease outlet resistance have been unsuccessful. In those patients who have inadequate urine storage due to involuntary bladder contractions, decreased compliance, or stress incontinence with adequate or inadequate emptying, it may also be used if the dysfunction can be converted solely or primarily to one of emptying by pharmacologic or surgical means (Wein et al., 1976). Lapides (Lapides et al., 1974, 1976) deserves enormous credit for first applying the concept of self-IC to large groups of outpatients with voiding dysfunction. Subsequently, he and his co-workers and many others have demonstrated the long-term efficacy and safety of such a regimen. IC requires a cooperative, well-motivated patient or family. The patient must have adequate hand control (or a family member willing to catheterize), and adequate urethral exposure must be obtained. It is advantageous to have a special urologic nurse who instructs the patients and/or families in the regimen; provides them with understandable written instructions to refresh their memory regarding technique, precautions, and danger signals; and who provides continuing support for patients who call with questions or problems referable to their regimen. Teaching self-IC requires an approach that communicates acceptance of the procedure by the instructor. Many patients are initially extremely reluctant to perform any procedure on themselves that involves the genitalia. Patients need a thorough explanation of the advantages of IC along with assurance that it is simple and will not tie them to their homes nor to an absolute time schedule. Additionally, proper selection of equipment for the patient's intelligence and financial level will increase patient acceptance of and compliance with the self-IC program. Initially reticent patients are continually amazed by the ease with which such a regimen is established.

For adult male patients, 14 or 16 F red rubber catheters are generally used. In some cases (for example, in patients with impaired fine motor skills), stiffer plastic catheters may be easier for the patient to insert. These are also commercially available in a disposable form. A notable advantage to the red rubber catheters is their longevity. They can be reused indefinitely and boiled for sterilization if desired. For patients without insurance it is almost necessary to use them. Disposable plastic female catheters, now manufactured by several companies, are recommended for female patients. They are inexpensive, very convenient, and can be obtained under most insurance plans. These 14 F 6-in. catheters are easy to handle. Female patients may catheterize themselves on the toilet without a mirror, making IC less confusing, cleaner, and quicker. Red rubber or Robinson catheters may also be used for female patients if desired. For the patient's convenience, liquid cleansing agents are usually easier to handle in the form of cotton balls soaked in the agent. These can be easily carried in a small jar. Any water-soluble lubricant is suitable for lubricating the catheter prior to insertion.

Continuous Catheterization

Indwelling urethral catheters may be used for short-term bladder drainage, and careful such use of a small-bore catheter (for a short time) does not, in our opinion, seem to adversely affect the ultimate outcome. Occasionally, an indwelling catheter is a last resort type of therapy for long-term bladder drainage. Virtually all patients with an indwelling urethral catheter have bacteriuria after a certain period of time. A contracted, fibrotic bladder may be the ultimate result. Bladder calculi may form on the catheter or on the retention balloon. Urethral complications are relatively uncommon in females, but bladder spasm may occur, producing urinary incontinence. The temptation to use a large retention balloon should be resisted, as the continuous use of such a balloon combined with some pressure on the catheter may cause erosion of the bladder neck. A suprapubic trochar catheter may be initially more comfortable than a urethral catheter and obviates urethral complications in the male, the main advantage of this type of continuous drainage over longer periods. Bladder spasm with incontinence may, however, be more of a problem, and when blockage occurs, nursing personnel are more reluctant to change this type of catheter without physician assistance. Finally, it should be mentioned that Kaufman et al. (1977) reported development of squamous cell carcinoma of the bladder in six of 59 patients with spinal cord injuries who had long-term indwelling catheters. Four of these had no obvious tumor visible on endoscopy and the diagnosis was made by bladder biopsy. Five of these patients also had transitional-cell elements in their tumor. Broecker et al. (1981) surveyed 81 consecutive spinal cord injury patients with an indwelling urinary catheter for greater than ten years and, although they did not find frank carcinoma in any, found squamous metaplasia of the bladder in 11, and leukoplakia in one. Thus, periodic urinary cytology and cystoscopy, perhaps with random biopsy, especially with the new onset of gross hematuria, seems necessary in patients on long-term indwelling catheter drainage.

Urinary Diversion

Supravesical Diversion

Although commonly employed in the past for treatment of neurogenic voiding dysfunction, supravesical diversion is rarely indicated in any patient with only voiding dysfunction. Indications for performing supravesical diversion may include (1) progressive hydronephrosis and intractable upper urinary tract dilatation (which may be due to blockade of the ureterovesical junction caused by a trabeculated, thick bladder, or to vesicoureteral reflux that does not respond to conservative measures), and (2) recurrent upper urinary tract infections. Although the various techniques of supravesical urinary diversion are covered in other chapters of this book, it is important to note that urinary diversion cannot always prevent upper urinary tract deterioration. The initial results of the ileal conduit seemed encouraging in terms of upper tract preservation (Bricker, 1950). Unfortunately, long-term results have been disappointing (Schwartz and Jeffs, 1975; Pitts and Muecke, 1979; Dunn et al., 1979; Orr et al., 1981). The colonic conduit, which allows a reflux-preventing implantation of the ureters, was expected to produce better long-term results. Although earlier reports seemed to support this supposition (Mogg and Syme, 1969; Altwein et al., 1977; Althausen et al., 1978), long-term results seem to be equally disappointing (Elder et al., 1979).

Continent forms of diversion that may be applicable to patients with voiding dysfunction involve the application of a continent abdominal wall stoma (Koch pouch, ileocecal reservoir, or Mainz pouch) (Goldwasser and Webster, 1985). Severe scoliosis and kyphosis are relative contraindications to conduit stomal diversion because of difficulty in fitting a stomal bag. However, this problem does not exist with continent stomal diversion (Ashken, 1982). On the other hand, continent stomal diversion requires that the patient be able to perform intermittent catheterization or that dependable assistance is available for catheterizing the stoma. Currently, there are no reports of long-term results in patients with these forms of continent diversion, and little is known about their long-term effects on the upper tracts. The subject of bladder reconstruction and substitution is covered more completely elsewhere in this book.

THERAPY TO FACILITATE URINE STORAGE

Inhibiting Bladder Contractility/Decreasing Sensory Input/ Increasing Bladder Capacity

Timed Bladder Emptying

This is actually a form of bladder conditioning (Opitz, 1984). Although it is not a sophisticated concept, like many we use it seems to work quite well in some circumstances. The idea is to completely or partially empty the bladder on a frequent enough schedule so as to keep the intravesical volume below that at which storage failure results. This may involve only frequent voiding with a limited fluid intake in the patient with detrusor hyperactivity. It may involve a more complicated coordination of an IC schedule with bladder volume in the patient with a detrusor hyperreflexia and sphincter dyssynergia whose status has been converted to that of relative emptying failure, but only if the bladder is emptied periodically (before the threshold for hyperreflexia or decreased compliance causing storage failure or upper tract damage is reached).

Pharmacologic Therapy

Anticholinergic Agents

Because at least a major portion of the neurohumoral stimulus for physiologic bladder contraction is acetylcholine-induced stimulation of postganglionic parasympathetic cholinergic receptor sites on bladder smooth muscle, atropine and atropine-like agents will depress true detrusor hyperreflexia of any etiology (Pedersen and Grynderup, 1966; Blaivas et al., 1980; Jensen, 1981a). In such patients the volume to the first involuntary contraction will generally be increased, the amplitude of the contractions decreased, and the total bladder capacity increased, with a proportionate reduction in symptomatology. Interestingly, bladder compliance in normal individuals and in those with detrusor hyperreflexia, where the initial slope of the filling curve on cystometry is normal prior to the involuntary contraction, does not seem to be significantly altered (Jensen, 1981a). The effect of these agents on intravesical pressure during filling in those patients who exhibit only decreased compliance has not been well studied. In patients with detrusor hyperreflexia, although significant clinical improvement may be achieved, only partial inhibition generally results, because of the phenomenon of atropine resistance. (See Section I for a complete discussion.) Atropine only partially antagonizes the bladder response to either pelvic nerve stimulation or direct electrical stimulation. Atropine does, however, completely inhibit the response of the bladder smooth muscle to exogenously administered acetylcholine. At present, there is no completely accepted explanation for this relative atropine resistance, but the most attractive theory is that a major portion of the neurotransmission mediated by parasympathetic (pelvic) nerve stimulation is noncholinergic and nonadrenergic. In other words, part of the excitation caused by pelvic nerve stimulation is secondary to release of a transmitter other than acetylcholine or norepinephrine. Most of the drugs discussed under the heading of inhibiting bladder contractility are agents that inhibit muscarinic cholinergic receptor sites. These agents, though helpful, leave much to be desired in terms of efficacy in certain situations, and there certainly exists a potential pharmacologic basis for attempting to further inhibit bladder contractility by inhibiting the various other types of receptor sites thought to be responsible for the noncholinergic portion of the contractile response elicited through pelvic nerve efferent impulses. Unfortunately, clinically useful agents of this type are either unavailable (as in the case of ATP) or have not been shown to produce consistently useful clinical effects, at least at this time.

The potential side effects of all antimuscarinic agents include inhibition of salivary secretion (dry mouth), blockade of the iris sphincter muscle (pupillary dilation), blockade of the ciliary muscle of the lens to cholinergic stimulation (blurred vision for near objects), tachycardia, drowsiness, and inhibition of gut motility (Weiner, 1980). Those agents that possess some ganglionic blocking activity may also cause orthostatic hypotension at high doses. Antimuscarinic agents are generally contraindicated in patients with narrow-angle glaucoma and should be used with caution in patients with significant bladder outlet obstruction, as complete urinary retention may be precipitated.

Although atropine sulfate is available as a 0.5-mg tablet form, and it and all related anticholinergics are well absorbed from the gastrointestinal tract, propantheline bromide is the oral agent that is most commonly used to produce an antimuscarinic effect in the lower urinary tract. The usual adult oral dosage is 15 to 30 mg every 4–6 hours. Oral administration in the fasting state rather than with or after meals is preferable from the standpoint of bioavailability (Gibaldi and Grundhofer, 1975). The clinical efficacy can generally be predicted by the observation of the effect of a parenteral dose on the cystometrogram (Blaivas et al., 1980). The parenteral preparation is no longer available in the United States, and atropine or glycopyrrolate may be used instead. There seems to be little difference between the antimuscarinic effects on bladder smooth muscle of propantheline and those of other antimuscarinic agents. Although there are obviously many other considerations that account for the activity of a given dose of a drug at its site of action, there is no oral drug available whose direct antimuscarinic binding potential, at least in vitro, approximates that of atropine better than the long available and relatively inexpensive propantheline bromide (Levin et al., 1982).

It would seem that an agent with a significant ganglionic blocking effect as well as such an action at the peripheral receptor level might be more effective in suppressing bladder contractility. Methantheline has a higher ratio of ganglionic blocking to antimuscarinic activity than does propantheline, but the latter drug, clinical dose per dose, seems to be at least as potent in each respect (Weiner, 1980). Methantheline does have similar effects on the lower urinary tract, however, and some clinicians still prefer it—in doses of 50–100 mg four times a day—over other anticholinergic agents (Lapides and Dodson, 1953; Hebjorn, 1977).

Musculotropic Relaxants (Antispasmodics)

These agents fall under the general heading of direct-acting smooth muscle depressants, whose "antispasmodic" activity reportedly is directly on smooth muscle at a site that is metabolically distal to the cholinergic receptor mechanism (Finkbeiner et al., 1978). Although all three of the agents to be discussed do relax smooth muscle in vitro by a papavarine-like activity, all have been found in addition to possess variable antimuscarinic and local anesthetic properties. There is still a question as to how much of their clinical efficacy is due simply to their atropine-like effect. If in fact any of these agents do exert a clinically significant inhibitory effect that is independent of an antimuscarinic action, there exists a therapeutic rationale for combining their use with that of a relatively pure antimuscarinic agent.

Oxybutynin chloride has been described as a moderately potent anticholinergic agent with a strong independent musculotropic relaxant activity, and local anesthetic activity as well (Lish et al., 1965; Finkbeiner et al., 1978; Fredericks et al., 1978). This agent has been used successfully to depress detrusor hyperreflexia in patients with neurogenic bladder dysfunction (Thompson and Lauvetz, 1976). A randomized double-blind control study in 30 patients with detrusor instability comparing oxybutynin, 5 mg three times daily, and placebo was carried out by Moisey et al. (1980). Of 23 patients who completed the study with oxybutynin, 17 had symptomatic improvement and nine had evidence of urodynamic improvement—mainly an increase in bladder volume at first contraction and an increase in total bladder capacity. The recommended adult dose of oxybutynin is 5 mg three to four times daily. The potential side effects are the same as those of propantheline.

Dicyclomine hydrochloride is also reported to possess a direct relaxant effect on smooth muscle in addition to an antimuscarinic action (Johns et al., 1976; Downie et al., 1977; Khanna et al., 1979). An oral dose of 20 mg, three times daily, in adults has been reported to increase bladder capacity in patients with detrusor hyperreflexia (Fischer et al., 1978). Our own experience suggests that the individual dose must often be raised to at least 30 mg to achieve a good clinical effect. The potential side effects are antimuscarinic ones. Flavoxate hydrochloride is another compound that has been reported to have a direct inhibitory action on smooth muscle in addition to anticholinergic and local analgesic properties (Kohler and Morales, 1968). Favorable clinical effects have been noted in patients with urodynamically documented detrusor hyperreflexia. However, Briggs et al. (1980) reported essentially no effect of this agent on detrusor hyperreflexia in an elderly population, an experience that would coincide with our own subjective impression of limited clinical efficacy in situations in which other less expensive agents have failed (Benson et al., 1977). However, as with all agents in this group, a short clinical trial may be worthwhile. The recommended adult dose is 100–200 mg three to four times daily. Reported side effects are rare and are primarily antimuscarinic in nature.

Polysynaptic Inhibitors

Baclofen has been discussed previously in the section about agents that decrease outlet resistance secondary to striated sphincter dyssynergia. It has also been shown to depress detrusor hyperreflexia secondary to a spinal cord lesion (Roussan et al., 1975; Kiesswetter and Schober, 1975). Taylor and Bates (1979), in a double-blind crossover study, reported it to be very effective also in decreasing daytime and nighttime urinary frequency and incontinence in patients with idiopathic detrusor hyperreflexia. Cystometric changes were not recorded, however, and it should be noted that considerable improvement was also obtained in this study with placebo.

Calcium Antagonists

The rationale underlying the potential use of calcium antagonists for the inhibition of bladder contractility has been described previously (see Section I). The calcium antagonist nifedipine has been shown to be an effective inhibitor of contraction induced by several mechanisms in human and guinea pig bladder muscle (Forman et al., 1978; Sjogren and Andersson, 1979). It is also capable of completely blocking the noncholinergic portion of the contraction produced by electrical field stimulation in rabbit bladder (Husted, Sjogren, and Andersson, cited by Husted et al., 1980). Nifedipine more effectively inhibited potassium-induced than carbachol-induced contractions in bladder strips, whereas terodiline, an agent with both calcium antagonistic and anticholinergic properties, had the opposite effect (Husted et al., 1980). However, terodiline caused a complete inhibition of the response of rabbit bladder to electrical field stimulation. This agent in low concentrations seemed to have mainly an antimuscarinic action, whereas at higher concentrations a calcium antagonistic effect became evident. In vitro experiments appeared to show that these two effects are at least additive with regard to bladder contractility. Whether the calcium antagonistic properties of terodiline contribute to its clinical effectiveness in vivo and whether the drug is actually more effective than standard antimuscarinic agents alone remain to be established. Rud et al. (1980) reported that in oral dosages of 12.5 mg 2 or 3 times daily it produced a marked decrease in the number of hyperreflexic contractions in a group of seven women with urgency incontinence and two with nocturnal enuresis. Bladder capacity was approximately doubled, and the amplitude of the contractions was decreased. In a double-blind crossover study in 12 women with motor urge incontinence, Ekman et al. (1980) reported an increase in bladder capacity and in the volume at which the sensation of urgency was experienced in all but one of the patients treated with terodiline, whereas placebo treatment had no effect on either objective or subjective parameters.

Palmer et al. (1981) reported a double-blind placebo trial with a single 20-mg daily dose of flunarizine in 14 females with urinary frequency, incontinence, and urodynamically proved detrusor instability. A statistically significant decrease in urgency was produced in the flunarizine-treated group, but there was no change in the frequency of micturition. Although there was a trend toward improvement of cystometric parameters, this was not statistically significant at the $P \leq .05$ level. The side effects produced in patients who have been treated with calcium antagonists for voiding dysfunction have been small in number, but it should be noted that the potential side effects of these agents can be considerable and consist of hypotension, facial flushing, headache, dizziness, abdominal discomfort, constipation, nausea, rash, weakness, and palpitations. Although work in this area is obviously in its infancy, this class of agents may yet prove to be a promising alternative or addition to existing treatment for the inhibition of bladder contractility.

β-*Adrenergic Agonists*

The presence of β-adrenergic receptors in human bladder muscle has prompted attempts to increase bladder capacity with β-adrenergic stimulation. Such stimulation can cause significant increases in the capacity of animal bladders, which contain a moderate density of β-adrenergic receptors (Larsen and Mortensen, 1978). In vitro studies show a strong dose-related relaxant effect of β_2-agonists on the bladder body of rabbits, but little effect on the bladder base or proximal urethra (Khanna et al., 1981). Terbutaline (Bricanyl), in oral dosages of 5 mg three times daily, has been reported to have a "good clinical effect" in some patients with urgency and urgency incontinence, but no significant effect on the bladders of neurologically normal humans without voiding difficulty (Norlen et al., 1978). Although these results are compatible with those in other organ systems (β-adrenergic stimulation causes no acute change in total lung capacity in normal humans while it does favorably affect patients with bronchial asthma), few if any adequate studies are available on the effects of β-adrenergic stimulation in patients with detrusor hyperactivity.

α-*Adrenergic Antagonists*

Jensen has reported an increased α-adrenergic effect in the bladders of patients he characterized as "uninhibited" (1981b). Short-term and long-term administration of prazosin have been reported by him to increase bladder capacity and decrease the amplitude of contractions in this category of patients (Jensen, 1981b, 1981c). Rohner et al. (1978) found a change in the normal β response of canine bladder body to an α response after bladder outlet obstruction. Perlberg and Caine (1982) studied the in vitro response of bladder dome muscle from patients with obstructive prostatic hypertrophy and found an α-adrenergic response to noradrenaline (instead of the usual β-adrenergic response) in 23% of 47 patients. They speculated as to a potential relationship between irritative symptoms in these patients and this altered adrenergic response. They further theorized that at least some of the symptomatic improvement in irritative symptoms seen in patients with benign prostatic hypertrophy treated with α-adrenergic blocking agents may be due to a direct effect of these agents on bladder muscle, rather than their effect on outflow resistance. Although highly speculative, this potential avenue of therapy seems worthy of further study, though it should be noted that considerable improvement was obtained also with a placebo.

Prostaglandin Inhibitors

As mentioned previously, prostaglandins are one class of compound with a potentially important role in excitatory neurotransmission in the lower urinary tract. Thus, there exist multiple mechanisms whereby inhibitors of prostaglandin synthesis might decrease bladder contractility.

Cardozo et al. (1980) reported such effects in a double-blind placebo study of 30 women with detrusor instability, with which they used the prostaglandin synthetase inhibitor flurbiprofen at a dosage of 50 mg three times daily. Abnormal bladder activity, however, was not abolished in significantly more drug-treated than placebo-treated patients, and actual bladder capacity likewise showed no change. It was concluded that the drug did not abolish detrusor hyperreflexia, but delayed the intravesical pressure rise to a greater level of distention. Forty-three per cent of the patients experienced side effects from the drug, primarily nausea, vomiting, headache, indigestion, gastric distress, constipation, and rash. Cardozo and Stanton (1980) reported symptomatic improvement in patients with detrusor instability given indomethacin, another prostaglandin synthetase inhibitor, in dosages of 50–200 mg/day. This was a short-term study with no cystometric data, and the drug was compared only with bromocriptine. The incidence of side effects was high, although no patient had to stop treatment because of these. It is interesting that this category of agents has proved to be useful in primary dysmenorrhea, a condition felt to be related to a high level of menstrual endometrial prostaglandin synthesis (Chan et al., 1981). Numerous prostaglandin inhibitors exist, most of which fall under the heading of nonsteroidal anti-inflammatory drugs. The most common such agent, aspirin, is only a relatively weak inhibitor of prostaglandin synthesis.

Tricyclic Antidepressants

Some authors have found tricyclic antidepressants, particularly imipramine hydrochloride, to be particularly useful for facilitating urinary storage (Milner and Hills, 1968; Petersen et al., 1974; Raezer et al., 1977; Castleden et al., 1981). These agents have been the subject of a voluminous amount of highly sophisticated pharmacological investigation to determine the mechanisms of action responsible for their varied effects (Hollister, 1978; Baldessarini, 1980; Richelson, 1983). Most of the investigations have had the aim of explaining their antidepressant properties, and consequently have been carried out primarily on central nervous system tissue. The results, and the conclusions and speculations inferred from them, are extremely interesting, but it must be emphasized that it is essentially unknown whether they apply to or have relevance for the lower urinary tract.

All of these agents possess varying degrees of at least three major pharmacological actions: they have central and peripheral anticholinergic actions at some—but not all—sites; they block the active transport system in the presynaptic nerve ending that is responsible for the reuptake of the released amine neurotransmitters serotonin and noradrenaline; and they are sedatives, an action that occurs presumably on a central basis but is perhaps related to their antihistaminic properties. There is also evidence that they desensitize α_2 receptors on central noradrenergic neurons (Spyraki and Fibiger, 1980). Paradoxically, they have also been shown to block α-adrenergic receptors and serotonin receptors. Many such compounds are available and have been categorized as to their relative potency insofar as their multiple effects are concerned.

Imipramine has prominent systemic anticholinergic effects (Baldessarini, 1980). However, it appears to have only a weak antimuscarinic effect on bladder smooth muscle (Dhattiwala, 1976; Olubadewo, 1980; Levin et al., 1983). A strong direct inhibitory effect on bladder smooth muscle does exist, however, which is neither anticholinergic nor adrenergic (Dhattiwala, 1976; Benson et al., 1977; Fredericks et al., 1978; Olubadewo, 1980). This may be due to a local anesthetic–like action at the nerve terminals in the adjacent effector membrane, an effect that seems to occur also in cardiac muscle (Bigger et al., 1977), or to an inhibition of the participation of calcium in the excitation-contraction coupling process (Olubadewo, 1980). Clinically, the drug seems effective in decreasing bladder contractility and in increasing outlet resistance (Cole and Fried, 1972; Mahony et al., 1973; Raezer et al., 1977; Castleden et al., 1981). In trying to correlate mechanism of action with clinical effect, one might postulate that the increase in outlet resistance is due to a peripheral blockade of noradrenaline reuptake, which would tend to produce or enhance an α-adrenergic effect in the smooth muscle of the bladder base and proximal urethra. Theoretically at least, the latter action, if indeed it occurs in the lower urinary tract as it does centrally, might also tend to stimulate predominantly β-adrenergic receptors in bladder body smooth musculature, an action that would further facilitate urine storage by decreasing the excitability of smooth muscle in that area.

Castleden et al. (1981) began therapy in elderly patients with detrusor instability with a single 25-mg nighttime dose, which was increased every third day by 25 mg until either the patient was continent, had side effects, or a dose of 150 mg was reached. Six of ten patients became continent and, in those who underwent repeated cystometry, bladder capacity increased by a mean of 105 ml and bladder pressure at capacity decreased by a mean of 18 cm H_2O. Maximal urethral pressure increased by a mean of 30 cm H_2O. Although our subjective impression (Raezer et al., 1977) was that such effects became evident only after days of treatment, some patients in this series became continent after only 3–5 days of treatment. Our usual adult dosage of imipramine for voiding dysfunction is 25 mg, four times daily; half that dose is given in elderly patients. In our experience the effects of imipramine on the lower urinary tract are often additive to those of the atropine-like agents. Consequently, a combination of imipramine and propantheline is sometimes especially useful for decreasing bladder contractility (Raezer et al., 1977). If imipramine is to be used in conjunction with an atropine-like agent, it should be noted that the anticholinergic side effects of the drugs may be additive.

When used in the generally larger doses employed for antidepressant effects, the most frequent side effects of this group of agents are those attributable to their systemic anticholinergic activity. Allergic phenomena, including rash, abnormal liver function, obstructive jaundice, and agranulocytosis may also rarely occur. Side effects on the central nervous system may include weakness, fatigue, a parkinsonian effect (a fine tremor most noted in the upper extremities), and a manic or schizophrenic behavioral picture. Sedation may also result from an antihistaminic effect. Postural hypotension may be seen, presumably on the basis of α_1 receptor blockade.

Antidepressants can be shown electrophysiologically and hemodynamically to have a depressant effect on the myocardium shortly after their institution (Burgess and Turner, 1980; Muller and Schultze, 1980). However, Veith et al. (1982) have pointed out that in the animal studies showing a direct myocardial depressant effect, this occurs at plasma concentrations that are in the toxic range for humans. This group of investigators followed 24 depressed patients with heart disease treated for four weeks and found that tricyclic antidepressants had no effect on left ventricular ejection fraction at rest or during maximal exercise. The mean daily dose of imipramine in their series was 129 mg and they suggest that such antidepressant doses can be used in depressed patients with pre-existing heart disease, except for those with severely impaired myocardial performance, without an adverse effect on ventricular rhythm or hemodynamic function. Whether cardiotoxic effects will prove to be a legitimate concern in patients receiving somewhat smaller doses for lower urinary tract dysfunction remains to be seen, and is a potential matter of concern.

If imipramine or any of the tricyclic antidepressants is to be prescribed for the treatment of voiding dysfunction, the patient should be thoroughly informed of the usual indications, the potential side effects, and, in the United States, of the fact that this drug is not approved by the FDA for this purpose. The onset of significant side effects (severe abdominal distress, nausea, vomiting, headache, lethargy, and irritability) following abrupt cessation of high doses of imipramine in children (Petti and Law, 1981) would suggest that the drug should be discontinued gradually, especially in patients receiving high doses. Tricyclic antidepressants can also cause excess sweating of obscure etiology and a delay of orgasm and orgasmic impotence, whose cause is likewise unclear (Baldessarini, 1980). The use of imipramine is contraindicated in patients receiving monoamine oxidase inhibitors, as severe central nervous system toxic effects (hyperpyrexia, seizures, and coma) can be precipitated.

Dimethyl Sulfoxide

Dimethyl sulfoxide (DMSO) is a relatively simple, naturally occurring organic compound that has been used as an industrial solvent for many years. Among its properties is its ability to penetrate the intact skin, transporting chemicals along with it for absorption into the bloodstream. It has multiple pharmacological actions (membrane penetrant, anti-inflammatory, local analgesic, bacteriostatic, diuretic, cholinesterase inhibitor, collagen solvent, vasodilatory) and is used for the treatment of arthritis and other musculoskeletal disorders [*Medical Letter*, 1980; Council on Scientific Affairs, 1982]. The only formulation approved for use on human bladder is a 50% solution; a 70% solution is generally used topically for musculoskeletal disorders.

Stewart and Shirley (1976) reported symptomatic improvement in 75% of patients with interstitial cystitis following a course of treatment with this agent and an improvement in bladder capacity in 80% of these patients. Generally, one 50-ml intravesical instillation is carried out every other week for a total of six treatments. The solution is allowed to remain in the bladder for 15 minutes, after which it is expelled by spontaneous voiding. Fowler (1981) reported results with dimethyl sulfoxide in 20 patients with early interstitial cystitis; three complete and 16 partial symptomatic remissions were achieved. However, functional bladder capacity, measured at the termination of therapy in 18 cases, was observed to increase by more than 25% in only four patients. In ten patients with severe detrusor hyperreflexia, Anderssen et al. (1981) were able to demonstrate no subjective or objective effects of the drug. The unpleasant garlic-like odor of dimethyl sulfoxide is its primary side effect and makes double-blind placebo studies impossible. Cataracts have been reported in experimental animals but not in humans; eye evaluation is, however, recommended with chronic therapy. As a last resort, this drug has been used by some clinicians in the frustrating patient with the urgency-frequency syndrome but without objective evidence of true interstitial cystitis or detrusor hyperreflexia. Although anecdotal improvement is sometimes reported, few—if any—formal reports of the results of such therapy exist. Currently, we use this drug only for the treatment of interstitial cystitis.

Biofeedback, Bladder Retraining

Cardozo and associates (1978, 1980) used biofeedback-assisted training in the treatment of a group of patients with idiopathic detrusor hyperreflexia and consequent symptoms of urinary incontinence, urgency, and frequency. With a detailed explanation of the problem and of the procedure, subtracted detrusor pressure data were converted to auditory and visual stimuli. The patients were asked to try to "control" the rise in intravesical pressure by any maneuver they found helpful. In between weekly sessions, they kept a diary to record the occurrence of urgency, frequency, and incontinence. Twenty-seven of 32 female patients completed the study. According to subjective data, 11 were cured, 11 improved, and 5 were considered failures of therapy. Objectively, the corresponding numbers were 12, 4, and 11. In this series, the treatment was most effective in patients with mild to moderate detrusor instability and was not helpful in severe cases, defined as a large detrusor contraction simultaneous with the first sensation of the desire to void.

Frewen (1978, 1980) used "bladder drill retraining" in patients with cystometrically documented idiopathic detrusor instability and urgency incontinence. Each patient was given a detailed explanation of the presumed causation of the symptomatology along with a written description. A micturition chart, on which was recorded the times of and intervals between urination, the volume produced, and the degree of incontinence, served as the biofeedback data. In this study, three quarters of the patients were hospitalized for an average stay of ten days. Supportive therapy with sedatives and anticholinergics was used in all patients. The objective cure rate was 82.5%. In a later study, 30 consecutive patients with urgency and/or frequency, ten of whom had urgency incontinence, were treated on an outpatient basis. Provocative cystometry was carried out in 22 of these patients, only eight of whom showed detrusor instability. At the conclusion of 12 weeks of treatment, 24 of the 30 patients were subjectively free of urinary symptoms. However, of the eight patients with bladder instability, only three showed objective disappearance of detrusor hyperreflexia.

Pengelly and Booth (1980) compared the results of bladder training in 25 patients (of 28 who completed their protocol) with a group of historical controls. All patients had cystometrically proved detrusor instability without obvious cause. Drug therapy was either stopped before admission to the study or remained constant throughout its duration. The overall symptomatic assessment of the patients in the treatment group showed that 7 were cured, 12 improved, 5 showed no change, and 1 was worse. The corresponding figures in the control group were 1, 7, 16, and 1. According to cystometric data, 8 patients in the treatment group were cured, 3 were improved, 12 showed no change, and 2 were worse. In the control group the corresponding figures were 0, 4, 17, and 4. Poor prognostic factors were a history of nocturnal enuresis after the age of 10 years, isometric bladder contraction above 100 cm H_2O during voluntary interruption of micturition, and failure to show any improvement within the first two weeks of treatment.

Elder and Stephenson (1980) reported the results of a Frewen-type regimen in the treatment of 21 of 27 patients who completed their study. All patients initially had symptoms of increased frequency, urgency, and urgency incontinence. Cystometric studies showed that 7 had detrusor instability, 11 had "reduced compliance," and 3 had normal filling curves. In addition to the bladder training program, 18 of 21 patients were admitted to the hospital for their initial therapy, which in all cases included an anticholinergic (emepronium bromide) and a tricyclic antidepressant (a combination of nortriptyline and fluphenazine). Of the three patients with normal cystometric filling curves, two were symptomatically cured and one was improved. In 5 of the 11 patients with "reduced compliance" there was a reversion of the cystometrogram to normal; all five of these women were symptomatically cured. In six patients the filling curve was unchanged; symptomatically, two of these were cured, three were improved, and one was unchanged. None of the seven patients with detrusor instability showed any change in the bladder filling curves. However, symptomatically, three were cured, while two were improved.

Although it is impossible to isolate the various factors in each of these studies, the value of some type of biofeedback data as an adjunct to the patients' training and conditioning seems obvious. Although in the United States hospitalization for such a regimen is apt to be disallowed because of objections to the cost by third-party insurance carriers, the combination of thorough explanation with continued support and perhaps adjunctive pharmacologic therapy, along with feedback data, certainly seems justified as a trial in these often extremely difficult and frustrating cases.

Bladder Overdistention

Cystodistention involves prolonged stretching of the bladder wall using a hydrostatic pressure equal to systolic blood pressure. Smith (1981) has summarized the experience at his center and detailed the technique used. The procedure is a modification of the original cystodistention procedure described by Helmstein. The bladder is distended to systolic blood pressure for four successive periods of 30 minutes. After each distention, the bladder is emptied and its capacity measured. An indwelling catheter is left overnight. For repeat distentions, longer periods are used. Distention is usually carried out under continuous regional (epidural) anesthesia. Improvement, when it occurs, is generally attributable to ischemic changes in the nerve endings or terminals in the bladder wall (Sehn, 1978). Thus, the procedure can be grouped under the general heading of those procedures designed to produce bladder denervation. Potential complications include bladder rupture (5%–10%), hematuria, and retention. We have been unimpressed with the results of this procedure in patients with storage failure secondary to neuropathic detrusor hyperactivity. Pengelly et al. (1978) studied 46 patients with urinary symptoms associated with detrusor hyperreflexia and came to similar conclusions. Of 43 patients fully reevaluated urodynamically, none showed a conversion from detrusor hyperreflexia to normal bladder behavior. Only four patients were symptomatically improved, while five patients reported that their symptoms worsened.

Electrical Stimulation

Electrical stimulation, applied through removable anal and vaginal devices and peripherally through patch electrodes, has been used to facilitate urine storage by an inhibition of bladder contractility (Glen, 1975; Godec and Krolg, 1976; Erlandson and Fall, 1977; Merrill, 1979; Plevnik and Janež, 1979; Godec et al., 1981). When effective, this is primarily by an inhibitory pudendal to pelvic nerve reflex. In cats, this depression of bladder contractility also involves a pudendal to hypogastric reflex with further inhibition mediated through a peripheral β-adrenergic effect on the bladder smooth muscle (Erlandson and Fall, 1977). There is much disagreement in the literature regarding the mechanisms involved, the optimal parameters for electrical stimulation, the necessity for chronic vs. acute stimulation, the criteria for patient selection, and the actual cure or improvement rates. Optimal criteria for successful use in a cooperative patient include the following: (1) preservation of the morphology of the urinary tract, (2) preservation of the sacral reflex center, (3) a low degree of peripheral denervation of the pelvic floor musculature, (4) positive urodynamic and neurophysiologic responses to test stimuli, and (5) ability to empty satisfactorily when the stimulus is turned off or with intermittent catheterization. In what authors term "properly selected cases" of detrusor incontinence, initial rates of cure or improvement as high as 50% are seen. McGuire (1983) reported 16 patients with involuntary contractions of varying etiologies treated with common perineal or posterior tibial nerve stimulation. Twelve patients were dry, three improved, and one "possibly improved." The parameters used were 5–8 V, 2–10 cycles per second, and a pulse width of 5–20 msec. It is very important when using this therapeutic option to make sure that the stimulation delivered by the device selected coincides with that desired. Even so, this modality has been much less successful in our hands than in others.

Interruption of Innervation

Central

Historically, central (subarachnoid) block was not used solely for urologic indications but was used to convert a state of severe somatic spasticity to flaccidity and to abolish autonomic dysreflexia (Bors, 1957; Comarr, 1959; Bors and Comarr, 1971). As a byproduct, a reflex neurogenic bladder was converted acutely to an areflexic one that could be emptied by methods described previously or by IC. In 8 of 29 patients in Gibbon's series (1966) and in 7 of 11 patients in that of Misak et al. (1962), a flaccid bladder developed that emptied without further surgical or medical treatment. Additional therapy, when necessary, was directed at increasing intravesical pressure and decreasing outlet resistance. The obvious disadvantage of this type of procedure is a lack of selectivity, with unintended motor or sensory loss other than related to the urinary bladder. Impotence was very common, and in those patients with some residual motor or sensory function, these were often significantly altered or lost. Additionally, as will be further discussed in a subsequent section, the conceptually simple result of an areflexic bladder, although it may be produced acutely, very often is not maintained on a long-term basis after decentralization. Such patients often develop decreased compliance, resulting in significant storage problems.

Peripheral (Sacral Rhizotomy or Selective Sacral Rhizotomy)

In most cases bilateral anterior and posterior sacral rhizotomy or conusectomy will also convert a hyperreflexic, hypertonic bladder to an autonomous one (Meirowsky et al., 1950; Misak et al., 1962). Adequate emptying was achieved in 23 of 28 such patients treated by Misak et al. (1962), but 13 required subsequent catheterization because of persistent vesicoureteral reflux or hypersensitivity to or technical difficulty with the required collecting device. Erections were lost or impaired in 85% of patients who were potent preoperatively. A temporary impairment of bowel function, lasting 6–12 weeks, also occurred postoperatively.

Selective sacral nerve section was introduced as a treatment to increase bladder capacity by abolishing only the motor supply responsible for uninhibited contractions, leaving sphincter and sexual function intact. The initial use of this procedure followed the observation by Heimburger et al. in 1948 that the third sacral anterior root provides the dominant motor innervation of the human bladder. To enhance the clinical response and minimize side effects, differential sacral rhizotomy should be preceded by stimulation and blockade of the individual sacral roots with cystometric and sphincterometric control. Rockswold, Bradley, and Chou (1973) and Torrens and Griffith (1974) described their experiences with differential sacral rhizotomy. Of Torrens' nine cases, two were unequivocal failures, two were successes, and five were "improved." No significant postoperative disturbance of bowel or sexual function occurred.

Although technique refinements, such as percutaneous radiofrequency selective sacral rhizotomy (Mulcahy and Young, 1978), have occurred, there is still much argument as to the place of these procedures within a plan of treatment for detrusor hyperactivity. Torrens (1985) quotes successful results in collected groups of patients that range from 48% in patients with idiopathic instability (presumably urodynamically documentable involuntary bladder hyperactivity without neurologic disease) to 81% in patients classified as having a paraplegic bladder. However, as he points out, what is meant by "success" varies from one series to another and from one patient to another. These procedures are seldom used today, and certainly should be preceded by urodynamic and urologic evaluation of the effects of selective nerve blocks before their performance, especially in patients without fixed neurologic disease or injury. Even then, unintended effects on pelvic and lower extremity sensory or motor functions may occur, with disastrous sequelae. Needless to say, the informed consent before such a procedure should be the responsibility of an experienced neurosurgeon.

Perivesical (Peripheral Bladder Denervation)

There are a number of procedures that fall into the category of those intending to achieve a peripheral parasympathetic decentralization of the bladder. As will be evident from neuroanatomic considerations discussed in the previous chapter, such attempts achieve, at best, partial peripheral denervation. The reported success rates for many of these procedures are high enough to make one wonder why they are not more commonly utilized. There seem to be a number of reasons for this. First, many clinicians feel that standard and more conservative methods are often successful in managing bladder hyperactivity in these patients. In their hands the success rates of peripheral bladder denervation in patients who fail vigorous but nonsurgical attempts at therapy are much lower than those reported. Second, there is almost a total lack of long-term follow-up in any of these procedures, and "postoperative assessment" usually means within a few months of the procedure.

Transvaginal partial denervation of the bladder was originally described by Ingelmann-Sundberg in 1959. This procedure has been utilized mostly for the treatment of refractory urge incontinence, and in Ingelmann-Sundberg's hands, success rates of up to 80% have been achieved (Ingelmann-Sundberg, 1980). Mundy (1985) cites reports of the successes of others in 50%–65% of cases.

Cystolysis is a term used to describe extensive perivesical dissection and mobilization with division of the superior vesical pedicle and the ascending branches of the inferior vesical pedicle (Leach et al.,

1983). At the conclusion of this procedure, the bladder is completely mobilized from all surrounding attachments except for the ureters, a portion of the inferior vesical pedicle that contributes blood supply to the ureter, and the completely mobilized urethra. The intent originally was to provide relief of bladder pain in patients with refractory interstitial cystitis. The procedure was originally reported by Worth and Turner-Warwick (1973) and was used by Freiha and Stamey (1980) in a small heterogenous group of patients with symptomatic bladder hyperactivity. Leach et al. (1983) originally reported that 28 of 32 patients so treated experienced partial or complete relief of their preoperative pain. Permanent retention occurred in seven of their 32 cases, and in six patients, intractable frequency continued.

Supratrigonal transsection of the bladder (cystocystoplasty) was first reported by Turner-Warwick and Ashken (1967) as a method of achieving a similar peripheral neural decentralization of the bladder body. Mundy (1985) has cited the encouraging reports of others, and reviewed his larger experience. Of 104 patients with a follow-up of 1–5 years, 74% were cured, 14% were improved, and 12% were failures. Between 20–32 months, 10% of the group initially judged to have a satisfactory response suffered relapse, giving a long-term subjective success rate of 65%. Thirty-five percent of those who claimed to be symptomatically cured had reverted to stable detrusor behavior, prompting Mundy to comment that a symptomatic cure did not necessarily mean a urodynamic one, and a symptomatic failure did not necessarily mean a urodynamic failure.

Augmentation Cystoplasty

Enterocystoplasty is the most major of surgical procedures for the treatment of storage failure secondary to bladder dysfunction. Originally, this procedure was used primarily for the treatment of bladder contraction secondary to tuberculosis or other types of fibrosis (Smith et al., 1977). The original UCLA experience included some patients with neurogenic bladder dysfunction, and the indications of the procedure were subsequently widened to produce very favorable results in this group of patients who had failed more conservative management (Linder et al., 1983). Although controversy exists regarding the optimal method of bladder reconstruction, and regarding the amount of bladder to be removed, successful results have been reported by a number of clinicians, as long as the technique employed avoids making a diverticulum of the augmenting bowel patch (Bramble, 1982; Mundy and Stephenson, 1985). Goldwasser and Webster (1986) have nicely reviewed the subject and categorized success rates by dysfunction etiology. Positive results have been obtained in 80%–90% of patients with tuberculous cystitis, interstitial cystitis, and neurogenic bladder dysfunction, while the success rate in a small number of patients with radiation injury to the bladder has been in the neighborhood of 50%. Many of these patients will experience emptying failure afterward, and in most of these, preoperative prediction of this phenomenon is possible by careful urodynamic evaluation. Sphincter weakening procedures may then be employed, or IC may be used to obviate this problem. Storage failure secondary to bladder dysfunction and a significant sphincter component may be safely managed with augmentation cystoplasty in combination with the use of an artificial urinary sphincter. IC can even be performed safely under these circumstances.

Increasing Outlet Resistance

Physiotherapy

By periodically carrying out various pelvic floor exercises for several months, it is possible for at least females to increase pelvic striated muscle tone, and to control minor degrees of prolapse and sphincteric incontinence (Jeffcoate, 1975; Greenhill, 1979). Kegel's exercises are designed to improve the functioning of the pubococcygeus muscles. These exercises involve voluntary tensing of the perineal muscles approximately 20 times in the morning, afternoon, and evening to strengthen the perineal muscular, fascial, and elastic tissues. Patients are instructed to contract their perineal muscles as though interrupting the flow of urine and to squeeze the vaginal muscles while drawing up the perineum and rectum as though interrupting a bowel movement. Every effort should be made to motivate the patient to learn the exercise routine correctly and to practice it conscientiously and on a daily basis. In uncomplicated urinary stress incontinence, consistent exercise is said to bring symptomatic improvement within six weeks, although several months are required to bring all supportive and sphincteric structures to optimal capacity. In our experience, only the most minor degrees of sphincteric incontinence can be significantly improved in this way.

Electrical Stimulation

Intravaginal and anal electrical stimulation have been utilized to treat storage failure by increasing outlet resistance as well as by decreasing bladder contractility (see previous text). The mechanism involves indirect stimulation of the striated pelvic floor musculature through branches of the pudendal nerve (Erlandson and Fall, 1977; Merrill et al., 1975; Teague and Merrill, 1977). In cats, additional urethral closure is provided by a pudendal to hypogastric reflex that stimulates the smooth muscle of the bladder neck and proximal urethra via an α-adrenergic effect. In "properly selected cases," initial cure or improvement rates range as high as 50%–80%, figures that we have not been able to reproduce. One must remember to select the proper unit, as parameters for this type of stimulation differ from those employed to inhibit bladder contractility.

Pharmacologic Therapy

α-*Adrenergic Agonists*

The bladder neck and proximal urethra contain a preponderance of α-adrenergic receptor sites that, when stimulated, produce smooth muscle contraction. Such stimulation alters the urethral pressure profile by increasing maximum urethral pressure (MUP) and maximum urethral closure pressure (MUCP) (Ek et al., 1978). Various orally administered pharmacologic agents are available to produce α-adrenergic sitmulation with relatively mild side effects. Potential side effects of all of the agents that produce a peripheral α-adrenergic sympathetic effect include blood pressure elevation, anxiety, and insomnia due to central nervous system stimulation. They may also cause headache, tremor, weakness, dizziness, respiratory difficulties, palpitations, and cardiac arrhythmias. All of these agents should be used with caution in patients with hypertension, cardiovascular disease, and hyperthyroidism (Weiner, 1980).

Ephedrine is a noncatecholamine sympathomimetic agent that owes part of its peripheral action to the release of norepinephrine, but that also directly stimulates both α- and β-adrenergic receptors (Weiner, 1980). The oral adult dosage is 25–50 mg, four times daily. Some tachyphylaxis develops to its peripheral actions, probably as a result of depletion of norepinephrine stores. Pseudoephedrine is a stereoisomer of ephedrine that is used for similar indications with similar precautions (Wein, 1986). The adult dose is 30–60 mg, four times daily, and the 30-mg dose form is available in the United States without a prescription. Norephedrine chloride in a dose of 75–100 mg was shown to acutely increase MUP and MUCP in women with urinary stress incontinence (Ek et al., 1978). At a 300-ml bladder volume, the MUP rose from 82 to 100 cm H_2O and the MUCP rose from 63 to 95 cm H_2O. The functional profile length did not change significantly. A 14-day double-blind crossover study comparing the effects of norephedrine to placebo showed that reduction of urinary leakage with the drug as compared with placebo occurred in 12 of 22 patients. Diokno and Taub (1975) reported a good to excellent response in 27 of 38 patients with sphincteric incontinence treated with ephedrine sulfate. They noted that beneficial effects were most often achieved in those with minimal to moderate wetting, and that little benefit was achieved in patients with severe stress incontinence. Obrink and Bunne (1978), however, noted that 100 mg of norephedrine chloride twice daily did not improve severe stress incontinence sufficiently to offer an alternative to surgical treatment. They further noted in their group of ten such patients that the MUCP was not influenced at rest or with stress at low or moderate bladder volumes.

Phenylpropanolamine hydrochloride shares the pharmacologic properties of ephedrine and is approximately equal in peripheral potency while causing less central stimulation (Weiner, 1980). Utilizing doses of 50 mg, three times daily, Awad et al. (1978) found that, after four weeks of therapy, 11 of 13 females and six of seven males with stress incontinence (severity not noted) were significantly improved. MUCP was increased from a mean of 47 to 72 cm H_2O in the empty bladder and from 43 to 58 cm H_2O with a full bladder. Fifty milligrams of phenylpropanolamine was combined with 8 mg of chlorpheniramine (an antihistamine) and 2.5 mg of isopropamide (an antimuscarinic) as a sustained-release capsule used primarily for relief of symptoms of allergic rhinitis (Ornade). Using one capsule twice daily, Stewart et al. (1976) found that, of 77 women with urinary stress incontinence, 18 were completely cured, 28 were much better, 6 were slightly better, and 25 were no better. In 11 men with postprostatectomy stress incontinence, the numbers in the corresponding categories were 1, 2, 1, and 7. Subsequently, Montague and Stewart (1979) carried out urethral profilometry in 12 women with moderate to marked stress incontinence and six women with no history of incontinence. The MUP increased more than 20% in 11 of the incontinent women and only 1 in the continent group. Rees and Ransley (1980) reported on the use of Ornade in 83 children with daytime wetting from a variety of causes. Of 24 children with bladder neck incompetence, 41% were cured, 29% had minimal symptoms, and 12% were improved. Interestingly, of 31 patients with bladder instability, the corresponding improved percentages were 24%, 24%, and 20%. The latter beneficial effect may have been due to the anticholinergic agent in the preparation. Treatment had to be discontinued in eight children because of side effects; 23 other children had mild and transient side effects. Major surgery was avoided by drug treatment in four children. The formulation of Ornade has now been changed, such that each capsule contains only 75 mg of phenylpropanolamine and 12 mg of chlorpheniramine. It is also available as a liquid.

Phenylpropanolamine is no longer a drug that can be obtained only by prescription in the United States. It is readily available as a component of many appetite suppressants, and a readily available and inexpensive source of this agent is available simply by asking patients to obtain a particular brand that contains 50–75 mg of phenylpropanolamine with no caffeine and with a minimum of extra ingredients.

Although some clinicians report spectacular cure and improvement rates with α-adrenergic agonists in patients with sphincteric urinary incontinence, our own experience coincides with those who report that treatment with such agents often produces improvement but rarely total dryness in cases of severe or even moderate stress incontinence. A clinical trial is certainly worthwhile, however, and will at the least assure the patient that the possibility of one type of nonsurgical therapy has been explored.

β-*Adrenergic antagonists*

Theoretically, β-adrenergic blocking agents might be expected to "unmask" or potentiate an α-adrenergic effect, thereby increasing outlet resistance. Gleason et al. (1974) reported success in treating certain patients with stress urinary incontinence with propranolol, a β-adrenergic blocking agent, with oral doses of 10 mg four times daily. The beneficial effect, however, became manifest only after 4–10 weeks of treatment, a difficult fact to explain on a pharmacologic basis. Although such treatment has been suggested as an alternative method of drug therapy in patients with hypertension and sphincteric incontinence, few—if any—subsequent reports of such efficacy have appeared, and others have reported no significant changes in urethral profile pressures in normal women after β-adrenergic blockade (Donker and Van der Sluis, 1976). Though 10 mg four times a day is a relatively small dosage of propranolol, it should be recalled that the major potential side effects of the drug are related to the drug's therapeutic β-blocking effects. Heart failure may develop as well as an increase in airway resistance, and asthma is a contraindication to its use. Abrupt discontinuation may precipitate an exacerbation of anginal attacks and rebound hypertension (Weiner, 1980).

Estrogen

Salmon et al. first reported the use of estrogen in the treatment of stress urinary incontinence in 1941. Raz et al. (1973) found that a daily dose of 2.5 mg of Premarin (conjugated estrogens) improved stress incontinence and increased urethral pressures in postmenopausal patients, effects that they attributed to mucosal proliferation with a consequently improved "mucosal seal effect" and to enhancement of the α-adrenergic contractile response of urethral smooth musculature to endogenous catecholamines. Schreiter et al. (1976) reported similar benefits after ten days of treatment with daily divided doses of 6 mg of estriol. They showed also that the effects of estrogen and of exogenous α-adrenergic stimulation were additive. Hodgson et al. (1978) reported that the sensitivity of the rabbit urethra to α-adrenergic stimulation was estrogen dependent, as castration caused a decreased sensitivity, and treatment with low levels of estrogen reversed the defect.

Rud (1980a) studied the effects of 4-mg daily doses of estradiol and 8-mg daily doses of estriol on 30 women with an average age of 61 years, 24 of whom had stress urinary incontinence. Profilometry parameters were recorded at a bladder volume of 200 ml using microtransducer technique. Small but statistically significant changes occurred in the MUP (59–63 cm H_2O), functional urethral length (25–28 mm), and actual urethral length (33–37 mm). No statistically significant change occurred in urethral closure pressure (37–39 cm H_2O). Eight of the 24 incontinent patients experienced subjective and objective improvement, 9 experienced subjective improvement only, and 7 experienced neither subjective nor objective improvement. There was no correlation between subjective or objective improvement and the previously mentioned urodynamic measurements. However, in 18 patients pressure transmission to the urethra was recorded during cough, and in seven of these this improved. All of these had subjective improvement and five were shown to be objectively dry. Rud pointed out that it is hard to believe that the small changes in urodynamic measurements, even though statistically significant, are directly related to resumption of continence. He noted also that the increased pressure transmission ratio might be due to factors outside the urethra—either in the striated musculature of the pelvic floor or in the periurethral vasculature or supporting tissues. Interestingly, he found no changes in urodynamic measurements in five continent and three stress-incontinent females with cystic glandular hyperplasia treated with a single injection of 1,000 mg of intramuscular progesterone, except that the pressure transmission ratio was lower in the three patients in whom this was measured.

Rud (1980b) also studied profilometry during the menstrual cycle in six females. There was no change in any profilometric values during the menstrual cycle and no correlation between estrogen levels and MUP. It may be, as he suggested, that at physiological levels estrogens have little influence on urodynamic measurements related to continence, and that only pharmacological doses cause urodynamically significant changes; further, pharmacological doses may alter responses to other exogenous autonomic stimulation, particularly α-adrenergic, as the previously described laboratory experiments by Hodgson et al. (1978) would suggest.

Beisland et al. (1981) administered 80 mg of estriol intramuscularly every four weeks in combination with an oral dosage of phenylpropanolamine of 50 mg twice daily to a group of 13 patients with what they described as an incompetent urethral closure mechanism, that is, proximal sphincter hypofunction. Patients with genuine stress incontinence were excluded. These patients had a poor urethral pressure profile and a low MUCP. All patients, however, had adequate transmission of increased abdominal pressure to the bladder and to the urethra. Eight of these patients became continent, and four showed improvement. The average MUCP increased from 24.6 to 43.6 cm H_2O ($P<.005$). In the one patient in whom MUCP did not change, the clinical condition likewise was unchanged.

Levin et al. (1981) have shown that parenteral estrogen administration can change the α-adrenergic receptor content and the autonomic innervation of the lower urinary tract of immature female rabbits. Whether these experiments have any clinical significance is unknown. Certainly, estrogen therapy seems capable of facilitating urinary storage in some female patients by increasing outlet resistance, and there is evidence of an augmentative or perhaps additive effect with α-adrenergic therapy in this regard. Whether the levels achieved by the commonly used oral or parenteral estrogen preparations or by estrogen vaginal creams (which simply provide a convenient vehicle for systemic absorption) actually increase the α-adrenergic receptor content of the smooth muscle of the bladder outlet or the "mucosal seal effect" is still a matter for speculation and is currently under study.

The potential long-term effects of such treatment must be carefully considered, however, in the light of the current controversy over whether estrogen therapy predisposes to the development of endometrial carcinoma. At the very least, if a beneficial effect on the lower urinary tract is achieved by a regimen that uses estrogenic therapy alone or in combination with other therapy, the lowest maintenance dose of estrogen therapy possible should ultimately be used, one which it is to be hoped is below that used for replacement therapy in menopausal and postmenopausal women.

Vesicourethral Suspension

Fixation of the vesicourethral junction in a physiologic position has been observed to correct genuine stress urinary incontinence in the female in 85%–90% of cases. Although the origins of this procedure are steeped in uromythology, an approach employing a retropubic exposure seems to have been reported first by Hepburn (1920), who anchored the bladder neck of a young girl to the periosteum of the pubis for the treatment of urethral prolapse. Bonney (1923) seems to have been one of the first clinicians to correlate correction of stress urinary incontinence with elevation and fixation of the vesicourethral junction. As far as the timing of the first true description of a retropubic vesicourethral suspension procedure for stress urinary incontinence, there is some disagreement. Williams (1974) described an operation involving retropubic mobilization of the vesicourethral junction with paired catgut sutures placed through the bladder wall and the pubic periosteum. The Marshall-Marchetti-Krantz operation was not reported until 1949, but was actually first reported as being done initially in 1944 (Marshall et al., 1949).

Innumerable modifications of the Marshall-Marchetti-Krantz procedure and innumerable other procedures designed to fix the vesicourethral junction in a physiologic position have been described, enough to convince these authors that: (1) there is not a "best" procedure for correcting genuine stress urinary incontinence; (2) a good surgeon who understands the pathophysiology of incontinence and who intelligently arrives at a diagnosis of genuine stress urinary incontinence in a given patient will have surgical success with any one of a number of methods with which he or she is comfortable; (3) there is a substantial lack of agreement as to what these procedures are actually designed to do; and (4) substantial disagreement exists as to the urodynamic effects of these various procedures. All of these operations seem to have in common the fact that they do indeed restore the physiologic position of the bladder neck-proximal urethral area, allowing transmission of intra-abdominal pressure increases to urethral as well as bladder pressure. This seems to us to be the common denominator shared by all these procedures, although other authors have cited other factors that they feel are important in correcting stress urinary incontinence, notably, increasing urethral closure pressure, increasing functional urethral length, restoring bladder neck competence, and increasing support to the bladder neck. A brief description of some of these procedures follows.

The Marshall-Marchetti-Krantz operation (Fig 59) most commonly is carried out by approximating the periurethral and vaginal fascia to the back of the cartilaginous portion of the pubic symphysis. Although the original procedure was done through a horizontal suprapubic incision, a vertical incision may yield better exposure in patients who represent failures of previous pelvic surgical procedures. It should be noted that the original procedure (Marshall et al., 1949) involved mobilization of the urethra to within 1 cm of the meatus, and employed three no. 1 doubled chromic sutures inserted equidistant from each other on either side of the urethra, the sutures catching the deep vaginal wall and the lateral wall of the urethra. A similar suture was placed lateral to the vesicourethral junction, and additional sutures placed in the vaginal wall to bolster the repair. Additional sutures were also placed between the musculature of the lower and lateral bladder and the posterior rectus sheath to further close the space of Retzius. Most surgeons who perform this operation do so in a fashion similar to that pictured here, and perform the surgery utilizing absorbable sutures. Some surgeons prefer to open the bladder to facilitate suture placement, some use nonabsorbable sutures, and some, who consider urethral lengthening to be the primary therapeutic goal, place sutures only between the bladder and rectus fascia (Lapides, 1971).

Retropubic colposuspension was first described by Burch in 1961, and was designed to accomplish repositioning and fixation of the vesicourethral junction without the need for retaining sutures in the pubis (Fig 60). The suture placement generally commences distally at the level of the vesicourethral junction, although some surgeons prefer a midurethral level. Fixation is to Cooper's ligament. Some feel that this operation gives broader support to the urethra and bladder base, and avoids the risk of urethral compression. Potential enteroceles in the pouch of Douglas must be obliterated by successive purse-string sutures in this area (Stanton, 1986).

The needle suspension procedure was first introduced by Pereyra in 1959. Numerous modifications of this procedure have evolved, and currently there are two modifications in common use by urologists in the United States, both of which involve endoscopic control to make sure that the suspending sutures are not passed through the lumen of the bladder or urethra. The Stamey procedure (Fig 61) utilizes the in-

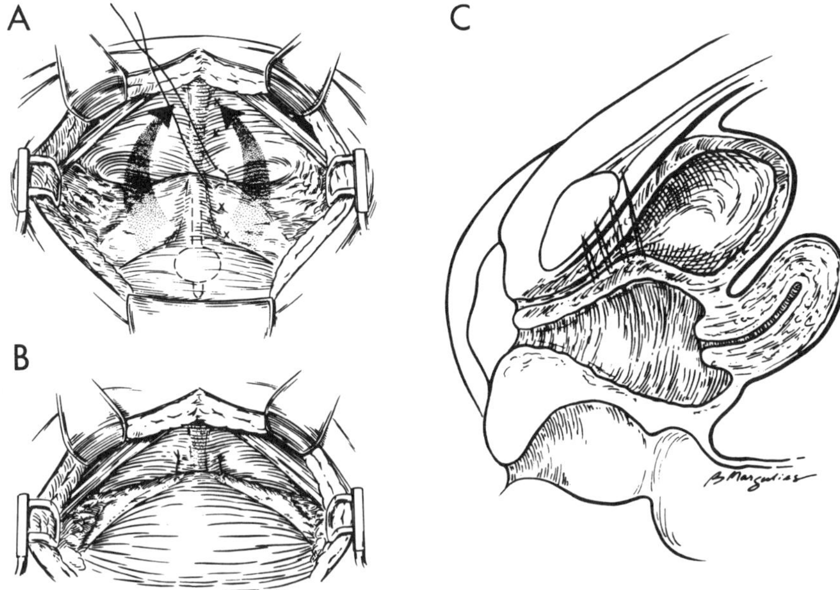

FIG 59.
The Marshall-Marchetti-Krantz (MMK) procedure. This procedure corrects stress urinary incontinence by approximating the periurethral and vaginal fascia to the underside of the pubic symphysis with three or four pairs of sutures. **A,** this shows the placement of the sutures in the periurethral and vaginal fascia and at the level of the vesicourethral junction. The *large, stippled, upward-curved arrows* point out the sites of suture attachment on the underside of the pubic symphysis. The orientation of this view is retropubical, as the surgeon would see it. Accurate placement of the sutures is important to achieve satisfactory suspension, and in order to ensure good fixation, it is helpful to take a double bite through the periurethral fascia and anterior vaginal wall, taking care not to put the suture through the vaginal mucosa. Insertion of the sutures is facilitated by elevation of the anterior vaginal wall. It is usually helpful for the surgeon to use his left hand to do this while placing the sutures with the right hand. **B,** this is the retropubic view after the sutures have been tied individually, commencing with the more distal pair. While the surgeon is tying the sutures it is helpful to have the assistant elevate the vaginal wall. The most proximal suture may need to be passed through the insertion of the rectus abdominal muscle. **C,** lateral view showing correction of the anatomic abnormality contributing to stress urinary incontinence by the MMK procedure. Here, the most proximal sutures are shown passing through the insertion of the rectus abdominus muscle. (From Webster GD: The urethra, in Paulson DF (ed): *Genitourinary Surgery*. New York, Churchill Livingstone, 1984. Used with permission.)

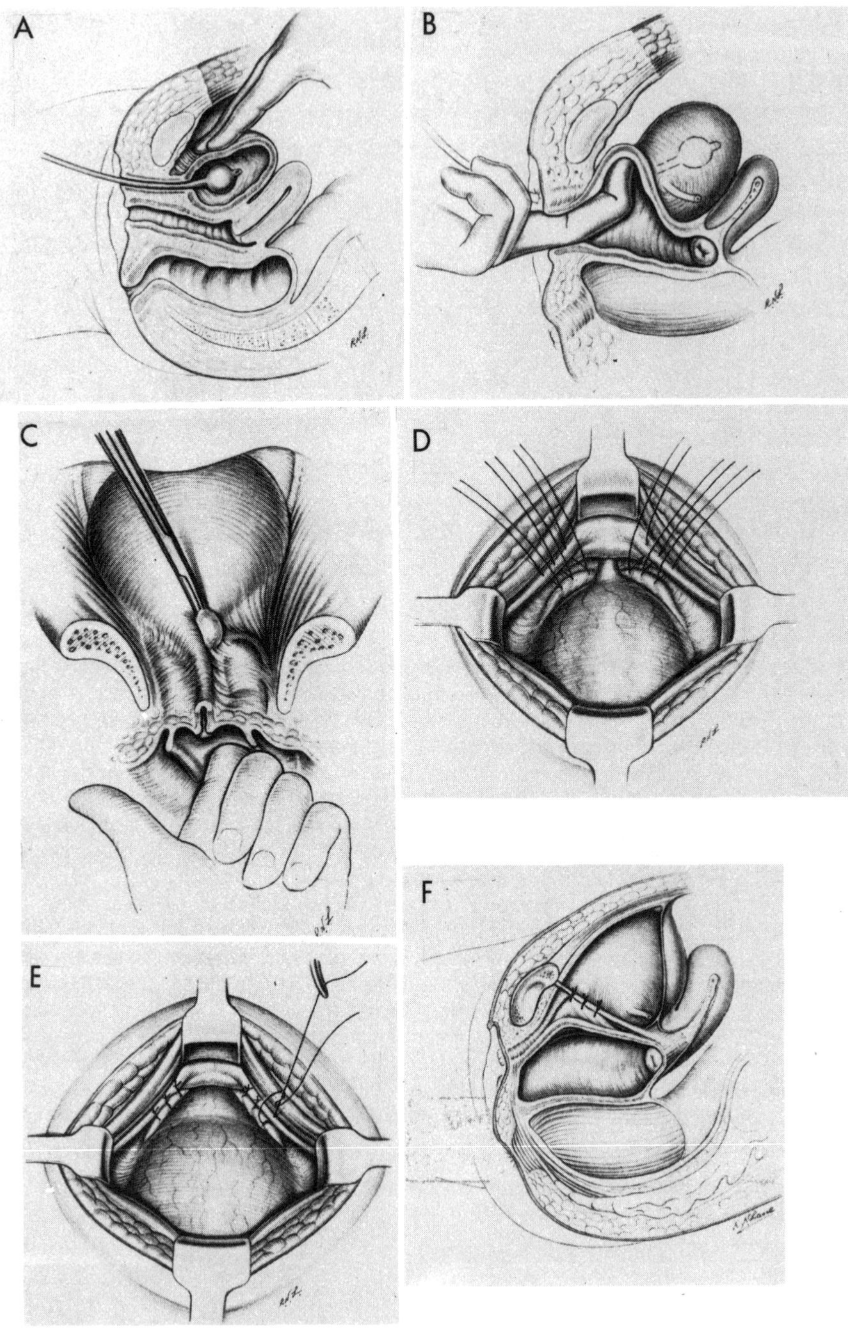
A
B
C
D
E
F

tact tissues lateral to the vesicourethral junction as the primary source of support for the suspension of the bladder neck. The Raz needle suspension (Fig 62) perforates the retropubic space between the pubic bone and the endopelvic fascia, freeing the endopelvic fascia from its lateral pubic attachments. The suspension sutures are placed through the edge of the lateral vaginal wall, incorporating the endopelvic fascia in this area (Hadley et al., 1985). Each of these modified Pereyra procedures has a large number of ardent supporters, and the results in the treatment of stress incontinence, when performed by experienced operators, seem to be similar to the best results achieved by modifications of the Marshall-Marchetti-Krantz procedure or the Burch procedure. However a comparison of long-term success rates, reports of which are few in number even concerning the older procedures, will be necessary before any valid statements regarding relative merit can be made.

Bladder Outlet Reconstruction

Reconstruction of the bladder neck is one method of restoring sphincteric continence in patients with a fixed, open bladder outlet. Other alternatives involve mechanical compression of the bladder outlet and include sling procedures, periurethral polytef injections, and the use of an artificial sphincter. Bladder neck reconstruction for the treatment of urinary incontinence was introduced by Young in 1907,

---

FIG 60.
The Burch colposuspension. **A,** sagittal section showing blunt finger dissection in the retropubic space of Retzius, between symphysis pubis and anterior surface of bladder and urethra. **B,** sagittal section showing upward pressure in the lateral vaginal fornix, to aid the surgeon in the abdominal section. **C,** retropubic view, from area of pubis, but with pubis removed. With the operator's finger still in the vagina and elevating the lateral vaginal fornix, the bladder base is dissected medially off the paravaginal fascia. **D,** retropubic surgeon's view showing three pairs of sutures in place but not tied. Some surgeons use heavy absorbable sutures, while others use nonabsorbable sutures. The sutures are inserted into the paravaginal fascia and then to the nearest point on the ipsilateral iliopectineal ligament. The most distal (caudal) sutures are inserted opposite the bladder neck and not lower. The next two sutures are inserted more proximally (cephalad) alongside the bladder base. The lateral vaginal fornix should be elevated toward the iliopectineal ligament as the corresponding suture is being placed through the ligament, so as to position the suture accurately. **E,** this illustrates tying of the sutures, showing approximation of the paravaginal tissue to the iliopectineal ligaments. **F,** sagittal section showing elevation of the bladder neck and bladder base on a shelf of paravaginal fascia, sutured to the iliopectineal ligament. (From Stanton SL: Colposuspension, in Stanton SL, Tanagho EA (eds): *Surgery of Female Incontinence.* Berlin, Springer Verlag, 1986. Used with permission.)

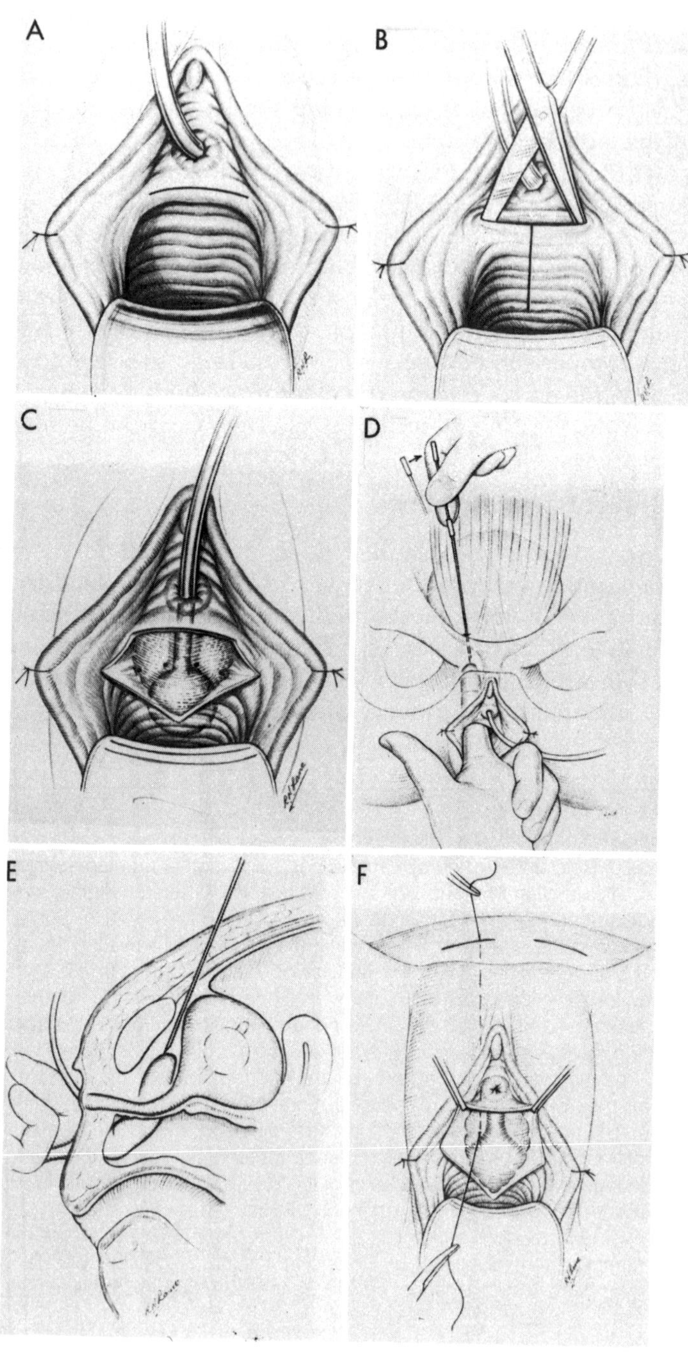
A
B
C
D
E
F

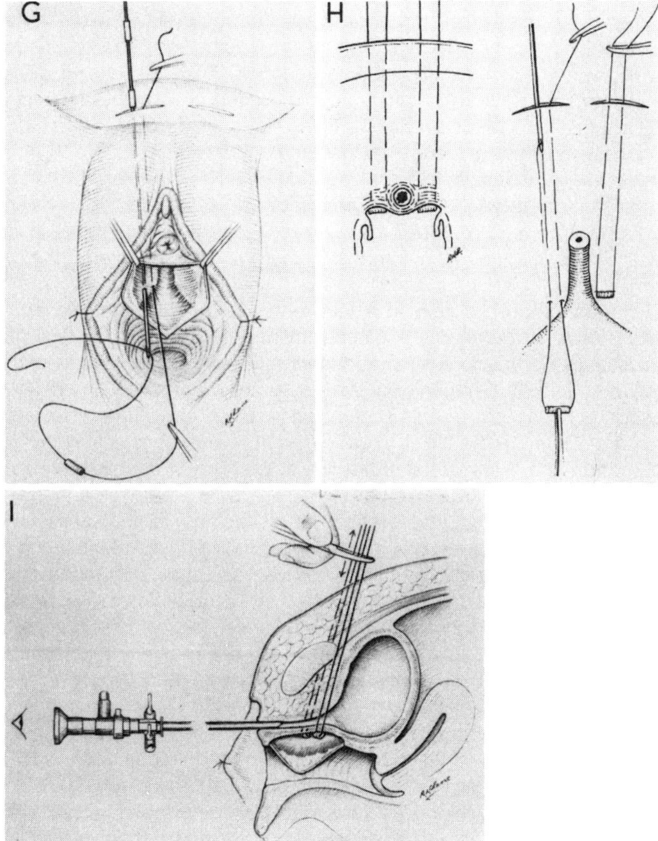

FIG 61.
The Stamey procedure. **A,** a transverse incision is made below the urethral meatus at the level of the vaginal wall. If the urethra is 2.5 cm or less, the incision is begun just below the meatus. If the urethra is longer, the incision can be made closer to the bladder neck. There is generally a convenient fold of tissue at least 2 cm from the bladder neck, and the incision may often be made at this level. **B,** the vaginal wall is carefully separated by dissection from the urethra and trigone. The tips of the scissors must be directed posteriorly toward the floor at all times to avoid entering the bladder. Adequate exposure is generally achieved by simply spreading the Metzenbaum scissors laterally in a posterior direction, and then incising this anterior flap in the midline. The Foley catheter balloon should be easily palpable within the incision, thereby determining exactly the location of the bladder neck. **C,** the two dots on either side of the urethrovesical junction indicate the sites of suture placement. Dissection of the fascia between the vaginal wall and the overlying urethra and trigone should be avoided. This pubovesicocervical fascia, together with the overlying endopelvic fascia, is the primary source of support of the bladder neck in this type suspension. **D,** two suprapubic incisions, 3–5 cm long, are made to the left and

Continued.

FIG 61 (cont.).
right of the midline, at the upper border of the pubic symphysis. These are carried down to the rectus fascia. This is generally done at the beginning of the procedure, and the incisions are packed with antibiotic soaked sponges. After the vaginal dissection, this coronal view shows a 15° angled Stamey needle passed through the right anterior rectus fascia and turned toward the undersurface of the pubic symphysis. This avoids any intestinal perforation and allows guidance alongside the urethrovesical junction. After the needle perforates the rectus fascia, it is not long before its tip will be felt by the finger shown in the vaginal incision at the point of the bladder neck. **E,** sagittal view showing location of the needle point on the tip of the index finger. Once the needle is in place, the right-angle cystoscope is used to make sure that the needle has not entered the bladder and that it has not been placed submucosally or intramuscularly. Vertical motion of the needle will tell the surgeon endoscopically whether the needle is exactly positioned at the level of the bladder neck. If the needle is placed improperly, it should be repositioned. **F,** a heavy monofilament nylon suture is threaded through the eye of the needle and the needle withdrawn suprapubically. Both ends of the suture are clamped. **G,** the Foley catheter is reintroduced, and the special needle once again passed 1 cm lateral to the first passage, and a Dacron or Gore-Tex sleeve is threaded on. It is important to maintain the position of the second passage 1 cm lateral to the first at the level of the bladder neck. After the suture is threaded through the Dacron or Gore-Tex bolster, the needle is then withdrawn suprapubically, pulling the second pass of the suture with it, thereby establishing the suspended loop with the buttress vaginally, reinforcing the pubocervical and endopelvic fascia. The bolsters should settle easily into the vaginal space at the side of the bladder neck. **H,** the identical procedure is then repeated for the incision on the opposite side, so that the two suspending sutures, each with its buttress, are located on either side of the bladder neck. The two loops, as pictured, support a shelf of pubovesicocervical fascia on either side of the bladder neck. **I,** the panendoscope is then introduced and used to observe the point of urethral closure when each suspending loop is pulled up suprapubically. Closure generally occurs exactly at the bladder neck with the suspending loops symmetrically placed. The vaginal incision must be closed first before tying the suspending sutures. If the rectus fascia is weak, each suture is passed through a small oval of Silastic, and tied over this, which then rests directly on the rectus fascia. (From Stamey TA: Endoscopic suspension of the bladder neck, in Stanton SL, Tanagho EA (eds): *Surgery of Female Incontinence.* New York, Springer-Verlag, 1986. Used with permission.)

---

and was subsequently modified by Dees (1949) and Leadbetter (1964). Procedures utilizing the Young-Dees principle involve construction of a neourethra from the posterior surface of the bladder wall and trigone. In the male, the prostatic urethra affords additional substance for closure and increase in outlet resistance. The Leadbetter modification involves proximal reimplantation of the ureters to allow more extensive tubularization of the trigone. Long-term success rates of between 60% and 70% have been achieved (Leadbetter, 1985). Tanagho (1969, 1981) has described a procedure based on a similar concept but using the anterior bladder neck to create a functioning neourethral sphincter. A success rate of 70% has been reported.

Surgical Mechanical Compression

Periurethral Polytef Injection

The injection of polytef paste periurethrally to increase urethral resistance was first reported by Berg (1973), and its use has been promoted and developed primarily by Politano and co-workers (Politano et al., 1974; Politano, 1982; Vorstman et al., 1985). Most clinicians inject the polytef paste transurethrally, and an ingrowth of fibroblasts is stimulated, which produces a bolstering effect, but does not stricture the urethra. Good results have been reported by Politano's group in up to 70% of patients. Schulman et al. (1983) reported a 70% cure rate in 56 women with stress urinary incontinence, with an additional 16% showing marked improvement. Lim et al. (1983) described cure in 21% and benefit in an additional 54% of 28 females so treated. Deane et al. (1985) described four cures and two improvements in six females with genuine stress incontinence, and five cures and six improvements in 22 females with bladder neck incompetence at rest. They were able to achieve only one improvement in eight males with postprostatectomy incontinence. Malizia et al. (1984) have expressed concern regarding the potential of distal embolization of the polytef particles, such as they observed in laboratory animals. They recommended against its use in children until long-term effects were further investigated. However, clinically significant instances of such embolization have not been reported in patients so treated up to this point.

Sling Procedures

The suburethral sling procedure, as cited by Ullery (1953), was first reported by vonGiordono in 1907. Since that time, a considerable number of procedures utilizing this principle have been described, employing either autologous or alloplastic material. These procedures have been used for patients with all types of stress incontinence, and they are quite effective in patients with recurrent stress incontinence and pelvic floor weakness, especially after repeated unsuccessful surgeries. Among urologists, McGuire (1978, 1981, 1985) has written most extensively about this procedure and feels that its use should probably be restricted to patients with poorly functional or nonfunctional urethral sphincter mechanisms, as opposed to those with stress incontinence because of urethral hypermobility. The procedure does involve elevation and fixation of the urethra in a normal retropubic position, and thus can be used as a treatment for genuine stress incontinence. How-

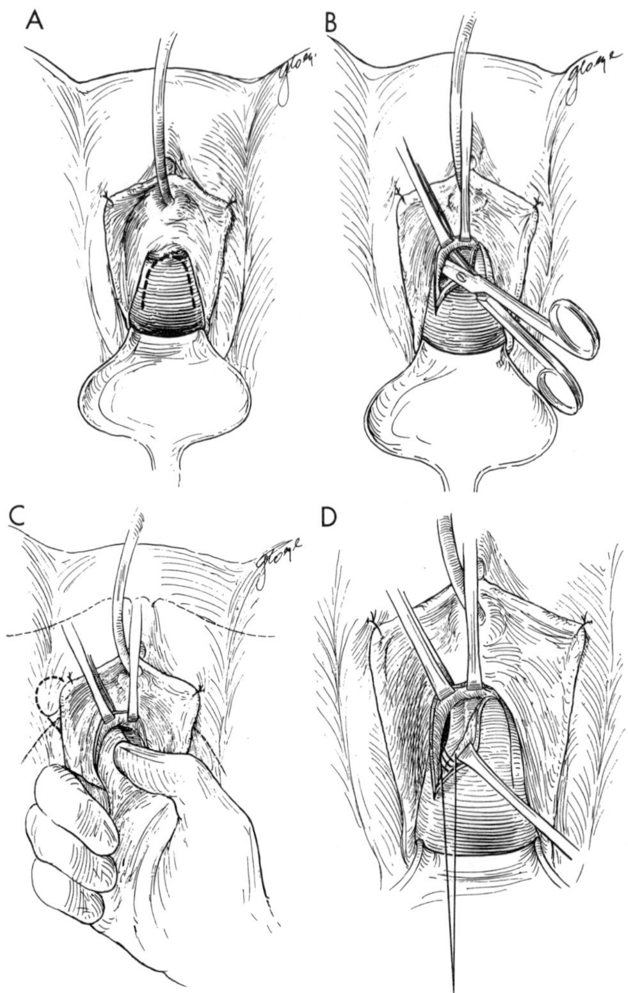

FIG 62.
The Raz bladder neck suspension. **A,** in the dorsal lithotomy position, a Foley catheter is inserted into the bladder and a posterior vaginal retractor is used to expose the anterior vaginal wall. Traction on the catheter facilitates identification of the level of the bladder neck. An inverted-U incision is made in the anterior surface of the vaginal wall. The apex should cross the level of the midurethra. **B,** a plane is created underneath the vaginal wall and advanced to the endopelvic fascia. Dissection proceeds laterally toward the pubic bone. The retropubic space is entered either bluntly or sharply between the pubic bone and the endopelvic fascia. **C,** the index finger is used to enter the retropubic space and to mobilize the urethra and the bladder neck. The endopelvic fascia is gently freed from its lateral attachments to the pubic bone. If the retropubic space is entered in the proper

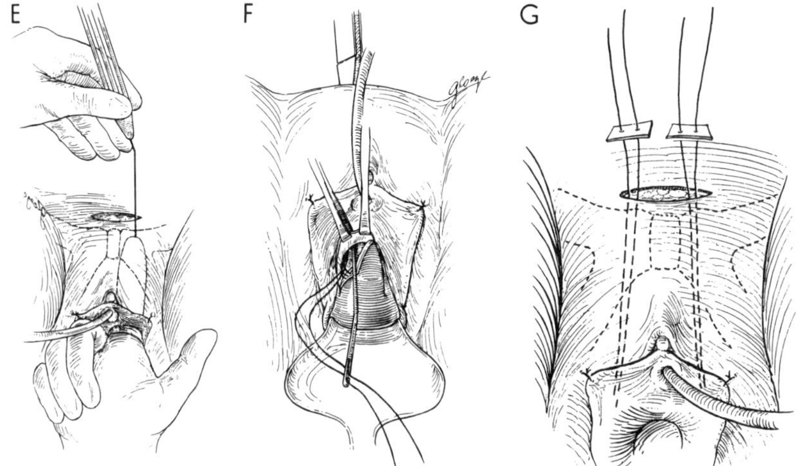

plane, bleeding should not be troublesome. The mobilization should be extended down to the level of the ischial tuberosity to adequately mobilize the vaginal wall, bladder neck, and urethra. With scar tissue, achievement of sufficient mobility may require sharp dissection of the paraurethral and perivaginal tissues. **D,** a no. 1 Prolene helical suture is secured to the vaginal wall (excluding the epithelium) and endopelvic fascia. The suture should include at least three separate passes. After each pass, traction should be placed on the suture to test the tissue integrity and the holding power of the suture. **E,** through a transverse suprapubic incision, the anterior rectus fascia is exposed. Through this fascia the suspension needle is guided into the retropubic space and out of the vaginal introitus under finger guidance. We pass the needle twice on each side, the needle enters into the rectus fascia betin about 1–2 cm apart. Through the area in which the endopelvic fascia has been penetrated, the finger should be able to contact the needle immediately after its passage through the rectus fascia. Penetration by the bladder should therefore not occur. **F,** the two ends of each Prolene suture are threaded through the eye of the needle and withdrawn through the suprapubic incision. The identical procedure is repeated on the contralateral side; 4–5 cm of rectus fascia should lie between the Prolene sutures in the suprapubic incision. **G,** the two ends of each Prolene suture then exit through the rectus fascia approximately 1 cm apart, with 4–5 cm, of rectus fascia separating the sutures on the two sides. Endoscopic examination is then carried out to make sure there has been no perforation of the bladder or urethra. Indigo carmine and furosemide (Lasix) is given, and efflux should be seen from both ureters. With the endoscopic instrument withdrawn to the level of the midurethra, the bladder neck should elevate and close during upward traction on the Prolene sutures. Considerable force should not be necessary to accomplish this. If it is, this generally means that further mobilization is necessary. The vaginal incisions are then closed. The two ends of each suture on each side are then tied to one another. If the rectus fascia is weak these can be first threaded through a small piece of Silastic mesh, as pictured. After each suture is secured individually, they are tied to one another across the midline. (From Hadley HR, Zimmern PE, Staskin DR et al: Transvaginal needle bladder neck suspension. *Urol Clin North Am* 1985; 12:291. Used with permission.)

ever, the noncircumferential compression afforded by the sling is optimal treatment for patients with no urethral closing function of any kind and those with poor urethral smooth muscle function. One of three general types of urethral dysfunction generally forms the indication for this procedure: (1) total failure, usually resulting from direct injury to the urethra or sloughing of the urethral musculature; (2) severe weakness of the urethral smooth musculature, usually as a result of neural injury or following radical pelvic surgery; and (3) fixation and rigidity of the urethra, usually due to prior operative procedures. Although originally described through a retropubic approach, a combined vaginal and abdominal approach (Fig 63) often facilitates the procedure. The vaginal access to and dissection of the retropubic space for sling placement is similar to that provided by the Raz-type suspension procedure. Success rates of up to 90% with the pubovaginal sling operation have been reported. Many patients have difficulty resuming volitional voiding after surgery, and permanent self-intermittent catheterization may be required. Additionally, detrusor instability may occur after the procedure or be exacerbated by it, if pre-existent. Adjustment of the proper sling tension requires considerable operator experience or necessitates intraoperative urethral pressure profilometry. An increase in urethral pressure in the area of the urethra subjacent to the sling of 10 cm H_2O has given consistently good postoperative results in McGuire's experience.

Artificial Sphincter

Control of sphincteric urinary incontinence with implantable prosthetic devices has evolved rapidly over the past 15 years (Berry, 1961; Kaufman, 1970; Foley, 1947; Rosen, 1976). Clearly the most significant contribution was the introduction in 1973 by Scott et al. of a totally implantable artificial sphincter mechanism that could be used in adults and children of both sexes. Through biomechanical evolution, device improvements have led to the currently used AS 800 device (manufactured by American Medical Systems, Minnetonka, Minn.), which is composed of an inflatable snap-on cuff, a pressure-balloon reservoir, and a control assembly (Fig 64). Constructed of silicone rubber, this hydraulic device is filled with iso-osmotic contrast medium. Cuff closing pressure is regulated by the elasticity in the wall of the balloon and is partially dependent on the volume of fluid within the balloon. Fluid flow through the system is mediated by the pump and a series of unidirectional valves within the control assembly. On the side of the con-

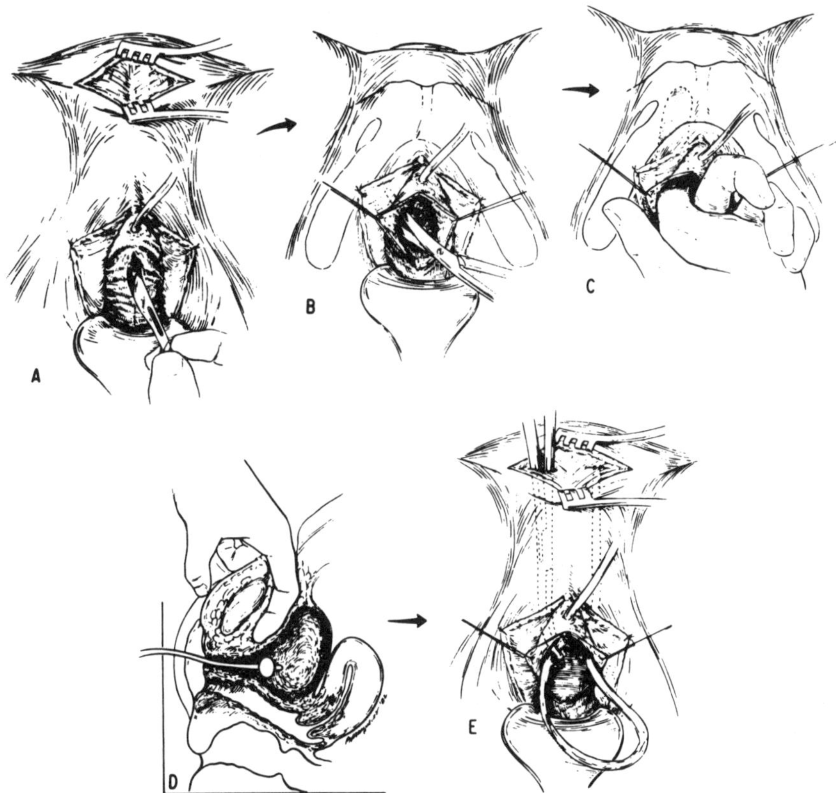

FIG 63.

Fascial sling procedure. **A,** in this variation, a combined vaginal and abdominal approach is used. **B,** after reflecting the vaginal wall from the urethra, the paraurethral musculofascial tissue is dissected into the retropubic space at the level of the bladder neck. This approach is very similar to that used in the Raz suspension procedure. **C,** this space is further digitally dissected, as in the Raz procedure. **D,** rarely, a retropubic dissection is also necessary, as pictured. **E,** the fascial sling, which may be obtained from rectus or external oblique fascia, or fascia lata, is looped around the urethrovesical junction, and fixed to the rectus fascia suprapubically. As mentioned in the text, the tension of the sling must be carefully adjusted to provide the minimum necessary to achieve the desired goal of elevation or compression. (From Webster GD: The urethra, in Paulson DF (ed): *Genitourinary Surgery.* New York, Churchill-Livingstone, 1984. Used with permission.)

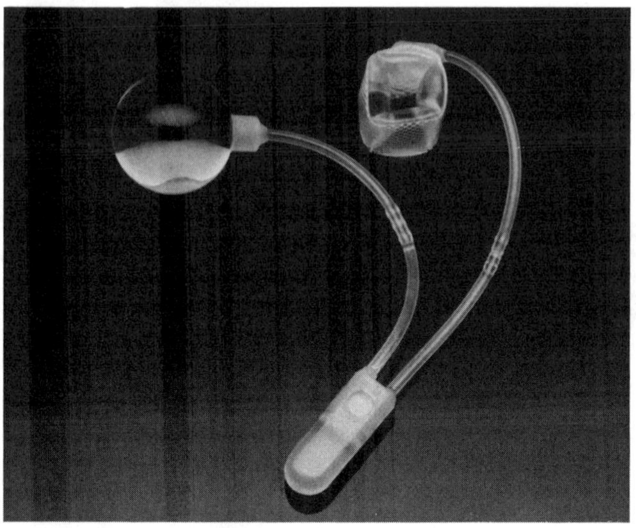

FIG 64.
The AS 800 artificial sphincter mechanism.

trol assembly is a small button that allows for manual activation and deactivation of the sphincter mechanism.

Balloon pressures have been manufactured that, under normal clinical situations, will provide for enough cuff closing pressure to ensure urinary continence but similarly will not damage the underlying tissue of the urethra or bladder neck.

Too much pressure will result in tissue ischemia and ultimate pressure necrosis with erosion of the cuff into the lumen of the underlying urethra or bladder neck. This generally is manifested by recurrent incontinence and concurrent infection around the implanted sphincter. Device removal is required for adequate healing; however, another device may be implanted later.

Identification of candidates for implantation requires a thorough neurourologic workup to properly establish the unique aspects of the patient's incontinence. Specific criteria for implantation have been established (Barrett, 1986), with most patients having true sphincteric incontinence with normal detrusor contractility and compliance. Ideal candidates are individuals with incontinence related to radical prostatectomy or transurethral resection of the prostate (TURP), neurogenic etiologies such as myelomeningocele, previous pelvic trauma, and females with failed conventional anti-incontinence procedures.

Surgical implantation of the device involves the implantation of the cuff around the bulbous urethra of adult males (Fig 65) and around the bladder neck in females and children (Fig 66). Bladder neck cuff placement may be technically challenging in patients with previous bladder neck or pelvic surgery. Dissection of the vesical rectal plane or the vesicovaginal plane, which is required for cuff placement, is carried out inferior to the point of entry of the ureters into the posterior aspect of the bladder. The pressure balloon reservoir is placed in a pocket underneath the fascia of the anterior abdominal wall and the pump control assembly is positioned in a convenient location in the subcutaneous tissues of the scrotum or labia.

The device remains in a deactivated configuration for 6–8 weeks to allow for complete healing around the pump and cuff. Device activation is carried out manually by merely compressing the pump chamber firmly. The device may again be deactivated by compressing the button on the site of the control assembly.

Results of implantation of 221 patients with the AS 800 device followed for up to three years would indicate 95% of the patients are acceptably dry. Mechanical reliability based on life-table analysis projects a 97% survivorship at three years. Although the initial results appear reasonable, the long-term results will help establish more accurately the exact role of the artificial sphincter in treating severe incontinence.

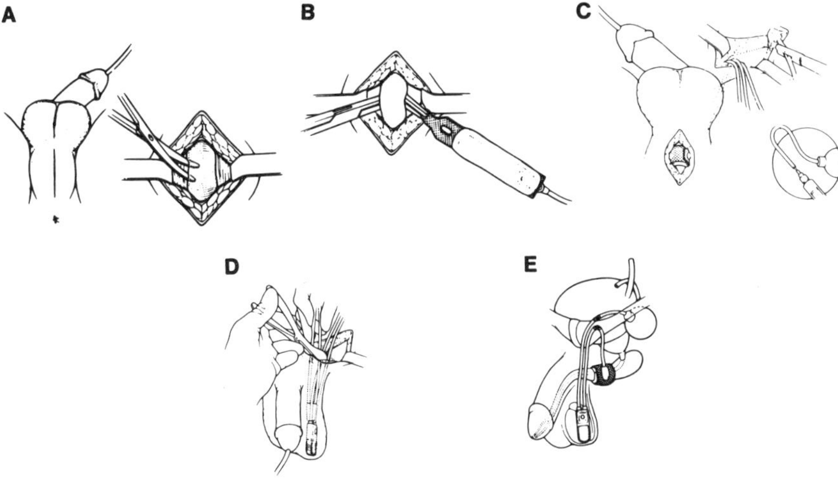

FIG 65.
Implantation of the artificial sphincter cuff around the bulbous urethra.

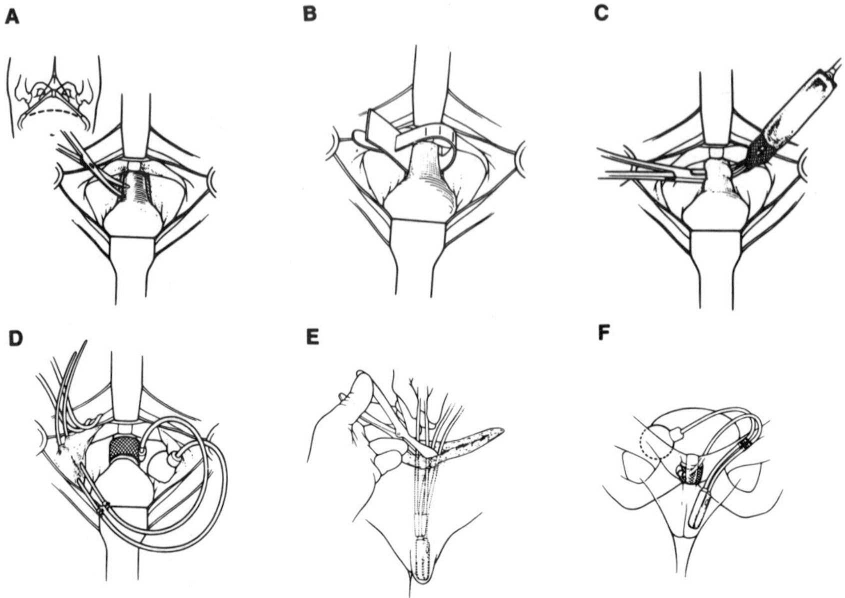

FIG 66.
Implantation of the artificial sphincter cuff around the bladder neck.

Nonsurgical Mechanical Compression

Nonsurgical occlusive devices have been used for the control of female incontinence for years. The status of these devices is somewhat confusing. Published reports are rare, and usually include a description of the particular device with "success" rates ranging from 70%–90%. Yet, there seems to be little enthusiasm for their use in general, or for any particular device, on the part of any clinician when questioned in person. Historically available devices are well described by Edwards (1975) and by Stanton (1978). "New" ones periodically appear and then characteristically disappear after adequate clinical trials. The idea is to maintain light but firm compression of the urethra with an intravaginal device. Although the concept seems simple, its execution apparently is not. Were a compression device available that was easy to apply, stayed in position for extended periods of time, was reasonably comfortable to wear, was extremely and continuously effective in preventing urinary leakage, and was easy to remove or deflate when micturition was necessary, it would obviously constitute a distinct advance in the treatment of female urinary incontinence.

Nonsurgical occlusive devices for the male are external and compress the penile urethra by squeezing the penis from two sides. Their main disadvantages include bulk, discomfort (in those with sensation) and, potentially, pressure necrosis of the urethra, especially in those patients with impaired sensation.

Continence achieved with urethral compression is applicable only to those patients with low-pressure bladders. Although any pressure system can theoretically be occluded, continued obstruction of a high-pressure system can result in disastrous lower and upper urinary tract sequelae.

Circumventing Storage Failure

Antidiuretic Hormone–Like Agents

A novel approach to the treatment of urinary frequency occurring within a specific period of time has been the use of synthetic antidiuretic hormone (vasopressin) analogues. Desmopressin acetate (DDAVP) has been used effectively in patients with central diabetes insipidus to increase the osmolality of urine and decrease its volume (intranasal spray administration of 5–20 μg produced 8–20 hours of antidiuresis in eight patients with central diabetes insipidus) (Robinson, 1976). The drug is well tolerated in both adults and children (Kosman, 1978). For diabetes insipidus, the usual adult dosage is 0.01-0.04 mg daily as a single or divided dose. (Desmopressin has a much greater antidiuretic potency than lysine or arginine vasopressin, a more prolonged duration of action [generally 8–10 hours], and virtually no pressor activity.) For children, the usual dosage range is from 0.005 to 0.03 mg daily. Large doses may cause transient headaches, nausea, and a slight increase in blood pressure. Fluid intake should be adjusted during this therapy to avoid hyponatremia and water intoxication.

The drug has been used to decrease the frequency of nocturnal enuresis. In one study of 22 children, the number of wet nights per two weeks for desmopressin-treated children was 4.2 compared with 10.9 for those given a placebo. In 19 of 22 patients the response during desmopressin therapy was better than that during placebo (Birkasova et al., 1978). A single nighttime dose of 10–40 μg was used. Ramsden et al. (1982) completed a double-blind crossover trial of desmopressin and a placebo in 21 adult patients with nocturnal enuresis who were wet more than 20 nights per month. The total number of nights wet on the active drug was statistically less than that on placebo (91 vs. 167). Sixteen patients had fewer nights wet on treatment with active drug, two showed improvement with placebo, and three showed no difference. Eight patients on the active drug became entirely dry or had only one night wet, compared with only one patient on placebo. The authors noted that three patients who had been taking active drug remained entirely dry. The dosage used was 20 mg intranasally at bedtime. Side effects were few and minor.

Hilton and Stanton (1982) used a nighttime dose of 20 mg intranasally in a double-blind placebo study of 25 female patients with nocturnal urinary frequency. The number of mean episodes per night decreased from 3.17 in the pretreatment group to 1.94 in the group treated with active drug, as compared with 2.61 in the placebo-treated group. The nocturnal urinary output, as expected, also decreased significantly in the drug-treated group. One patient already receiving treatment for hypertension with a diuretic became hypertensive with a diastolic pressure of 110 mm Hg (entrance pressure was 80 mm Hg). The authors emphasize that hypertension, ischemic heart disease, and congestive failure should all be considered contraindications to the use of this type of medication. A double-blind placebo-controlled study was also carried out in a group of 21 males with benign prostatic hypertrophy and significant nocturia (Mansson et al., 1980). Active treatment consisted of 20 mg of drug administered intranasally. This produced a mean fall in nocturia from 2.60 episodes during the control period to 1.93, statistically significantly better than the response to placebo (2.31), but hardly a significant clinical change.

Although the overall results with this type of agent in patients other than those with central diabetes insipidus seem more statistically than clinically significant, this class of treatment may prove to be useful on a long-term basis in the occasional case of nocturia or enuresis that has proved refractory to all other forms of therapy or in acute situations in which a decrease in intravesical volume and consequent urinary frequency is desired for a limited period of time.

External Collection Devices

Unfortunately, no satisfactory external collecting device has been devised for the female, primarily because of the difficulties of fixation and leakproof collection. Absorptive padding, a collection device of sorts, is a last resort for many patients. The ideal substance is one that is highly permeable and absorbent. Immediately next to the patient is generally a layer of hydrophobic material, through which the urine passes into the absorbent pad, in turn surrounded by a waterproof material to keep the clothing dry. The hydrophobic material next to the patient will ideally keep her relatively dry and reduce chafing as much as possible.

External collecting devices for the male (Texas or condom catheter) are generally successful insofar as urine collection is concerned, but are unacceptable to many patients because of the visible equipment required, the incontinence, and the "leaks" of often foul-smelling urine that can result. They can also cause severe pressure necrosis of the penis, down to and including the urethra, especially in a patient with impaired sensation (Golz, 1981). A collecting device without a single discrete roller band or application ring would seem to offer at least a theoretical advantage for this reason.

Specific Voiding Dysfunctions Associated With Neurologic Disease

Discrete neurologic lesions generally affect bladder filling and urine storage and bladder emptying in a relatively consistent fashion, dependent on the area affected. Neurologic lesions above the brain stem that affect micturition generally result in involuntary bladder contractions with changes in the smooth sphincter and striated sphincter areas analogous to those that occur in normal micturition. Patients with complete lesions of the spinal cord above spinal cord level S2, after they recover from spinal shock, generally exhibit involuntary bladder contraction with smooth sphincter synergia but striated sphincter dyssynergia. Patients with significant spinal cord trauma below that level generally do not manifest involuntary bladder contractions per se. Detrusor areflexia is the rule initially, and, depending on the extent of neurologic injury, various forms of decreased compliance during filling may occur. Damage to the neurologic outflow from the lower thoracic and upper lumbar levels may result in an open smooth sphincter area, while the area of the striated sphincter generally retains a residual resting sphincter tone, but is not under voluntary control. Spotty lesions of the spinal cord and brain stem area generally result in involuntary bladder contractions with variable degrees of striated sphincter dyssynergia or synergia, depending on the severity of the disease and the intactness of the cortical and pontine-mesencephalic regulatory tracts. In this section the most common types of voiding dysfunction that occur with specific neurologic diseases or trauma are discussed.

AT OR ABOVE THE BRAIN STEM (SUPRASPINAL)

Cerebrovascular Disease

Cerebrovascular disease is about the third most common cause of death and the most common cause of disability in the United States and Europe. Arterial thrombosis, occlusion, and hemorrhage are the most common causes, leading to ischemia and infarction of variably sized areas in the brain, usually around the internal capsule. Transient ischemia has not been associated with any particular type of bladder dysfunction, but following an occlusive episode or a hemorrhagic episode of a cerebral vessel, focal neurologic deficits often occur and voiding dysfunction of a particular type may result (Kahn, 1981; Hald and Bradley, 1982; McGuire, 1984; Mundy and Blaivas, 1984). After the initial acute episode, acute urinary retention may occur. Following the variable degree of recovery of the neurological lesion, a fixed deficit becomes apparent over a few weeks or months. During this time the symptoms of bladder dysfunction generally become apparent. The most common long-term expression of lower urinary tract dysfunction after cerebrovascular accident is detrusor hyperreflexia. Sensation is variable, but generally intact, and thus the patient has urgency. The appropriate response is to try to inhibit the involuntary bladder contraction by forceful contraction of the striated sphincter. If this can be accomplished, only urgency results; if not, urgency with incontinence results. The increase in striated sphincter EMG activity during bladder filling is usually normal until just before the involuntary contraction occurs. A burst of striated sphincter activity will be seen when the patient voluntarily attempts to inhibit this voiding contraction. If one pays attention just to the tracings, and not to the patient, this is indistinguishable from true detrusor striated sphincter dyssynergia, when in reality it is an appropriate response for a patient who does not wish to soil himself, the urodynamic table, or the urodynamic technician ("pseudodyssynergia"—Wein and Barrett, 1982). Smooth sphincter synergia is the rule, and thus the disorder is one solely of filling and storage, occasioned by detrusor hyperactivity.

Mundy and Blaivas (1984) point out some important modifying factors that must be considered in the care of such patients. This problem generally occurs in an elderly population, some of whom have preexistent involuntary bladder activity during filling and/or outlet obstruction and/or stress incontinence. These individuals may not have sought medical attention because these problems were manageable, but the additional difficulty of a physical disability makes the situation intolerable. In other words, the bladder dysfunction may be primarily due to a pre-existent problem, and may exist with outlet pathology as well, and the entire voiding dysfunction may be adversely or beneficially affected by treatment regimens that concentrate on the detrusor hyperactivity alone. Another problem relates to the effect of the confusion and disorientation that often results after such a neurologic catastrophe and the fact that many such patients become depressed—especially if they have lost their independence and then require nursing home care. Vigorous pharmacologic treatment of the detrusor hyperactivity may make these associated problems worse. Finally, some patients with dementia will lose the awareness of the desirability of voluntary urinary control. These individuals may either have involuntary bladder contractions or not. In any case, they will simply void where and when they want, because they see no reason why they shouldn't. This is generally a reflection of dementia, and there really is no treatment for this, other than trying to circumvent this problem with a collection device or pads.

Concussion

Generally, when voiding dysfunction occurs following a closed head injury, there is an initial period of detrusor areflexia followed by recovery of unstable reflex detrusor dysfunction (McGuire, 1984). This is not a very common sequela of concussion, but when it occurs, the same considerations apply as for voiding dysfunction secondary to cerebrovascular disease.

Brain Tumor

Both primary and metastatic brain tumors have been reported to be associated with disturbances of bladder function (Hald and Bradley, 1982; McGuire, 1984). When voiding dysfunction results, it is related to the localized area involved. The most frequently involved area that results in bladder dysfunction is the superior aspect of the frontal lobe (Blaivas, 1985a). Resultant voiding dysfunction consists of detrusor hyperreflexia and urinary incontinence. These individuals may have a markedly diminished awareness of all vesical events and, if so, are totally unable to even attempt suppression of the micturition reflex. Smooth and striated sphincter activity is generally synergic in the absence of attempts to suppress the involuntary detrusor reflex.

Parkinson's Disease

This degenerative disorder primarily affects the pigmented neurons of the substantia nigra. This results in a relative dopamine deficiency and a predominance of cholinergic activity in the corpus striatum. Classical neurologic symptoms include bradykinesia, tremor, and skeletal rigidity. The annual prevalence is estimated at between 100 and 150 cases per 100,000 population, with onset between the ages of 45 and 65 years, and affecting men and women equally (Mundy and Blaivas, 1984; Blaivas, 1985a). Voiding dysfunction occurs in 25%–75% of patients, but—as with cerebrovascular disease—there may be preexisting detrusor or outlet abnormalities, and the symptomatology may be affected by the various treatments that are instituted.

Symptoms generally consist of urgency, frequency, nocturia, and urge incontinence. The most common urodynamic correlate is detrusor hyperreflexia (Murnaghan, 1961; Andersen et al., 1976; Pavlokis et al., 1983). Striated sphincter dyssynergia with detrusor hyperreflexia generally does not occur, but it is less clear whether these patients retain voluntary striated sphincter control (Blaivas, 1985a).

One of the significant problems that we and others (McGuire, 1984; Mundy and Blaivas, 1984) have had in dealing with these patients is deciding whether or not male patients have anatomic outlet obstruction secondary to prostatic enlargement and whether prostatectomy is indicated in these patients. In our experience, the considerations here are slightly different than they are for a patient with voiding dysfunction following a stroke who also has outlet obstruction. Generally, detrusor contractility seems to be unimpaired in stroke patients with involuntary bladder hyperactivity, and, in the absence of dyssynergia, poor flow rates and high residual urine volumes in the male generally indicate prostatic obstruction. Outlet reduction in these patients is generally beneficial, because the functional bladder capacity improves as a result of a decrease in the residual urine volume, and one feels more comfortable in treating these patients with agents to decrease bladder contractility if they do not have concomitant anatomic bladder outlet obstruction. Male patients with Parkinson's disease and the identical symptoms and urodynamic findings do not seem to fare as well after prostatectomy. Poorly sustained bladder contractions, sometimes with slow sphincter relaxation, may occur as a result of the neurologic disease, and in these individuals prostatectomy may result in no change or in a worsening of the voiding symptoms. Acontractile bladders are unusual in Parkinson's disease, and are generally seen only in women, in which case the situation is probably representative of a pre-existent problem and unrelated to the Parkinson's disease per se.

Shy-Drager Syndrome

This uncommon degenerative disorder results in atrophy of areas in the cerebellum, brain stem, peripheral autonomic ganglia, and thoracolumbar preganglionic sympathetic neurons (Blaivas, 1985a). Patients generally present with parkinsonian symptomatology coupled with orthostatic hypotension and anhidrosis. Voiding dysfunction generally consists of detrusor hyperreflexia, a bladder neck that is open at rest, and denervation of the striated sphincter. Areflexia or poorly sustained bladder contractions may occur, however, and with diminished smooth and striated sphincter tone, may make management of the voiding dysfunction quite difficult, especially if prostatectomy seems indicated.

SPINAL CORD LESIONS

Suprasacral Spinal Cord Injury

Traumatic spinal cord injury may occur as a consequence of injury by a high-velocity missile, fracture or fracture dislocation of the spinal column, or after sudden or severe hyperextension. Spinal cord bony segments are numbered by the vertebral level, and these have a differing relationship to spinal cord segmental level at different locations. The sacral spinal cord begins at about the spinal column level of T12–L1. The spinal cord terminates in the cauda equina at the spinal column level of approximately L2. In addition to trauma, spinal cord damage may be produced by vascular disease, arteriovenous malformations, myelopathy, arachnoiditis, or myelitis.

Over the past 25 years or so, the survival of the patient with spinal cord injury has improved dramatically. This has resulted from the development of specialized centers for the care of such patients resulting in a decreased number of potentially significant complications of all types. Urologic care and urologic surveillance have undergone decided improvements, but renal failure is still one of the most common late causes of death, at least in male patients. Although amyloid disease of the kidneys accounts for some of these, bladder and outlet dysfunction and urinary tract infection with urosepsis are still significant problems. Controlled and coordinated bladder emptying depends on an intact neural axis. Bladder contractility and the occurrence of reflex bladder contractions depends on an intact conus medullaris (sacral spinal cord segments) and its afferent and efferent connections. Complete lesions above this area but below the area of the sympathetic outflow generally result in detrusor hyperreflexia, absent sensation below the level of the lesion, smooth sphincter synergia, and striated sphincter dyssynergia. Lesions above the spinal column level of T6 (spinal cord level of T7 or T8) may result in smooth sphincter dyssynergia as well.

Following a significant spinal cord injury, "spinal shock" occurs. This refers to a decreased excitability of spinal cord segments below the level of the lesion (Hald and Bradley, 1982; Thomas, 1984; McGuire, 1984). This is synonymous with absent somatic reflex activity and a state of flaccid muscle paralysis below this level. Although classic teaching refers to generalized areflexia, Thomas (1984) points out that the most peripheral somatic reflexes of the sacral cord segments (the anal and bulbocavernous reflexes) may never disappear or, if they do, return within minutes or hours of the injury. Spinal shock includes a suppression of autonomic activity, and the bladder is acontractile and areflexic. The smooth sphincter mechanism generally functions, however, and EMG activity can generally be recorded from the striated sphincter (McGuire, 1984; Awad et al., 1977; Yalla et al., 1978). Because sphincter tone exists, urinary incontinence does not result, urinary retention is the rule, and intermittent catheterization (or continuous catheterization in some instances) is necessary to circumvent this problem. If the distal spinal cord is intact but simply isolated from higher centers, there will eventually be a return of detrusor contractility. At first such reflex activity is poorly sustained and produces only low-pressure changes, but the strength and duration of such involuntary contractions increases, producing involuntary voiding, usually with incomplete bladder emptying. The return of reflex bladder activity in such patients is generally manifested by involuntary voiding between intermittent catheterizations, and occurs along with recovery of lower extremity deep tendon reflexes. In evolving lesions every attempt should be made to preserve as low bladder pressure storage as possible, and to avoid any measures that might impair this, such as indwelling catheter drainage and any operations designed to decrease outlet resistance.

The characteristic fixed dysfunction that results when a patient has a complete lesion above the sacral spinal cord is detrusor hyperreflexia, smooth sphincter synergia (with lesions below T6), and striated sphincter dyssynergia. Neurologic examination shows spasticity of skeletal muscle distal to the lesion, hyperreflexic deep tendon reflex, and extensor plantar responses. There is impairment of superficial and deep sensation. Incomplete bladder emptying generally results, usually because of striated sphincter dyssynergia. The neurological center responsible for coordinating bladder and striated sphincter activity is in the pontine mesencephalic formation (see Section I) and any lesion between this area and the sacral spinal cord may interfere with this coordination. True dyssynergia, either continuous or intermittent, generally occurs, but in some instances there is simply a failure of relaxation without an increase in sphincter activity over baseline. Occasionally, incomplete bladder emptying may result from poorly sustained detrusor contractions. This seems to occur more commonly in lesions close to the conus medullaris than with lesions higher up (Hald and Bradley, 1984). Poorly sustained contractions may also be due to locally functioning reflex arcs, which result in detrusor inhibition from strong striated pelvic floor muscle contraction or are due to a loss of higher center mediated detrusor facilitation, which normally occurs after the initial increase in intravesical pressure during a bladder contraction (Thomas, 1984).

The involuntary bladder contractions may occur spontaneously or in response to external somatic stimulation of certain areas. Detrusor hyperreflexia with true striated sphincter dyssynergia is generally easily demonstrable urodynamically, and fluoroscopic studies generally demonstrate that, with the bladder contraction, the smooth sphincter area opens normally, and there is obstruction at the level of the striated sphincter, usually most pronounced in the region of the urogenital diaphragm. The primary urologic risk factor is high intravesical pressure. It is essential to know what the bladder pressures are prior to contraction during filling, to know the volume tolerated by the bladder at a safe intravesical pressure, and to recognize what the "leak point" is. To avoid upper tract sequelae, the pressures at volumes recovered by intermittent catheterization must be less than 40 cm H_2O, or pressures at the time of urinary leakage must be less than 40 cm H_2O. If bladder pressures are suitably low, or can be made low with nonsurgical or surgical treatment, intermittent catheterization can be continued as a safe and effective way of satisfying many of the goals of management. Alternatively, external sphincterotomy can be used in males to lower the leak point to an acceptable level.

Autonomic dysreflexia refers to the syndrome of exaggerated sympathetic activity in response to stimuli below the level of a spinal cord lesion (McGuire, 1984; Thomas, 1984; Hald and Bradley, 1982). It occurs most commonly in patients with lesions of the cervical spinal cord, but may occur with any lesion above T6. The syndrome consists of hypertension with headache and profuse sweating in the skin of the face and neck, and reflex bradycardia. The stimulus for this exaggerated response commonly arises from the rectum or bladder. This syndrome may be precipitated by instrumentation or by a change of a tube or catheter, and, in such cases, resolves quickly if the stimulus is withdrawn. Striated sphincter dyssynergia invariably occurs, and smooth sphincter dyssynergia is generally a part of the syndrome as well. Acutely, the hemodynamic effects of the syndrome may be managed with parenteral ganglionic or α-adrenergic blockade or with parenteral chlorpromazine (Thorazine) (McGuire, 1984). On a chronic basis, such episodes can be treated with α-adrenergic blocking agents or with chlorpromazine. To maintain volumes and pressures below which such changes will not occur may require more frequent intermittent catheterization or measures to decrease bladder hyperactivity or increase bladder capacity or measures to decrease outlet resistance so that leakage occurs at a lower pressure and lower volume.

Sacral Spinal Cord Injury

Following recovery from spinal shock, there is generally a depression of deep tendon reflexes below the level of the lesion with varying degrees of flaccid paralysis. Sensation is absent below the level of the lesion. Detrusor areflexia is the common initial result, and is generally accompanied by a competent but nonrelaxing smooth sphincter and a striated sphincter that retains some tone, but is generally not under voluntary control, and that shows absent or diminished EMG activity (Hald and Bradley, 1982; McGuire, 1984; Thomas, 1984). Although the classical description of this problem is that of a decent capacity bladder with high compliance, it is obvious that in many of these patients decreased compliance develops, and because such decreased compliance also develops in neurological lesions distal to the sacral spinal cord, this type of change most likely represents a response to decentralization. At a point at which bladder pressure becomes greater than urethral pressure, leakage results, and if this leak point is high enough, upper tract deterioration may occur. It is not uncommon for incomplete lesions to result at this level, and so varying degrees of bladder and sphincter(s) dysfunctions and combinations may occur. Neurourologic evaluation should be able to exactly characterize each of these patients, and management modalities are generally obvious, consistent with the goals and practicalities previously mentioned.

Multiple Sclerosis

Multiple sclerosis is one of the most common neurologic diseases causing voiding dysfunction (Blaivas, 1985b; Mundy and Blaivas, 1984;

Hald and Bradley, 1982; Blaivas et al., 1979; McGuire and Savastano, 1984; Andersen and Bradley, 1976; Schoenberg and Gutrich, 1980). The disease is due to focal neural demyelination, which causes impairment of nerve conduction. The slowing of nerve conduction results in varying neurologic abnormalities that tend to be subject to exacerbation and remission over time. The demyelinating process most commonly involves the posterior and lateral columns of the cervical spinal cord, the site of pathways that subserve bladder and outlet function. Fifty percent to 80% of patients with this disease complain of voiding symptoms at some time. Bladder involvement is part of the presenting symptom complex in approximately 10% of patients, and may constitute the sole initial complaint, either in the form of acute urinary retention of unknown etiology or in the acute onset of involuntary bladder contractions with urgency and frequency. Detrusor hyperreflexia is the most common urodynamic abnormality detected, and occurs in 50%–90% of cases (McGuire, 1984; Mundy and Blaivas, 1984; Blaivas, 1985b). Of patients with detrusor hyperreflexia, 30%–65% also have striated sphincter dyssynergia. Bladder areflexia may also occur, and in fact has been reported in 1%–40% of cases, but, of these, a substantial proportion progress to detrusor hyperreflexia. Smooth sphincter synergia is the rule.

Blaivas and Barbalias (1984) have identified certain risk factors referable to voiding dysfunction in patients with multiple sclerosis. These include an indwelling catheter, detrusor striated sphincter dyssynergia in men, and decreased compliance, resulting in sustained intravesical pressures greater than 40 cm H_2O. Because sensation is frequently intact, one must be careful to separate pseudodyssynergia from true striated sphincter dyssynergia. Also, there are some varieties of striated sphincter dyssynergia that are more worrisome than others (Blaivas et al., 1981), and it is those that are sustained—resulting in high bladder pressures of long duration—that are most associated with urologic complications.

PERIPHERAL NERVE LESIONS

Diabetes Mellitus

Peripheral and autonomic neuropathies are common in diabetes. The etiology is a metabolic derangement of the Schwann cell that results in segmental demyelinization and impairment of nerve conduction (Blaivas, 1985b; Mundy and Blaivas, 1984). Neuropathy tends to develop in middle-aged and elderly patients with long-standing or poorly controlled diabetes. The exact incidence is uncertain, as unselected patients generally do not complain of bladder symptoms. If specifically questioned, 5%–50% report symptoms of voiding dysfunction. Frimodt-Moller (1976a, 1976b) coined the term "diabetic cystopathy" to refer to involvement of the lower urinary tract by this disease. The insidious onset of impaired bladder sensation is usually the first manifestation of such involvement. There results a gradual increase in the time interval between voiding, which may progress to a point at which the patient voids only once or twice a day without ever sensing any real urgency. Ultimately, detrusor decompensation occurs; detrusor contractility is therefore diminished, and abdominal straining is necessary to initiate and maintain the voided stream, the strength and force of which are impaired. The typical urodynamic findings include impaired bladder sensation, increased cystometric capacity, decreased bladder contractility, impaired uroflow, and residual urine. The main differential diagnosis is generally from outlet obstruction, as both conditions produce a low flow rate. However, the flow pattern in diabetic patients is more commonly one of abdominal straining, and, of course, pressure/flow studies are easily able to differentiate the two. What one generally sees in these patients is actually the secondary manifestations of resultant bladder decompensation, and this could be obviated by early awareness of the problem and the institution of strictly timed voiding.

Tabes Dorsalis

Luetic involvement of the posterior sacral roots and the dorsal columns of the spinal cord may result in the loss of bladder sensation and the same sequelae as seen in the patient with diabetes and resultant voiding dysfunction (Hald and Bradley, 1982). Pernicious anemia may also result in a similar type of "sensory neurogenic bladder."

Herpes Zoster

Herpes zoster may affect the urinary tract by causing urgency and frequency, followed by urinary retention (Hald and Bradley, 1982). Invasion of the sacral spinal ganglia with the causative virus results in the typical skin eruption within the corresponding dermatomes. Endoscopic examination may reveal a similar type of vesicles within the vesical mucosa. This condition is generally self-limited and resolves spontaneously within a month or two.

Disk Disease

Most disk protrusions compress the spinal roots in the L4–5 or L5–S1 disk interspaces. Voiding dysfunction may occur as a result of a prolapsed disk, and, when present, generally occurs with the usual clinical manifestations of low back pain radiating in a girdle-like fashion along the involved spinal root areas (Hald and Bradley, 1982). The most consistent urodynamic finding is detrusor areflexia. The striated sphincter may be normal or show evidence of denervation. Patients with voiding dysfunction generally present with the onset of difficulty voiding, straining, or urinary retention. Laminectomy may not improve bladder function, and it may be difficult in these cases to separate causation as a result of the disk sequelae itself from changes secondary to the surgery.

Radical Pelvic Surgery

Voiding dysfunction is unfortunately relatively common after pelvic plexus injury. This most commonly occurs after abdominoperineal resection and radical hysterectomy. Neurologic dysfunction after these procedures is reported in 10%–60% of patients, and in 15%–20%, voiding dysfunction is permanent (McGuire, 1984; Mundy, 1984; Hald and Bradley, 1982). The type of voiding dysfunction that occurs is dependent on the specific nerves involved and the degree of injury, and on the pattern of reinnervation or altered innervation that results over time. Urinary retention, with varying degrees of sensory preservation, is generally the initial manifestation of such voiding dysfunction. The permanent pattern is generally a failure of voluntary bladder contraction, or impaired bladder contractility, with obstruction by residual striated sphincteric tone, which is not subject to voluntarily induced relaxation. Often, the smooth sphincter area is open and nonfunctional, a result—some think—of destruction of the terminal sympathetic nerve supply to this area. Alternatively, such an appearance in a patient whose bladder neck has not been operated on may result from increased intravesical pressure and obstruction at the level of the striated sphincter. Decreased compliance is common in these patients, and this, with the obstruction caused by fixed residual striated sphincter tone, results in the paradoxical occurrence of both storage and emptying failure. These patients often leak across the distal sphincter area and, in addition, are unable to empty their bladder, because although they have an increased intravesical pressure, they have nothing that approximates a true bladder contraction. Thus, they represent a combined problem of filling/storage and emptying. They often present with urinary incontinence, which is characteristically most manifest with increases in intra-abdominal pressure. This is usually most obvious in females, as the prostatic bulk in males often masks a deficit in urethral closure function. Alternatively, patients may present with variable degrees of urinary retention. Urodynamic studies may show decreased compliance, poor proximal urethral closure function, loss of voluntary control of the striated sphincter, and a positive bethanechol supersensitivity test. Upper tract risk factors are related to the "leak point," and the therapeutic goal is low-pressure bladder storage with periodic emptying. The temptation to perform a prostatectomy should be avoided unless a clear demonstration of outlet obstruction is possible. Prostatectomy will often simply decrease urethral sphincteric function and thereby result in occurrence, or worsening, of stress urinary incontinence.

Sacral Agenesis, Tethered Cord Syndrome, and Myelodysplasia

These are all discussed in the section Voiding Dysfunction in Children.

Other Voiding Dysfunctions and Related Topics

BLADDER OUTLET OBSTRUCTION

General Pathophysiology

Bladder outlet obstruction is one of the most commonly encountered disorders in urology. Surgical treatment of the most common variety, benign enlargement of the prostate, constitutes one of the most frequently performed operative procedures within the specialty. Generally, bladder outlet obstruction can be divided by etiology into fixed anatomic obstructions and functional obstructions. "Functional" in this case does not mean psychogenic, but simply indicates increased urethral resistance to the forces of bladder emptying by neuromuscular phenomena, which may be involuntary or voluntary. Anatomic causes of bladder outlet obstruction include prostatic enlargement (benign or malignant), bladder neck contracture, urethral stricture, and meatal stricture. Functional causes of bladder outlet obstruction include dyssynergia at the level of the smooth sphincter and at the level of the striated sphincter.

Bladder Response to Obstruction

The bladder responds to obstruction in a somewhat unpredictable fashion, but the dysfunction usually involves either a form of hyperactivity or a form of decompensation. Abrams (1985), although he does not entirely endorse the hypothesis that outlet obstruction causes involuntary bladder contractions, summarizes data that strongly suggest that outlet obstruction does cause detrusor instability. Gathering information from eight sources, he cites evidence that the incidence of detrusor instability in patients with outlet obstruction secondary to prostatism ranges from 53%–80%, with a mean of 62% in the series that he cites. Postoperatively, the incidence ranged from 0%–55% in these same series, with a mean of 24%. The fact that outlet obstruction in the form of prostatic enlargement is a major cause of bladder instability in the male is certainly supported by the high rate of instability preoperatively in such patients and the high reversal rate of this phenomenon following prostatectomy. This concept is widely endorsed (Hald and Bradley, 1982; Turner-Warwick, 1984; Jones and Schoenberg, 1983; McGuire, 1984b). Although the proof of cause and effect generally consists of retrospective correlation of the disappearance of this phenomenon after the relief of outlet obstruction, this nevertheless seems to be a reasonable argument, even though the disappearance of the phenomena generally takes between one and six months (and reversion to a normal cystometric accommodation limb and disappearance of all irritative symptoms may take as long as 12 months). In those instances in which the involuntary contractions seem to result from outlet obstruction, the exact pathophysiology is uncertain. Abrams (1985) points out that no series has demonstrated an association between the incidence of instability and the severity of obstruction. He also points out an increasing incidence of detrusor instability in "asymptomatic" elderly men. Chalfin and Bradley (1982) have presented evidence that there may be an increased input of stimuli that trigger detrusor reflex activity in the area of obstruction. In prostatic enlargement, this could be a result of anatomical distortion and/or compression of the abundant nerve endings in this area due to prostatic enlargement. Reversion to normal after prostatectomy could then be explained by a decompression phenomenon. Involuntary contractions occurring in response to outlet obstruction are looked on by some as a compensatory or protective mechanism to keep bladder and residual urine volumes small, thus preventing elongation of detrusor fibers by overdistention to a point at which they cannot contract efficiently (Jones and Schoenberg, 1983). These involuntary contractions may also occur on an irritative or neurologic basis. Perhaps the sensory tension receptors in the bladder wall are more prone to early activation when the bladder wall is under stress or when it has undergone the morphological changes of trabeculation or thickening. The most reasonable view of this phenomenon seems to be that although it can occur in response to outlet obstruction alone, its occurrence in most cases probably reflects a multifactorial origin—a response to a combination of neurologic, architectural, and strictly urodynamic factors related to pressure/volume changes within the bladder. All would agree that the phenomenon is much less common in response to urethral stricture disease and, although it may occur in response to smooth or striated sphincter dyssynergia, is much less common in response to these abnormalities as well. Regardless of arguments to the contrary, it is very important to keep in mind that the phenomenon of the production of involuntary bladder contractions in response to outlet obstruction is reproducible experimentally, as it has been clearly shown that in pigs, infravesical obstruction results in involuntary bladder contractions or decreased compliance in 80%–90% of animals (Jorgenson et al., 1983; Sibley, 1985).

Decreased bladder compliance during filling without discrete involuntary contractions is another interesting phenomenon that can likewise be caused by outlet obstruction (or simply coexist with it). In either case, its significance is the same as that of involuntary contractions, insofar as its detection prior to a procedure designed to correct the outlet obstruction is concerned. The possible relationship of this phenomenon to outlet obstruction has been the subject of much investigation. Benson et al. (1975) showed that increasing the degree of stretch on muscle strips from the bladder body changed the response to norepinephrine from the usual β or relaxation response to an α or contractile one. Rohner et al. (1978) recorded the same type of change of response to adrenergic stimulation after producing chronic bladder outlet obstruction in dogs. Perlberg and Caine (1982) showed that muscle strips from the bladder dome of 23% of patients with prostatic enlargement requiring surgery showed an α-adrenergic response instead of the normal β-adrenergic response. Decreased compliance during filling may result also from destruction of the viscoelastic properties of the bladder wall (see Chapter 27), generally resulting from infection, inflammation, and fibrosis. The clinical significance of all these forms of detrusor hyperactivity that occur in response to outlet obstruction is that they—and not the simple phenomenon of residual urine with a decreased functional bladder capacity—are often responsible for the clinical correlates of frequency, nocturia, urgency, and urge incontinence.

Detrusor hypoactivity, as opposed to hyperactivity, may also occur in response to significant infravesical obstruction (Hald and Bradley, 1982; McGuire, 1984; Turner-Warwick, 1984). The finding of residual urine is more a sign of detrusor decompensation than of the outlet obstruction that caused it. For this reason, the relief of outlet obstruction more commonly leads to satisfactory urodynamic resolution in patients with a low, as opposed to a large, residual urine volume (Hald and Bradley, 1982). Patients with outlet obstruction and decompensation of the detrusor muscle generally find it necessary to void with the aid of abdominal straining, easily detectable urodynamically.

Morphologically, the clinically detectable changes to bladder outlet obstruction are bladder muscle hypertrophy followed by connective tissue replacement with increased collagen deposits within the bladder wall (McGuire, 1984b). Smooth muscle hypertrophy and hyperplasia occur in response to outlet obstruction along with collagen deposition. Although the absolute amount of collagen increases, the collagen concentration decreases (Uvelius and Mattiasson, 1984). What regulates the degree of cellular hypertrophy in response to obstruction is unknown, but Gilpin et al. (1985) reported that the largest increases in cell size were observed only in patients with concomitant connective tissue infiltration. Whether the endoscopic appearance of trabeculation is more related to collagen deposition or muscular hypertrophy is a matter of discussion (McGuire, 1984b). Experimentally, models of bladder outlet obstruction vary with respect to the species employed and the degree or duration of the obstruction. Even so, general response patterns exist (Brent and Stephens, 1975; Uvelius et al., 1984; Levin et al., 1984). An initial dilation of the bladder is followed by concentric bladder wall thickening with variable degrees of smooth muscle hypertrophy/hyperplasia and collagen deposition. After one week of partial bladder outlet obstruction, the rabbit bladder shows a ninefold increase in mass. Although clinically this is felt to represent a compensatory response that maintains normal emptying (as defined by low residual urine volume, but with high intravesical pressures), experimentally the response of the obstructed bladder to cholinergic stimulation drops to 50% of control values, and the ability of such a bladder to expel urine in response to such stimulation drops to 28% of control values. These rapidly induced contractile and metabolic changes are partially reversible, as a two-week recovery period (following one week of obstruction) results in a decrease in bladder mass to only twice control levels, a return of the contractile and pressure responses to cholinergic stimulation to control levels, and a recovery of the ability of the bladder to expel its contents to 75% of control levels (Levin et al., 1984, 1985). Although it is difficult to compare experimental and clinical situations, this would seem to grossly correlate with the fact that after relief of outlet obstruction, some patients experience total resolution of their symptoms and exhibit normal pressure flow/emptying characteristics, while others experience only partial resolution of some or all of these parameters, suggesting that the reversibility of changes in the coordination of contraction and in pressure development may not occur in the same proportion.

Outlet Obstruction in the Male

Prostatic obstruction may be due to hyperplasia, carcinoma, or inflammation. Obstruction is defined by an elevated intravesical pressure and a subnormal flow rate during voiding. Many asymptomatic elderly males satisfy this definition, but without the usual symptom complex known as "prostatism" (Hald and Bradley, 1982; Andersen et al., 1978). When symptoms are associated with prostatic obstruction, they fall into two general categories: obstructive and irritative. The obstructive symptoms consist of hesitancy, a slow stream, prolonged urination, and a feeling of incomplete emptying. These are variable among individuals, and do not occur in any direct relationship to either pressure or flow parameters. However, they are clearly distinct from the irritative symptoms, which consist of frequency, nocturia, urgency, and urge incontinence. These findings are statistically related to detrusor hyperactivity, which, as we have just discussed, occurs either in response to outlet obstruction or along with it in a substantial percentage of cases. Frequency and nocturia can also occur on the basis of a substantial residual urine volume, with a resultant decrease in the functional bladder capacity. Bladder trabeculation can occur in response to either detrusor hyperactivity or obstruction without such hyperactivity (Andersen and Nordling, 1979, 1980; McGuire, 1984; Turner-Warwick, 1984; Hald and Bradley, 1982). The optimal neurourologic evaluation for the patient with suspected outlet obstruction secondary to prostatic enlargement differs markedly from center to center, and may vary from a history, physical examination, and endoscopic examination to sophisticated combined pressure/flow studies. It should be noted that significant outlet obstruction can exist in the presence of relatively normal flow rates, and that diagnoses can be made in this subgroup of patients only by pressure/flow studies that show grossly elevated intravesical pressures (Gerstenberg et al., 1982).

Other anatomic causes of bladder outlet obstruction in the male include sclerosis or fibrosis of the bladder neck, urethral stricture disease, and urethral valves. Functional causes of outlet obstruction in the male include smooth sphincter dyssynergia (sometimes called bladder neck dyssynergia or dyskinesia) and striated sphincter dyssynergia. Each of these can be secondary to neurologic or nonneurologic causes. We have previously discussed the neurologic causes of sphincter dyssynergia. Turner-Warwick deserves credit for defining the condition of dyssynergic bladder neck obstruction (Turner-Warwick and Whiteside, 1970; Turner-Warwick et al., 1973; Turner-Warwick, 1984). This syndrome characteristically occurs in males between the ages of 30 and 55 years who complain of long-standing obstructive and irritative symptoms. Many of these patients have been to see many urologists and have been diagnosed as having psychogenic voiding dysfunction because of a normal prostate on rectal examination, a negligible residual urine volume, and a normal endoscopic bladder appearance. In this group of patients, objective evidence of outlet obstruction is easily obtainable by uroflowmetry or/and pressure-flow studies. Secondary bladder changes may occur, manifested by detrusor hyperactivity or decompensation with residual urine volumes. Once obstruction is diagnosed, it is localized at the level of the bladder neck in these individuals either by micturitional urethral profilometry or by a formal videourodynamic study or cystourethrography during a bladder contraction that shows obstruction at the level of the bladder neck, prostatic enlargement having already been excluded endoscopically. The diagnosis may also be made indirectly by the finding of outlet obstruction in such a patient in the absence of a distal urethral stricture, prostatic enlargement, or evidence of striated sphincter dyssynergia. The etiology of this problem is unknown (Turner-Warwick, 1984). Bates et al. (1975) proposed that these patients had an abnormal arrangement of musculature in the bladder neck region, such that coordinated detrusor contraction caused bladder neck narrowing instead of the normal funneling. The occurrence of this problem in young, anxious, and high-strung individuals and its partial relief by α-adrenergic blocking agents have prompted some to speculate that it may in some way be related to sympathetic hyperactivity. Neither of these theories has ever been substantiated. When individuals with this problem develop prostatic enlargement, a double obstruction results, and Turner-Warwick has applied the term "trapped prostate" to this entity (Turner-Warwick, 1984). A patient so afflicted generally has a lifelong history of voiding dysfunction that has gone relatively unnoticed because he has accepted this as normal. Exacerbation of these symptoms occurs during a relatively short and early period of prostatic enlargement, and marked relief in these cases is generally effected by a "small" prostatic resection. As Turner-Warwick (1984) points out, such patients often note after outlet resection that they have "always" had some voiding problem, and that they have "never" voided so well as after their treatment.

Functional obstruction at the level of the striated sphincter in males and females occurs most commonly in association with neurologic disease, and such dysfunction has previously been discussed. It is easy to voluntarily produce obstruction in this area, and we do so routinely when obeying the command to stop voiding. This is, in fact, one form of pseudodyssynergia (Wein and Barrett, 1982), which must be distinguished from true involuntary functional obstruction at this level. Many believe that true detrusor striated sphincter dyssynergia, implying involuntary contraction of the striated sphincter during the emptying phase of micturition, occurs only in patients with neurologic disease. The existence of this entity in individuals without neurologic disease seems to be reported most commonly in children, but is reported in some adults as well, in whom the entity has been postulated to cause problems ranging from obstructive or/and irritative symptoms of obscure etiology to recurrent urinary tract infection (Van Gool and Tanagho, 1977; Raz and Smith, 1976; Kaplan et al., 1980; Hinman, 1974; Allen, 1977). It should be noted that it is very difficult to prove urodynamically that an individual has such an entity, and it should further be noted that diagnoses in most of the patients reported have been made on the basis of history, isolated flowmetry, isolated measurements of total intravesical pressure, and pelvic floor EMG activity. Unequivocal demonstration of this entity, in our opinion, requires simultaneous pressure-flow-EMG evidence of bladder emptying occurring simultaneously with involuntary striated sphincter contraction in the absence of any element of an abdominal straining component, either in an attempt to augment bladder contraction or as a response to discomfort during urination. Such reports do exist (Jorgensen et al., 1982; Gerstenberg et al., 1983), and seem to confirm the existence of the syndrome. The etiology is uncertain, and may represent a persistent transitional phase in the development of micturitional control or persistence of a reaction response to the stimulus of urethral pain during voiding long after the problem has disappeared (Jorgensen et al., 1982).

Outlet Obstruction in the Female

The frequency of infravesical obstruction in the female is rare when compared to incidence in the male. Farrar and Osborne (1984) cite a figure of 10% of females referred to urodynamic centers as having outlet obstruction. They report that the most common site of urodynamically proved outlet obstruction in the female is in the distal urethra, and that this condition usually results from a failure of this area to fully attain its potential caliber during voiding. The exact cause of this is uncertain, and authors note the apparent discrepancy of their conclusion with the fact that the distal urethra is rarely smaller than the 10–12 F size that seems necessary to produce significant obstruction. Nonneurologic striated sphincter dyssynergia is possible as an etiology, but as we have just discussed, this diagnosis is quite difficult to make. Whether findings such as these justify empiric urethral dilation in females with obscure voiding symptoms is doubtful, but it may explain the small number of patients that seems to obtain reproducible clinical and urodynamic benefit in response to such treatment.

Bladder neck obstruction in females is quite rare. Diokno et al. (1984) have clearly defined this entity in a small number of patients on the basis of urodynamic video-pressure-flow criteria. They point out that the diagnosis of obstruction in this situation must be based on the demonstration of a relationship between pressure and flow, and should not be made on the basis of a single isolated parameter or any study that does not include simultaneous measurements of such parameters. Once the diagnosis of obstruction has been made, the site of obstruction must be localized further, either by simultaneous (during flow) periurethral EMG recording and fluoroscopic monitoring or by micturitional urethral pressure profilometry. Even then, surgical treatment of this entity should obviously be approached with caution, as incontinence presents a significant risk.

URINARY INCONTINENCE

Definitions

Urinary incontinence is not a disease, but rather a symptom that can result from many different types of lower urinary tract dysfunction. The International Continence Society has defined urinary incontinence as a condition in which involuntary loss of urine is a social or hygienic problem and is objectively demonstrable (International Continence Society Committee on Standardization of Terminology). Such loss of urine can first of all be divided into loss that occurs through the urethra and through channels other than the urethra. We are concerned here only with urethral incontinence. The terminology used to describe various types of urethral urinary incontinence is somewhat confusing because symptoms, signs, physical conditions, urodynamic findings, and anatomic factors are sometimes mixed together to describe the situation. There are a number of terms, however, that seem to have general acceptance and are understood by all to mean certain things. The International Continence Society's Committee on the Standardization of Terminology is responsible for most of these definitions, and this committee now has input from the American-based Urodynamics Society. Stress incontinence can either denote a symptom, a sign, or a condition. The symptom of stress incontinence indicates the patient's statement of involuntary loss of urine when exercising physically. The sign denotes the observation of involuntary loss of urine from the urethra immediately on an increase in abdominal pressure. The condition of "genuine stress incontinence" (many criticize this term, but none have been able to come up with a better one) denotes involuntary loss of urine when the total intravesical pressure exceeds the maximum urethral pressure, but in the absence of detrusor activity ("subtracted bladder pressure": total intravesical pressure minus intra-abdominal pressure). Urgency incontinence refers to the involuntary loss of urine associated with a strong desire to void. Urgency incontinence may be subdivided into motor urge incontinence, which is associated with involuntary bladder contractions, and sensory urge incontinence, which is not associated with involuntary bladder hyperactivity. Reflex incontinence applies to the involuntary loss of urine due to abnormal reflex activity in the spinal cord in the absence of sensation. Overflow incontinence is the involuntary loss of urine when intravesical pressure exceeds the maximum urethral pressure due to an elevation of intravesical pressure associated with distention of the bladder, but in the absence of detrusor activity.

Incidence

True prevalence figures for urinary incontinence vary widely. There are reports that cite the occasional leakage of small quantities of urine in over half of healthy females when exercising (Nemir and Middleton, 1954; Wolin, 1969). However, because this is not a social or hygienic problem, this does not strictly qualify for inclusion. To cite another example, most urologists would agree that the incidence of urinary incontinence following radical prostatectomy is somewhere between 1% and 15%. Rudy et al. (1984) reported an incidence of 87%. This was based on detailed evaluation, and basically counted any leakage of urine as incontinence. In fact, only 13% of their patients had incontinence severe enough to warrant treatment. Three patients complained of incontinence in whom it could not be demonstrated by sophisticated urodynamic techniques, and two others had easily demonstrable incontinence despite a negative clinical history. Thus, in almost one-third of their patients, either the clinical or urodynamic assessment would have been incorrect had they been the only means of defining incontinence. Thomas et al. (1980) reported the prevalence of urinary incontinence in Great Britain, determining this by the number of incontinent patients under the care of various health and social service agencies in two London boroughs ("recognized" incontinence), and by a postal survey of 22,430 persons on the practice lists of 12 general practitioners in different parts of the country ("unrecognized" incontinence). Recognized incontinence occurred in 0.2% of women and 0.1% of men aged 15–64 years and in 2.5% of women and 1.3% of men aged 65 years and over. Unrecognized incontinence showed a prevalence of 8.5% in women and 1.6% in men aged 15–64 years and 11.6% in women and 6.9% in men aged 65 years and over. Feneley (1979) found the prevalence of recognized incontinence to be approximately 1% of a community population, and found the prevalence of unrecognized incontinence to be 2.0% in the male population aged 15–64 years and 5.7% in the male population aged 65 years and over. For females, the corresponding rates were 7.6% and 13.9%. Yarnell et al. (1981) carried out a small survey in women in South Wales and found that 45% admitted to some degree of incontinence. Some degree of stress incontinence was reported by 22% of women, urge incontinence by 10%, and combined incontinence by 14%. In most women the urinary loss was small and infrequent, but 5% experienced a loss sufficient to necessitate a change of clothes, and in 2.6% such loss occurred daily. Over 3% reported urinary incontinence that interfered with their social or domestic life, but only half of these had sought medical advice.

Pathophysiology

Very simply, discounting those individuals who, most commonly because of cerebral disease and dementia, do not recognize a need to urinate in a socially acceptable manner or place, the pathophysiology of urinary incontinence can be thought of as either primarily related to the bladder, to the outlet, or to both. Bladder hyperactivity may be manifested either as discrete involuntary contractions or as a more tonic decrease in the volume-pressure curve during filling (decreased compliance). Bladder-related incontinence may also occur in an individual without hyperactivity but with such hypersensitivity on filling that urinary incontinence results from an uncontrollable need to rid oneself of a painful bladder sensation that has occurred in response to filling. Incontinence primarily related to the outlet most commonly results from intermittent decreases in urethral pressure below that of bladder pressure, which occur during abdominal straining and are unrelated to bladder hyperactivity (another way of defining "genuine stress incontinence"). Episodic decreases in outlet pressure that are unrelated to increases in bladder pressure may also be responsible for urinary incontinence (urethral instability). Finally, the bladder outlet may simply have lost its closure potential and be nonfunctional. Although the incontinence in individuals so affected increases greatly with abdominal straining, the pathophysiology, and therefore the correction, is quite different. Virtually any combination of bladder- and urethra-related causes may exist, compounding the complexity of finding an adequate solution.

Outlet-Related Incontinence in the Female

Under this category we will consider genuine stress incontinence, the nonfunctional bladder neck and proximal urethra, and urethral instability. Urethral instability refers to a seemingly reflex-caused total loss of urethral closure pressure provoked by bladder filling without a corresponding increase in intravesical pressure (McGuire, 1978). Although others have subsequently reported significant urethral pressure variations during bladder filling, some in association with involuntary bladder contractions and some in association with stress incontinence (Ulmsten et al., 1982; Hindmarsh et al., 1983; Vereecken and Das, 1985), it is not clear whether this entity is really the same as that reported by McGuire. In McGuire's series it was clearly only the urethral instability that was responsible for the urinary incontinence that occurred, and it may have been that these patients were experiencing a reflex phenomenon related to their lower urinary tract without any component of increased bladder pressure because of bladder hypotonicity. The etiology of urethral instability is unknown, and it is unknown whether it is related to bladder instability. This is an entity that cannot be diagnosed by conventional urodynamic study, but obviously requires the performance of urethral pressure recordings. Additionally, there have been no systematic investigations regarding the treatment of this entity, but conceptually it would seem to make sense to try to raise the urethral pressure well above the threshold at which a precipitous decrease results from whatever stimulus is involved. Fossberg et al. (1981) have reported some success with this approach in individuals with sensory urge incontinence without bladder hyperactivity.

Many of the factors related to maintaining outlet continence have been discussed in Section I. These fall under three general categories: those related to urethral closure pressure, those related to urethral length, and those related to support of the urethral trigonal anatomy. Urethral length has been considered an important factor by some in the prevention of stress urinary incontinence. Lapides (1958) considered the normal functional urethral length in the female to be 3–4.5 cm, and felt that stress incontinence occurred when and because the functional length of the urethra was less than 3 cm in the erect position. Although this may be correct much of the time, there is considerable disagreement about whether there is more than a minimal change in the resting urethral pressure profile and functional urethral length following surgical correction of stress urinary incontinence. Also, there seems to be a minimal change in functional urethral length in the elderly between those patients who have stress urinary incontinence and age-matched controls. Factors such as these have led most people to believe that reduction of urethral length is rarely a factor per se in promoting stress urinary incontinence. Urethral closure pressure certainly contributes to a cough competent outlet, and any decreases in factors that contribute to urethral closure pressure, though they may not cause stress incontinence by themselves, in combination can certainly either result in stress incontinence or make a preexisting problem much worse. Alternatively, augmenting these factors may result in enough of an increase in urethral closure pressure to significantly ameliorate the problem. The smooth muscle of the outlet, as previously discussed, is estimated to account for 30%–50% of urethral closure pressure. The smooth muscle has inherent tonus and is responsive to pharmacologic stimulation, particularly α-adrenergic stimulation. Those factors that decrease smooth muscle tone and responsiveness include overstretching, trauma, α-adrenergic blockade, β-adrenergic stimulation, progesterone administration, and age. Factors that increase smooth muscle tone and responsiveness include stretch (up to a certain point), α-adrenergic stimulation, β-adrenergic blockade, and estrogen administration. The striated muscle of the outlet likewise has been estimated to account for 30%–50% of urethral closure pressure. As we have discussed, this striated muscle effect is not just confined to the urethra in the area of the urogenital diaphragm, as the striated muscle continues along the urethra from this level for a variable distance to the bladder neck. Striated muscle also possesses an inherent tonus and is capable of voluntary or reflex activity. The factors that decrease striated muscle tone and responsiveness include a section of the pudendal nerve (and perhaps the pelvic nerve), skeletal muscle blockade, age, trauma, and overstretching. Factors that increase striated muscle tone and responsiveness include pudendal nerve stimulation, and perhaps pelvic nerve stimulation as well. The vascular cushion effect refers to the turgor of the blood vessels in the urethral submucosa, and is estimated by Raz et al. (1972) to account for 20%–30% of urethral closure pressure, although others think its contribution is minor. Factors that decrease this effect include estrogen deficiency, trauma, and age. Factors that increase this effect include estrogen administration. This "inner urethral softness" (Zinner et al., 1980) acts as a framework of spongy tissue that supplements the pliability and elasticity of the urethral mucosa. The "mucosal seal effect" is due to the infolding of the urethral epithelium surfaces and the complete apposition of the surface folds for which the mucus secretion is necessary. Although the exact contribution of this mucosal seal effect to urethral closure pressure is unknown, the lack of it certainly increases the amount of compression pressure required to form a complete seal. Factors that decrease this effect include estrogen deficiency, trauma, and age, and factors that increase this effect include estrogen administration in an estrogen-deficient female. Staskin et al. (1985) have concisely summarized current concepts of the anatomic support and configuration of the urethral trigonal region. Pelvic support of the vesicourethral segment is contributed mostly by the pubourethral ligaments, which are condensations of the endopelvic fascia. The main support is from the posterior pubourethral ligaments, which extend from the inferior portion of the pubis to the midurethra. These prevent downward and posterior rotational displacement of the urethra. A "hammock" of levator ani muscle, covered by endopelvic fascia, supports the bladder and urethra in their intra-abdominal position. The pubourethralis, a division of this muscle, forms a sling around the proximal urethra as it passes through the pelvic diaphragm, and aids in preventing posterior displacement of the proximal urethra and bladder neck. The perineal musculature and fasciae provide additional inferior support, especially during abdominal straining. The fascia of the bladder and anterior vaginal wall fuse to form the pubocervical fascia. At the level of the bladder neck and proximal urethra, and at the level of the bladder and the fascial ring of the cervix, these two fasciae are densely adherent. Along the base of the bladder, the vesicovaginal space can be developed between these two fascial planes. The pubocervical fascia prevents herniation of the bladder and urethra into the vagina. The vagina provides a potential space for both anterior and posterior vaginal prolapse. Anterior vaginal prolapse may occur through the upper (cystocele), middle (trigonocele), or lower (urethrocele) third of the pubocervical fascia. The sacrouterine and cardinal ligaments support the uterus and cervix laterally and posteriorly, respectively, and provide direct and indirect supports to the bladder and urethra through these attachments. The primary function of these suspensory mechanisms is to support the upper urethra and urethrovesical junction and to provide a stabilizing effect to check the descent of these areas, which might otherwise be produced by an increase in intra-abdominal pressure.

The one factor that seems to be common to patients with genuine stress urinary incontinence is a failure of transmission of intra-abdominal pressure increases such that these increases do not act to occlude the proximal urethra. Enhorning (1961) was the first to urodynamically demonstrate this failure of abdominal pressure transfer to the upper urethra. Anatomically, the pathophysiology seems to involve downward and posterior rotational movement of the bladder neck and proximal urethra during intra-abdominal straining such that the bladder neck and proximal urethra descend to a position in which concomitant transmission of intra-abdominal pressure to these areas does not occur. The urethra is in a dependent position with respect to the bladder base, and the tensile forces of the full bladder open the bladder neck with stress and permit flow into the proximal urethra (Staskin et al., 1985). Whatever other factors contribute to decreases in urethral closure pressure, this abnormal descent of the bladder base and proximal urethra seems to be the only factor regarding which a consensus has been reached as an etiology common to all patients with genuine stress incontinence. All of the true vesicourethral suspension procedures previously discussed correct this problem by anchoring the vesicourethral junction in a physiologic position and preventing its descent during abdominal straining.

Many gynecologists, though not all, are fond of the "angle concept" in discussing stress incontinence and recommending various types of therapy. At rest with a full bladder, the bladder base lies parallel to or 1–2 cm above a line joining the lower sacral border to the lower border of the pubic symphysis. The posterior urethrovesical angle is equal to or less than 100°. With straining, a downward and backward displacement of 1–1.5 cm of the bladder base and proximal urethra occurs, but the posterior urethrovesical angle stays the same. The angle of inclination of the upper urethral axis to the vertical is approximately 35° or at least less than 45°. The classic gynecologic definition and classification of stress incontinence into type 1 and 2 was made on the basis of changes in these angles (Green, 1962, 1975, 1982; Hodgkinson, 1970). These diagnoses were made on the basis of a lateral cystogram, sometimes using a chain to visualize the path of the urethra. Type 1 incontinence referred to complete or nearly complete loss of the posterior urethrovesical angle, but with maintenance of the angle of inclination of the urethral axis. Type 2 incontinence referred to those patients who had loss of the posterior urethrovesical angle and an abnormal angle of inclination of the urethral axis—greater than 45°—and often even completely reversed—greater than 90°. The angle concept held that type 1 incontinence could be corrected by an anterior vaginal repair, which supported the urethra and the bladder neck, while a true suspension procedure was necessary for type 2, which actually comprised downward and backward rotational descent of the urethral axis. Although the angle concept provides some quantitative determination of the degree of failure of support of the vesicourethral segment, it is obvious to any who have studied women with voiding dysfunction that some who are continent have abnormal angles and some who have stress incontinence have normal angles. Stanton (1985) comments further that the angle concept is "unphysiological and mechanically unsound," implying support of the view that angle changes per se are not the cause of stress urinary incontinence, but simply are often a correlate of the changes that occur that cause failure of intra-abdominal pressure increases to the bladder neck/proximal urethra. We have found the diagrammatic conceptualization of Constantinou et al. (1981) to be an excellent teaching aid in explaining both the deficit in stress incontinence and just what it is that vesicourethral suspension procedures actually do (Fig 67).

The pathophysiology of classical stress urinary incontinence is corrected by any of the standard vesicourethral suspension procedures, all of which, when properly done, restore the anatomic and physiological position of the proximal urethra in such a fashion as to allow transmission of intra-abdominal pressure so that urethral closure pressure is enhanced at least to a similar degree, and sometimes to a greater degree. In doing so, proper support is provided to prevent rotational descent of the bladder neck and proximal urethra. Such correction assumes that the factors responsible for urethral closure pressure in the first place are physiologically intact and capable of translating these intra-abdominal pressure increases into increased urethral resistance. There are some patients who have gross incontinence during abdominal straining in whom a vesicourethral suspension may not be effective for correction. These patients, classified by McGuire as having type 3 stress incontinence (McGuire, 1984), have a nonfunctional bladder neck and proximal urethra, in the sense that there is no or poor closure pressure in this area. On an x-ray film with the patient erect and the bladder full, this area appears fixed in an open or relatively open position. The incontinence that is seen in patients with this finding is generally quite severe, although they often complain primarily of stress incontinence, i.e., incontinence with any increases in intra-abdominal pressure. They may state that they "leak" constantly, and they very well may, in the sense that almost any slight increase in intravesical pressure will cause urinary leakage. Often, they complain particularly of gravitational incontinence that occurs simply on assuming the erect

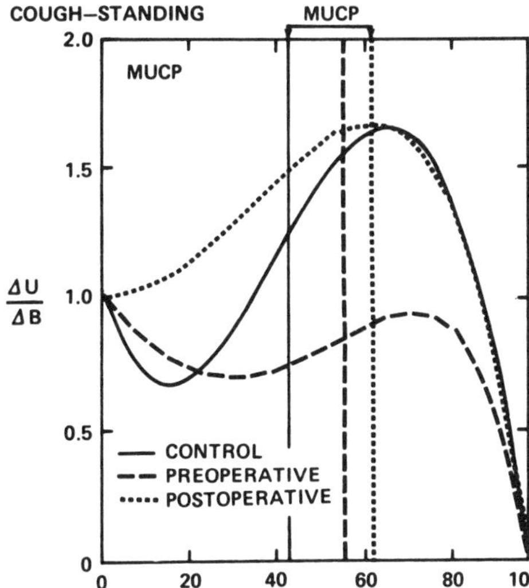

FIG 67.
Transmission of intra-abdominal pressure along urethra in normal females and in those with stress incontinence. Data shown were recorded in standing position with a soft perfusion urethral catheter. The vertical lines show position of the maximum urethral closure pressure (MUCP) expressed as a percentage of urethral length for comparison. Note that this maximum is most proximal in controls. Vertical axis shows the ratio of change in urethral pressure to change in bladder pressure. Note that in controls this is greater than 1 for most of urethral length. Note that in preoperative patients with stress urinary incontinence, this transmission ratio is less than 1 along the urethral length, making it easy to understand conceptually why stress incontinence occurs. Note that following correction, a transmission ratio of > 1 is restored for entire urethral length. (From Constantinou CE, et al: The impact of bladder neck suspension on the mode of distribution of abdominal pressure along the female urethra, in Zinner NR, Sterling AM (eds): *Female Incontinence: Progress in Clinical and Biological Research.* New York, Alan R Liss, 1981, pp 121–132. Used with permission.)

position. These patients often have a history of previous pelvic surgery, and the characteristic history includes three or more failed procedures for what was diagnosed as genuine stress incontinence. These patients have a particularly low urethral closure pressure in the first 1–2 cm distal to the bladder neck, and radiographically they exhibit a bladder neck and proximal urethra that never quite closes in the erect position with the bladder full, but such patients do not exhibit an increase in subtracted bladder pressure. Hypermobility of the vesicourethral segment is generally not a problem in these patients, as this segment is relatively fixed because of previous scarring and fibrosis.

Bladder-Related Incontinence in the Female

Bladder-related incontinence in the female may be related to phasic rises in detrusor pressure, either of neurologic (detrusor hyperreflexia) or nonneurologic (detrusor instability) causation. Such incontinence may also be related to an abnormal tonic rise in intravesical pressure (decreased compliance). The neurologic causes of involuntary bladder contraction have already been reviewed. The etiology of detrusor instability is obscure, especially in women, in whom outlet obstruction (a common cause in males) is very uncommon and more uncommon still as a cause of detrusor instability (Mundy and Stevenson, 1984; Mundy, 1985). Although some work has begun to elucidate neurophysiologic and neuromorphologic differences in the detrusor muscle in patients with bladder instability from those of normal subjects, the etiology of this troublesome and common clinical problem remains obscure. One subject that should be mentioned is the simultaneous occurrence of bladder instability and stress urinary incontinence. Detrusor instability per se is a common cause of urinary incontinence in females, and has been cited as one of the most common causes of failure of a suspension operation for stress urinary incontinence (Stanton et al., 1978; Webster et al., 1984). Whether these urodynamic findings really do indicate that such an operation is likely to fail is an important question, as an affirmative answer would mandate a very careful urodynamic evaluation in all such patients, and might well decrease the enthusiasm for corrective surgery in such patients who also have genuine stress incontinence. Many, ourselves included, have noted the occurrence of detrusor instability in patients with stress incontinence, but have repaired the stress incontinence anyway, hoping to ameliorate the involuntary bladder contraction component of the incontinence by nonsurgical means. More often than not, however, this does not constitute a problem, and McGuire and Savastano (1985) have documented their long-stated position that only a small number of women with both stress incontinence and detrusor instability and/or urge incontinence will still have symptomatic urinary loss as a result of persistent detrusor abnormalities at eight weeks after corrective surgery for the stress incontinence. They reviewed 603 women with urodynamically and radiographically diagnosed stress incontinence, 180 of whom had associated detrusor instability and/or urge incontinence. The overall incidence of detrusor instability was 30%. By eight weeks after surgery, only 25 patients, or 4% of the entire group, and only 14 of those with detrusor instability and/or urge incontinence at any time, were still troubled with incontinence due to that condition. Thus, in McGuire's experience, women with both stress incontinence and detrusor instability fare worse after operation with respect to total freedom from incontinence than those with only stress incontinence. However, 90% of women with stress incontinence and detrusor instability and/or urge incontinence were totally relieved of urinary incontinence at six months by an operation designed to treat only the stress incontinence. These data also suggest that, at least in some patients, stress incontinence and detrusor instability are causally related. Patients with stress incontinence who also have bladder-related incontinence because of decreased compliance do not seem to fare so well after surgery to correct just the stress incontinence. The decreased compliance generally does not change, and if it was refractory to nonsurgical therapy before a suspension operation, it will remain that way, at least in our experience. There are few published reports regarding the fate of such patients after only an operation for stress incontinence, probably because experience elsewhere has been the same as ours.

Urgency-Frequency-Incontinence in the Female Without Detrusor Hyperactivity or Outlet Incompetence

There are a number of patients who have symptoms that suggest involuntary bladder contractions, but who in fact have no detectable consistent pathology during the filling phase of micturition. Most of these patients report symptoms of urgency, frequency, dysuria, pressure, and incontinence in varying proportions. The treatment of this symptom complex is, initially at least, usually empirical and consists of one or a combination of the agents to decrease detrusor hyperactivity (Wein, 1985). The fact that most of these patients do not have involuntary contractions most likely accounts for the generally less than optimal results achieved only with this type of treatment (Rees et al., 1976; Ulmstein et al., 1977). Urodynamic evaluation of these patients may be entirely normal, may show only hypersensitivity during filling, or may show variations in urethral pressures. Fossberg et al. (1981) did report successful subjective results in 22 of 34 female patients with sensory urge incontinence, many of whom had wide urethral pressure variations during filling, with phenylpropranolamine (50 mg, twice daily). The ideal pharmacologic treatment for at least the urgency, frequency, and dysuria component of this symptom complex, which seems to be more sensory than motor in origin, would be an agent that produces topical anesthesia or hypoesthesia of the bladder and urethral mucosa. Although there are agents that are reported to have this action as their primary effect, the clinical results that have been obtained with

TABLE 27.
Possible Etiologies for Urgency-Frequency-Incontinence Syndrome

Lower urinary tract or genital infection, bacterial or nonbacterial
Meatal obstruction
Bladder outlet or urethral obstruction
Detrusor hyperactivity
Smooth sphincter dyssynergia
Striated sphincter dyssynergia
Urethral diverticulum
Urethral caruncle
Urethral carcinoma
Bladder carcinoma or carcinoma in situ
Bladder stone
Estrogen deficiency
Interstitial cystitis
Radiation cystitis
Tuberculous cystitis
Emotional factors
Decreased central or peripheral opioid/peptide influence
Nonlaminar turbulent distal urethral flow

such compounds in these circumstances, at least by us, have been poor. There is no doubt that, in at least some of these patients, the symptoms are psychosomatic. However, more likely reasons for the relatively poor treatment results in this group are (1) that current "state of the art" techniques and practices fail to detect pathophysiology from the myriad possibilities (Table 27) and (2) optimal treatment for some of these has not yet been defined.

Bladder-Related Incontinence in the Male

Detrusor hyperreflexia and detrusor instability in the male have previously been discussed, and the relationship between outlet obstruction secondary to prostatic enlargement and detrusor instability has received particular mention. Likewise, decreased compliance as a cause of urinary incontinence in the male has also been covered. Overflow incontinence has not yet been discussed and does represent a form of bladder-related incontinence that seems to be more common in the male than in the female, though it occurs in both. Overflow incontinence, although everyone "knows what it is," is in reality very poorly understood. The primary pathophysiology is actually a failure of emptying, leading to urinary retention with "overflow" incontinence, which results from either continuous or episodic elevation of the intravesical pressure over the urethral pressure. Overflow incontinence is said to result from outlet obstruction or from detrusor inactivity, either neurological or pharmacological in origin, or may be secondary to inadvertent overdistention of the bladder. Our subjective impression is that it generally occurs in patients whose bladder neck and proximal urethral resistance is somewhat decreased to begin with, or it occurs in patients in whom the detrusor is not totally decompensated. The treatment is obviously directed at the primary cause of the failure to empty, or at circumvention of this if correction of the primary cause is not possible or if irreversible bladder decompensation has in fact occurred.

Outlet-Related Incontinence in the Male

In theory at least, categories of outlet-related incontinence should exist in the male that are similar to those in the female, i.e., urethral instability, stress urinary incontinence, and a nonfunctional bladder neck and proximal urethra. In reality, there is little if any information regarding the topic of urethral instability in the male, and we personally have never seen a case analogous to that reported in the female. Stress-related incontinence does exist following neurological injury (this is discussed in the sections Voiding Dysfunction Following Radical Pelvic Surgery, and Myelodysplasia). The best known type of outlet-related incontinence in the male is post prostatectomy incontinence, best known perhaps because it is iatrogenic. In discussing this entity, we must first recognize that post-prostatectomy incontinence is not solely due to outlet-related reasons. A substantial proportion of these patients have bladder dysfunction (hyperactivity) that accounts for all or part of their symptoms. The incidence of bladder hyperactivity in patients with postprostatectomy incontinence has been variously reported as 55% (Mayo and Ansell, 1979), 40% (Abrams, 1980), 66% (Reid et al., 1980), and 38% (Yalla et al., 1982). Although many of these patients had not been studied urodynamically prior to surgery, it can be assumed that—because of the high incidence of bladder instability secondary to outlet obstruction in the male—a substantial proportion of them actually had the detrusor hyperactivity preoperatively. Thus, in most cases, it did not develop in response to the prostatectomy. Recognition of the abnormal bladder function is of utmost importance in the management of these patients, as satisfactory continence may most often be obtained with pharmacologic therapy alone when the patient has only a minimal amount or no element of sphincteric insufficiency.

Postprostatectomy incontinence is one of the most distressing complications that can befall the patient and the urologist. Caine and Edwards (1958) demonstrated quite conclusively that the continence mechanism after a nonradical prostatectomy is located between the verumontanum and the urogenital diaphragm. One can characterize the various types of prostatectomy, including radical prostatectomy, as to the potential anti-incontinence mechanisms left intact, and therefore as to the probability of urinary incontinence (related to the outlet) after prostatectomy. All types of prostatectomy essentially ablate the proximal sphincter mechanism (smooth muscle of the bladder neck and proximal prostatic urethra, as well as the nonmuscular elements of the wall of these structures). These hopefully leave intact enough of the distal sphincter mechanism (the smooth muscle of the urethra from the level of the verumontanum to the urogenital diaphragm, the striated muscle between the leaves of the urogenital diaphragm, the striated muscle that is applied along the outer wall of the urethra for a variable distance from the urogenital diaphragm to and beyond the apex of the prostate, and the nonmuscular elements of the urethral wall in that area) to produce continence in the absence of bladder hyperactivity and sensory urgency. Radical prostatectomy has the greatest potential for significant distal sphincter mechanism destruction, while transurethral prostatectomy generally results in the least disturbance of this mechanism. If one considers the potential damage to proximal or/and distal sphincter mechanisms with various types of prostatectomy, a correlation with the commonly quoted figures for incontinence after different types of prostatectomy is evident: transurethral prostatectomy for benign prostatic hypertrophy, 0.2%–1.4%; transurethral prostatectomy for carcinoma, 10%–20% (presumably because the distal sphincter mechanism is in some cases compromised by the carcinoma itself); suprapubic prostatectomy, 1%–6%; nonradical retropubic prostatectomy, 0.2%–2.6%; radical retropubic prostatectomy, 1%–87% (depending on the definition of incontinence); simple perineal prostatectomy, 1.9%–10.5%; and radical perineal prostatectomy, 2%–15%.

The evaluation of postprostatectomy incontinence should be carried out in a nonpanicky fashion. Incontinence associated with detrusor hyperactivity or sensory urgency will generally resolve within three months. Incontinence without urgency is more worrisome and less apt to resolve spontaneously. There is little excuse for a less-than-expert urodynamic evaluation of patients with these problems to ascertain the exact contribution of outlet and bladder-related factors. Although by no means foolproof, the following suggestions, which we have found useful, might help to avoid postprostatectomy incontinence:

1. When evaluating these patients, first remove all tags and tissue remnants protruding into the lumen, especially those at the level of the resected bladder neck and distal sphincter mechanism.
2. With a transurethral resection avoid capsular perforation, as it is very possible that extravasation of irrigating fluid through a capsular perforation can result in fibrosis and/or fixation with resultant dysfunction of the distal sphincteric mechanism.
3. It is sometimes necessary to resect prostatic tissue distal to the verumontanum. Be careful when doing this. The classical teaching to stop a resection at the level of the verumontanum is not because the so-called external sphincter is at this level, but because this generally gives a safe margin of sphincteric mechanism distal to this point (between the verumontanum and the urogenital diaphragm).
4. With an open prostatectomy for benign disease, try to divide the apical urethra at the verumontanum or close to it.
5. With the radical prostatectomy, try to maintain some sphincteric mechanism distal to the prostate, but do not sacrifice total removal of the prostate for this (leaving a "button" of prostatic tissue is not a radical prostatectomy). If in doubt, create a pseudo–bladder neck.
6. Be careful of instrumenting the urethra after any type of prostatectomy in such a fashion as to potentially injure what is left of the distal sphincteric mechanism.
7. Remember that any patient whose proximal or distal sphincteric mechanism is already compromised is at greater risk from incontinence when another procedure in the area of the bladder neck and anterior urethra is carried out. Remember that any neuromuscular disease affecting the tone of the smooth or striated muscle of the distal sphincteric mechanism will predispose an individual patient to a greater chance of urinary incontinence after even a well-done transurethral resection. This may include any neuromuscular disease, diabetic neuropathy, or alcoholic neuropathy. Remember also that a patient who has had a transsphincteric urethroplasty or who has a rigid urethral stricture in this area is at greater risk for urinary incontinence following a prostatectomy.

Incontinence in the Elderly

This is a common and distressing problem for elderly patients, their families and friends, and for the health professionals who care for them. This subject, of immense social and economic importance, has recently been reviewed by Ouslander (1981), Williams and Pannill (1982), Farrar (1984), and Resnick and Yalla (1985). The following represents a summation of salient points from these excellent reviews. Studies in Great Britain and Europe have fixed the prevalence of urinary incontinence in the hospitalized elderly at between 18% and 40% in men and at between 24% and 46% in women. In elderly persons living in the community, the corresponding figures are 5% to 25% in men and 7% to 42% in women. In the United States it is estimated that 28% to 50% of elderly nursing home–bound patients are incontinent of urine. It is estimated that over $8 billion per year in additional care is required for the 15% of incontinent elderly who are institutionalized. As with all statistics regarding incontinence, it is difficult to arrive at an exact, agreed-on prevalence in this population, simply because the definition of incontinence varies so widely from clinician to clinician, and may or may not include the implication of social or vocational disability. The subject of incontinence in the elderly requires somewhat different considerations than incontinence in other age groups. First of all, there is a large segment of the elderly who may be classified as having "transient incontinence." Transient incontinence is most often associated with acute medical conditions, psychological responses, or iatrogenic factors, particularly associated with the administration of various types of pharmacologic agents. Restricted mobility and impaction of stool are also common causes of transient incontinence. Appropriate early management can often prevent this type of incontinence from becoming an established problem. Such transient incontinence may represent as much as 50% of the total number of cases of incontinence in the elderly. Another type of problem, not particular to the elderly, but certainly more common in this group, consists of "functional" incontinence. This refers to the inability of a normally continent person to reach the toilet in time to avoid an accident. The reason may be an illness—commonly a musculoskeletal limitation—that prevents an appropriately quick response to a need to void, or it may be a failure—either on an organic, cerebral or psychological basis—of the individual to appreciate the social necessity for voiding in the right place at the right time, or it may represent spiteful behavior associated with depression, suppressed hostility, or anger. Bladder hyperactivity, usually with sensation (urge incontinence), is the most common of urodynamically definable conditions contributing to incontinence in the elderly, and is estimated to occur in between 40% and 70% of elderly incontinent patients. Involuntary voiding without stress or sensation (reflex incontinence) may occur as well, either because of interruption of sensory pathways, spinal cord disease, or cortical damage that can both cause detrusor hyperreflexia and also diminish the awareness of bladder filling. Stress incontinence in the elderly is much more common in the female than in the male who has not undergone prostatectomy. Nonsurgical management of these patients is often beneficial and extremely gratifying. Overflow incontinence represents an easily diagnosable problem in these patients. If this is secondary to outlet obstruction with an intact detrusor, surgical treatment is often successful. If the detrusor is decompensated, intermittent catheterization, if practical or available, will totally obviate the problem.

THE PAINFUL BLADDER AND URETHRA

Evaluation and management of patients afflicted with purely sensory disorders of the lower urinary tract is a frustrating and challenging experience for the urologist. These disorders, as such, defy precise definition, and have been aptly characterized by the term "a hole in the air," attributed to Tage Hald (George, 1986). These patients often complain bitterly of symptoms suggestive of lower urinary tract dysfunction, without an obvious infectious cause or urodynamic correlate, but occasionally with endoscopic abnormalities; however, these abnormalities are by no means constant. As George (1986) so concisely puts it, "these patients constitute the very substance of the 'hole in the air'; the boundary is formed by those who have been identified and abstracted by due clinical process."

Interstitial Cystitis and the Urethral Syndrome in the Female

Hunner (1915) first described a painful bladder condition manifested by frequency, nocturia, urgency and suprapubic pain in a group of young female patients whose endoscopic examination revealed ulcers on the vesical mucosa. Subsequently, it has become evident that the classical finding of a scarred, contracted bladder that splits and bleeds on distention is present only in about 10% of cases of interstitial cystitis. The onset of the disease is commonly subacute and full development of the symptom complex takes place over a relatively short time (Hald and Holm-Bentzen, 1986). Many women can pinpoint exactly the time and the circumstances under which the symptoms first developed. Many times, the symptoms initially seem to be similar to those of urinary tract infection, of which many of these women have a repeated history. However, the symptom complex, though initially thought to be due simply to another infection, "never disappears." The most common symptoms of the patient with "classic" interstitial cystitis are pain, frequency, nocturia, and urgency because of suprapubic discomfort. In most cases, voiding relieves the pain somewhat, but the pain recurs with bladder filling. The patients are usually females between 30 and 70 years old, although men and children of either sex constitute approximately 10% of cases (Hald and Holm-Bentzen, 1986). The incidence of the disease varies with the investigator. Oravisto (1975) found the occurrence in Helsinki to be 18 per 100,000 women. Kinder and Smith (1958) found only 27 cases in more than 17,000 urological registrations in London.

One of the problems in gathering data about this disease entity is the total lack of a precise or agreed-on definition. The symptom complex is certainly not specific for whatever this entity is. Urodynamic investigation is generally unrevealing except for the presence of hypersensitivity during filling. Occasionally, patients will exhibit decreased compliance during filling, and in our experience, these are usually "classic" cases, with a long duration of disease, and with fibrosis of the bladder wall. Endoscopic findings vary widely. Classical Hunner's ulcers are rarely seen, but bleeding on refilling the bladder following cystoscopic distention is common. The bleeding may result from petechial hemorrhage, ecchymoses, or free bleeding from vessels, and is estimated by Hald and Holm-Bentzen (1986) to occur in up to 90% of patients. Messing and Stamey (1978) described glomerulation (discrete rounded petechial mucosal hemorrhage) as a manifestation of early interstitial cystitis. It should be noted, however, that such endoscopic findings are seen after cystoscopic filling and emptying of the bladder in patients with other inflammatory bladder conditions but few symptoms, and in patients undergoing endoscopic examination for periodic surveillance (e.g., bladder tumors) without either definable disease or symptoms. The etiology of the disease has variously been considered to be infectious (bacterial and nonbacterial), traumatic, and autoimmune. Dixon and Hald (1986) have nicely summarized the varied pathological findings, and also the recent attempts to implicate a defective bladder urothelium in the pathogenesis of this disease, an idea originally suggested by Gordon et al. (1973). They summarize the available pathologic evidence, which suggests that the disease is associated with a pancystitis. The bladder wall is frequently thickened and the perivesical tissues are infiltrated. There is frequent thinning of the mucosal lining, and in some areas the mucosa may be denuded. The areas of ulceration are frequently covered by a layer of fibrin. An intense reaction occurs in the subepithelial connective tissue beneath the areas of mucosal thinning. The lamina propria is edematous, congested, and contains dilated capillaries and perivascular hemorrhages. A diffuse cellular infiltration of all areas of the bladder wall by lymphocytes exists, but this is most evident in the lamina propria. Mast cell infiltration in the muscle coat ("detrusor mastocytosis") has been proposed as a diagnostic feature by Larsson et al. (1982), and this has been adopted as a diagnostic feature by others. However, there is no agreement as to this criterion among many other clinicians (Messing and Stamey, 1978), particularly in "early" cases. Parsons et al. (1983) have proposed a theory of pathophysiology involving a defect in the protective layer of glycosaminoglycans (GAG) lining the mucosa of the urinary bladder, allowing a marked increase in bladder urothelial permeability, allowing the "leakage of urine" into the bladder wall, thereby inducing a local inflammatory response. Dixon and Hald (1986) could not support such a theory implicating a defective glycocalyx, as they detected no structural differences in the GAG layer in patients with interstitial cystitis from that in controls. However, they mention the possibility that abnormalities of bladder urothelial permeability may occur because of other reasons, perhaps defective "urothelial tight junctions," with resultant urine "leakage" into the bladder wall. Attempts to formulate any sort of a meaningful review of this disease are hampered by the fact that there is absolutely no agreement on a definition of the disease, or any sort of way to grade its severity. The disease is often defined on the basis of symptoms alone without endoscopic or pathologic findings; it may be defined on the basis of symptoms with endoscopic findings but without specific pathology, or on the basis of pathologic findings with symptoms but with or without typical endoscopic findings. Doubtless, responses to treatment differ among patients in these various categories, probably accounting for the wide variations and disagreements regarding successful results with hydrodistention, intravesical instillations of dimethyl sulfoxide and sodium oxychlorosene (Clorpactin), surgically or laser-induced "denervation," synthetic GAG therapy, and biofeedback.

The urethral syndrome in the female is another imprecisely defined entity that to most urologists is a diagnosis of exclusion for those patients with frequency and/or urgency and/or dysuria without evidence of any pathological process in the urinary or genital tract. George (1986b) has nicely summarized the clinical features. Frequency by day is the primary complaint of most patients who describe a constant, unpleasant sensation in the area of the urethra that is only temporarily relieved by voiding. Nocturia is generally of mild degree, and never reaches the levels experienced by patients with true interstitial cystitis. Patients complain that their voiding is typically slow and hesitant, and in fact the measured flow rate, even with an adequate volume, may indeed be low.

However, the diagnosis of obstruction should certainly not be made only on the basis of flowmetry, but the diagnosis of obstruction in this syndrome must include pressure-flow documentation. Any positive finding uncovered during the course of a search for infectious, inflammatory, or urodynamically definable pathologic characteristics should be treated specifically. Unfortunately, this leaves a large number of patients who must be treated either by biofeedback, reassurance and encouragement (really a form of biofeedback, but simply practiced by the urologist in the course of his or her office hours), empiric pharmacologic therapy, and a host of other treatments, generally directed toward the urethra or the surrounding structures. Schmidt (1985) and Tanagho have come up with a very interesting theory of striated sphincter dysfunction as a cause for the urethral syndrome. Treatment of such dysfunctional striated sphincter activity, in their hands, has been successful in ameliorating the clinical condition, and such treatment has ranged from simple reeducation—with or without pharmacologic therapy—to various forms of neurostimulation, to fatigue, to presumed erratic behavior of the striated sphincter.

Prostatodynia in the Male

Prostatodynia is a term that was formulated to describe a syndrome in the male that is somewhat similar to the urethral syndrome in the female (Drach et al., 1978). This describes a patient with ill-defined discomfort in the prostatic area, but with no evidence of true acute or chronic prostatitis, and with no evidence of infectious or inflammatory findings in the expressed prostatic secretions. This syndrome of chronic genital discomfort, which often includes symptoms of irritative voiding dysfunction, typically occurs in tense and anxious persons (Osborn, 1986). In a series of 37 such patients in whom the diagnosis had been established by clinical, bacteriologic, and urodynamic screening (with no identifiable pathology), Osborn (1986) reports the somatic symptoms as consisting of perineal pain (76%), pain after ejaculation (56%), suprapubic discomfort (55%), penile pain (44%), orchialgia (35%), and loin pain (17%), with voiding symptoms consisting of a postmicturition dribble (35%), hesitancy (26%), a persistent nagging urethral sensation (23%), and a necessity of straining to void (17%). The pathophysiology is obscure, and etiologic considerations have ranged from undiagnosed bacterial, trichomonal, or chlamydial infections to what is described as tension myalgia of the pelvic floor striated musculature, occurring primarily in persons with a tendency to a tense, neurotic personality (Segura et al., 1979). Specific disorders that are uncovered in the evaluation of these patients, whether infectious, inflammatory, or urodynamic, are treated with some rationale. In the remainder of patients, which is unfortunately quite large, empiric anti-infective therapy, often long-term, is often employed, sometimes with equally empiric therapy to either decrease bladder contractility or decrease outlet resistance.

Pediatric Voiding Dysfunction

With the Assistance of Jeffrey Woodside, M.D.*

A full spectrum of voiding abnormalities is seen in pediatric patients (Allen and Bright, 1978). Urologists, pediatricians, and primary care clinicians are charged with the responsibility of defining the characteristics of voiding problems in children early so as to prevent subtle but potentially significant deterioration of the bladder and upper urinary tract. Certain congenital abnormalities that are obvious at birth, such as myelodysplasia or urogenital sinus abnormalities, signal the potential for underlying voiding dysfunction (Bauer et al. 1982). In such instances, it has been shown that an early assessment of the neurourologic status of the patient allows for placement of the patient into either a therapeutic or a regular surveillance group (McGuire et al., 1981; Bauer et al., 1984). Such a program greatly decreases the likelihood of insidious vesical deterioration and upper tract disease as the child matures (Raezer et al., 1977).

Unfortunately, not all children with the potential for voiding problems can be identified early. Many patients have no apparent problem with urination. Thus, parents and physicians are unable to note subtle changes in voiding activity until retention, marked incontinence, or urosepsis develops. Typically, children are poor historians and are unlikely to communicate a subtle voiding problem to their parents or physicians. Also, because they do not perceive voiding changes to be abnormal, significant micturitional abnormalities may go undetected for some time. This does not mean that all children with the most mundane alterations in urination require extensive neurourologic evalua-

*Professor of Urology, University of New Mexico.

tion. However, awareness of the potential for serious underlying disease does mandate the need for a thorough understanding of the peculiarities of voiding dysfunction in children. Knowledge of normal and abnormal micturition physiology, the indications and reliability of diagnostic testing modalities, and a current concept of therapeutic alternatives is necessary for all practitioners caring for children with voiding disturbances. The symptoms and conditions indicating further investigations of a child's neurourologic status are listed in Table 28. However, clinical experience and intuition must also be included as important ingredients in the decision-making process as to which child should undergo further investigation of vesicourethral function.

It is the goal of this presentation to outline a practical approach to the problem of vesicourethral dysfunction in children. Diagnostic modalities will be presented, with references to their relative importance and usefulness in the pediatric age group. Certain conditions common to vesicourethral dysfunction in children will be discussed and the nuances relative to their diagnosis and management will be reviewed.

NORMAL VESICOURETHRAL MATURATION

In the newborn child, urination is a reflex event. It is regulated by a relatively simple spinal reflex (Bradley et al., 1974). When the detrusor becomes distended by urine, stretch receptors in the wall of the detrusor evoke a sensory impulse conducted to the spinal cord by autonomic afferent fibers, which in turn evoke an autonomic efferent stimulus that causes contraction of the detrusor smooth muscle. This

TABLE 28.
Indications for Pediatric Neurourologic Investigation

Urosepsis
Retention
Hematuria
Dripping incontinence
Overt neurologic disease (including trauma)
Painful urination
Straining or squatting during urination
Secondary enuresis
Frequency and urgency incontinence
Encopresis
Polydipsia
Urogenital sinus abnormality

spinal reflex mechanism is coordinated by a simultaneous relaxation in the periurethral striated skeletal muscle sphincter during the voiding reflex sequence, and probably requires an intact brain stem (deGroat, 1975; deGroat and Saum, 1971; deGroat and Theobald, 1976; El Badawi and Schenk, 1968, 1971, 1974). This mechanism has been described in detail and is outlined elsewhere in this text; however, in very young children this reflex mechanism lacks the inhibitory influence from central nervous system areas above the brain stem. Although there is little volitional control of voiding, the functions of urine storage and continence are maintained and it is the relative state of bladder fullness and bladder wall distention that triggers the detrusor contraction and subsequent bladder emptying.

Goellner and co-workers (1981) studied the various aspects of micturition during the first 3 years of life. They pointed out that most children sleep approximately two-thirds of the day and that almost half of the voidings occur during the sleep period. During the first 12 months, the number of voidings averages 20 per day. As the child matures, the frequency of voiding decreases but the volume increases to approximately four times that of the newborn infant. It has been suggested that the increase in voided volume and the decrease in voiding frequency are a function of a subtle assumption of the central (above brain stem) neurologic control of urination (Yeates, 1973). However, physiologic studies indicate that the change in voided volume–frequency relationship during the first 3 years of life is related more to fluid volume ingested for body weight and the changing functional volume of the child's bladder.

It would seem reasonable to conclude that both factors influence enhanced urinary control. By the end of the third year, most children are able to have some conscious control over urination. However, enuresis and daytime accidents do occur. At the age of 4 years, bladder volume is adequate and central urinary control is complete in most individuals. The degree of neuromuscular maturation that occurs is most dramatic on the assumption of voluntary control of the external (skeletal muscle) urethral sphincter and voluntary control of detrusor contractility. Both of these functions are related to neurologic organization of the centers in the midbrain and cerebral cortex. There is no question that there are some neurologically normal children who have a temporary delay in the maturation of these functions and may well exhibit significant voiding dysfunction at the ages of 4, 5, or 6 years and who eventually "outgrow" their problem. As with adults, for normal coordinated voiding to occur in the child, the brain stem must be intact, allowing for adequate contraction of the detrusor smooth muscle and vesicourethral segment and a simultaneous relaxation of the skeletal muscle sphincter at the bladder outlet. During the period of maturation, if one area of maturation lags behind the other, discoordinated voiding patterns may be seen.

PEDIATRIC NEUROUROLOGIC EVALUATION

History and Physical Examination

For all practical purposes, neurourologic tests should not be ordered for a child with suspected vesicourethral dysfunction without first pursuing a complete history and physical examination. A history suggestive of subtle central nervous system disease, such as a traumatic birth, neonatal anoxia, convulsive disorder, and head or back trauma, may explain many voiding abnormalities despite the absence of apparent outward neurologic disease.

During the initial interview with the child and parents, an assessment should be made of the fluid ingested in a 24-hour period. Historical approximations of this volume may be misleading, however, and when clinically related to a voiding problem such as diabetes insipidus, the child or parents should bring a documented list of volumes ingested and voided.

The voiding history itself may well hold the clue as to which of the various available tests will offer the best opportunity for an accurate and cost-effective diagnosis. In the very young child, parents should be questioned about their observations of diaper wetness, number of diapers used, diaper rash, dripping loss of urine, leakage while crying, stream characteristics, straining during urination, and apparent pain or discomfort when voiding. The older child may be asked questions about painful urination, urgency, frequency, and unusual voiding positions, although corroboration from parents is often necessary for information related to enuresis, soiling, and the problem of malodor.

Aside from the potential damage to the bladder and upper tracts, vesicourethral dysfunction in children, especially when incontinence is involved, may have a dramatic impact on the psychologic and sociologic adjustment of the child or family as a unit. During the initial interview, an assessment should be made regarding the impact of the "voiding problem" on the child and parents. This information is important not only diagnostically, because psychogenic voiding dysfunction must be excluded, but also therapeutically, because eventual selection of therapeutic alternatives depends greatly on the psychosocial status of the patient and family.

The physical examination should be directed to those conditions that may foretell underlying neurologic diseases or suggest the more immediate problem of bladder overdistention and hydronephrosis. In the absence of overt neurologic problems, the examination should first be directed toward the integrity of the spinal column by looking for clues to vertebral dysrhaphism. Hairy patches, depressions, or dimples over the spine or sacral area may indicate underlying dysrhaphism or sacral agenesis. A rough estimate of intact reflex arc activity can be evaluated by evoking deep tendon reflexes in the lower extremities, and also a rough estimate can be made of sensory neurologic integrity of the abdomen, perineum, and lower extremities. Further neurologic assessment should be left to a pediatric neurologist, and any clues that may be uncovered during the initial physical examination may lead to a consultation that would include more specificity.

After the initial history and physical examination have been completed and a urinalysis is obtained, a determination must be made as to the severity of the "voiding problem." Does it require further evaluation or can the child and parents be reassured that the symptoms are normal variants and there is no threat to the unseen portions of the urinary tract? Clinical judgment becomes the most important indicator at this time. Children with those conditions listed earlier will be evaluated further. However, in those children who cannot be placed in a particular category, one must weigh the relative costs and degree of invasiveness involved in additional tests against the risk of failing to diagnose a potentially serious vesicourethral abnormality.

Urodynamics

In many children, a satisfactory evaluation for the cause of a voiding abnormality can be made with various combinations of uroradiographic studies and cystoscopy. The voiding cystourethrogram is most efficient in evaluating the detrusor and bladder outlet. Vesicoureteral reflux, ureterocele, urethral valves, ureteral ectopy, and fistula all may be related to voiding difficulties and must be excluded before an abnormality of intrinsic vesicourethral function can be implicated as the cause of a particular voiding problem. It is also not unusual to have a combination of abnormalities (e.g., vesicoureteral reflux and detrusor hyperreflexia) that simultaneously produce an abnormal voiding symptom (Blaivas et al., 1977).

Once structural abnormalities have been excluded, a urodynamic evaluation should be considered to more accurately define voiding dynamics (Bauer, 1984). The goals of urodynamics in children are to define the nature and cause of voiding symptoms, help determine the best mode of therapy, and provide a means to assess therapeutic progress (Gierup, 1970). The urodynamic parameters available to most clinicians include (1) uroflow determination, (2) cystometry, (3) pelvic floor skeletal muscle EMG, (4) urethral pressure profilometry, and (5) combined studies—which include simultaneous measurements of various combinations of the aforementioned studies, with or without abdominal pressure recordings. For all practical purposes, videourodynamics, in which multiple voiding parameters are recorded in sequence with voiding cystourethrography, are only occasionally indicated in children, and the availability of such urodynamic equipment is rarely found outside the medical center environment (Mundy et al., 1982). For that reason, only the most complex voiding disorders in children would require videourodynamic assessment.

As the urodynamic test becomes more complex, the degree of invasiveness tends to increase. With children, invasiveness increases the possibility of alienating the patient and thereby introducing an unacceptable degree of artifact into the study. Therefore, it is generally best to begin the urodynamic testing sequence with a minimally invasive examination, yet one that will produce reliable data relative to the abnormal voiding symptom. At the beginning, the examiner should ask the question, "What do we want to know?" Do the symptoms suggest a detrusor abnormality or an outlet abnormality, or could it be a combination of both problems?

In some patients, the use of sedation, such as intramuscular meperidine (1 mg/kg), has been proposed to decrease discomfort and anxiety during urodynamic testing (Evans et al., 1979). Others report reliable results in children by using nitrous oxide anesthesia (Koff et al., 1980).

Uroflowmetry

When dealing with children, patient cooperation is essential for the recording of any urodynamic parameter, and because uroflowmetry is the least invasive of all urodynamic tests, many clinicians prefer to use this procedure as an initial screening tool. This, of course, requires that the child be of an age to follow instructions and void in a fashion that is typical for that particular individual. For all practical purposes, this eliminates children much younger than the age of 4 or 5 years. If the uroflow characteristics that are recorded are normal, more invasive urodynamic testing may not be necessary subsequently. On the other hand, when uroflow is abnormal, the additional tests may be tailored to concentrate on the specific voiding abnormality.

Not infrequently, the volume voided may be insufficient to accurately assess the flow rate and pattern. Although some degree of invasiveness is introduced into the study, an accurate test may be obtained by filling the child's bladder through a small catheter with body-temperature sterile water to a point of comfortable bladder fullness (Barrett, 1984). The catheter is removed and the child is instructed to void. An accurate residual volume measurement may also be obtained by calculating the difference between the volume voided and the volume instilled in the bladder.

Many clinicians prefer to record pelvic floor or abdominal skeletal muscle EMG activity during uroflowmetry (Barrett and Wein, 1981; Barrett, 1980; Maizels and Firlit, 1979). This technique requires the placement of electrodes on or in the muscles of the perineum and abdominal wall (Koff and Kass, 1982). Normal micturition occurring in the absence of pelvic floor EMG activity confirms the relaxation of the external urethral sphincter during a detrusor contraction (Fig 68). A lack of coordination between detrusor contractility and simultaneous external sphincter relaxation is manifested by an interrupted flow pattern and corresponding bursts of EMG activity. Straining to void produces concomitant contractions in the abdominal and perineal skeletal muscles that may or may not produce significant outflow obstruction. When obstruction is evident, the flow rate will be decreased and EMG activity will be increased.

Regardless of the exact methodology used, which may be modified to suit the needs of the clinician and child, uroflowmetry offers a cost-effective means of assessment for significant underlying vesicourethral dysfunction.

Cystometry

Although moderately invasive and dependent on a cooperative child, cystometry in children can provide enlightening information regarding detrusor contractility and detrusor compliance (Merrill et al., 1972). Every investigator has preferences regarding the age of the child to be investigated, catheter size, infusion medium, rate of filling, and the need for simultaneous EMG recording (Gleason et al., 1977). The amount of information obtained from childhood cystometry is directly related to the degree of interest and care directed to the test by the clinician. Moreso than with adults, cystometry in children requires a

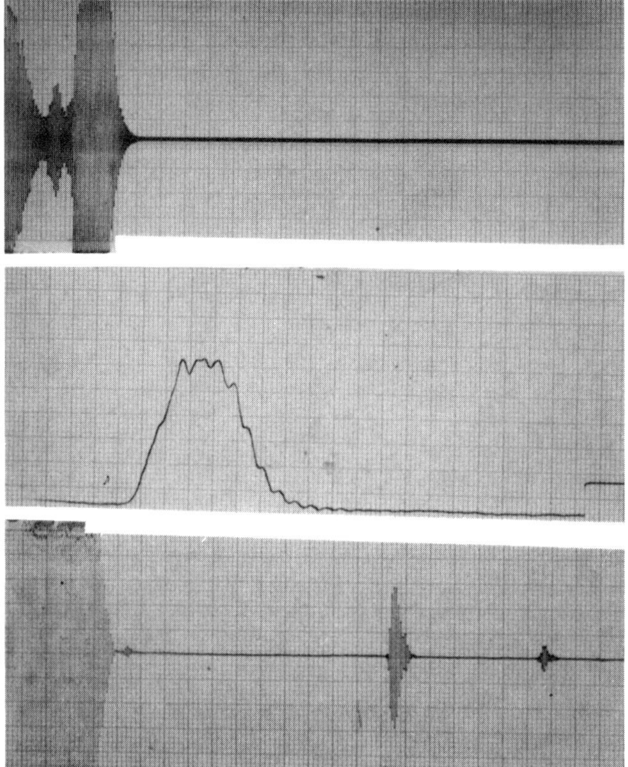

FIG 68.
Uroflow rate with abdominal wall EMG *(top)* and urethral sphincter EMG *(bottom)*. The flow rate *(middle)* is normal, with a peak rate of 30 ml/sec (flow rate scale, 0–50 ml/sec). Both the abdominal wall musculature and the urethral sphincter appropriately relax during voiding.

gentle hand and the ability to abate the fears of the child during the testing sequence. Extremely young children who undergo cystometry may be surprisingly cooperative, especially if there are associated neurologic deficits; however, others may require sedation or even light general anesthesia (Fig 69).

Many younger children, especially males, require the use of small intraurethral catheters (5–8 F) to infuse the bladder during cystometry. When water is used as a testing medium, larger tubes are preferred so as to decrease the erroneous pressure increases that occur during moderate infusion rates (5–100 ml of water per minute). Alternatively, carbon dioxide may be conveniently used without fear of false pressure

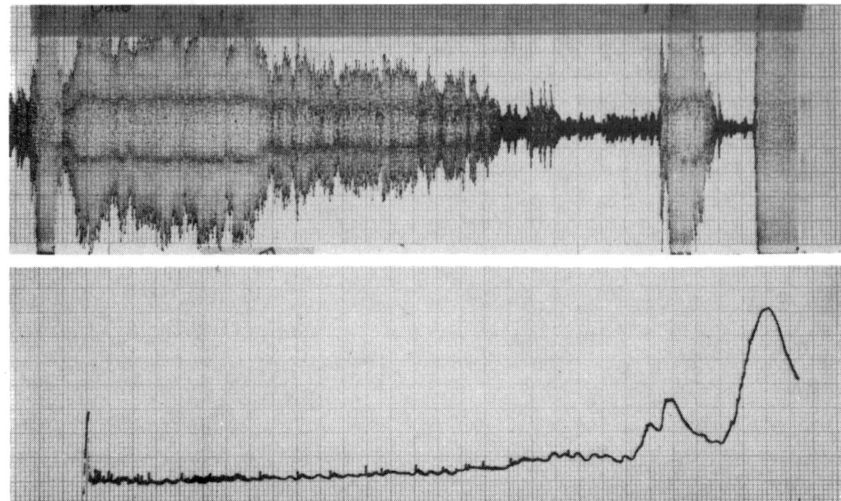

FIG 69.
A normal CMG-EMG in a 12-year-old girl. The tonus limb reflects normal compliance *(bottom)*, and EMG activity *(top)* is noted to decrease during detrusor contractions that are under voluntary control. Electrocardiographic patch electrodes were used to record EMG activity.

increases, even at high infusion rates. However, one should be aware of the alteration in detrusor compliance as the infusion rate is increased. Infusion rates higher than 100 ml of water or carbon dioxide per minute are unphysiologic and will produce a recording that may reflect a significant decrease in detrusor compliance. When testing for the possibility of detrusor instability, higher infusion rates may be used advantageously to provoke what may otherwise be an undetected hyperreflexic detrusor contraction. On the other hand, infusion rates that are too high and extremely unphysiologic may induce a detrusor contraction that ordinarily would not be seen during the child's normal voiding sequence. This is especially true in children under the age of 4 years in whom complete maturation of the inhibitory mechanism of micturition has not occurred. Therefore, the interpretation of cystometry data must take into account all such variables and care must be taken not to produce extreme unphysiologic conditions that may produce data that are overinterpreted and thus lead to erroneous conclusions regarding vesicourethral dysfunction (Grossman et al., 1977).

At times during cystometry it may be unclear as to whether an increase in intravesical pressure is related to a "true" detrusor contraction or is transferred from increases in intra-abdominal pressure during straining. The measurement of intra-abdominal pressure through a closed-catheter system placed in the rectum may clarify this source of artifact. Again, more invasiveness is required and additional pressure recording equipment is necessary. However, most modern urodynamic recording devices will provide the capability of simultaneously measuring rectal pressure, bladder pressure, and subtracted detrusor pressure (bladder pressure minus rectal pressure).

It is clear that some children are at risk of developing upper tract decompensation secondary to ureterovesical obstruction and/or reflux that is a result of excessively high resting or voiding pressure. In bladders that have decreased contractility and decreased compliance, the pressure at which the urine leaks out of the urethra has been shown to be of predictive value in defining the potential for upper tract decompensation. A measurement of "leak pressure" may be undertaken in children of all ages by merely infusing fluid through a small catheter and then noting the intravesical pressure at which the fluid leaks out of the urethra around the catheter. The critical pressure is at or near 40 cm H_2O (McGuire et al., 1983).

Urethral Pressure Profile

Static urethral pressure profilometry has only limited use in pediatric urodynamic testing. It was devised to assess the status of the bladder outlet and offer information relative to the inherent resistance of the continence mechanism. Its drawback centers on evaluation of tissues when they are static and equating this information to their function during the dynamics of voiding.

In most situations, information relative to the continence mechanism (combined smooth and skeletal muscle sphincters) can be obtained more accurately from other urodynamic tests or combinations thereof.

Urethral pressure profile measurement has occasionally been useful in following the function of artificial sphincter occlusive cuff pressures; however, radiographic studies are usually more diagnostic when there is a sphincter malfunction.

Sphincter Electromyography

In pediatric urodynamics, accurate recording of EMG activity in the pelvic floor skeletal muscles has been reliably produced by using surface electrodes such as the patch ECG electrodes that may be pasted on the skin overlying the perineal skeletal muscles. Not only is invasiveness reduced, but also the reliability of recording electrical activity in the muscles has been shown to be accurate. This type of electrical activity measurement can easily be recorded on a strip-chart recorder and combined with other urodynamic testing modalities such as cystometry or uroflow.

Combined Studies

During the initial screening urodynamic investigation, it may not be clear whether an obvious voiding defect is a result of a detrusor contractility abnormality or an outlet abnormality. A combination study of simultaneous cystometry (with or without rectal pressure measurement), uroflowmetry, and EMG is ideally suited to better define the voiding abnormality (Firlit et al., 1978). Children who are candidates for this relatively invasive test are those that fail to completely empty or those with interrupted voiding thought to be related to sphincter-detrusor dyssynergia. From the information gained from this study, a rough calculation of outflow resistance can be made when voiding pressure is compared to peak flow rate.

Cooperation from the child is necessary during combined studies, as a considerable amount of manipulation is necessary to set up for this test (Cook et al., 1977). EMG electrodes must be placed on the perineum or abdominal musculature, rectal pressure catheters must be inserted, and one or two urethral catheters must be placed for the infusion of fluid and the recording of pressure. For this study one has the option of inserting one catheter through which the water medium is infused and intravesical pressure is recorded. However, experience has shown that it is very convenient to insert into the bladder a small 4–5 F polyethylene feeding tube through which pressure is measured, followed by an 8 F catheter through which the water medium is instilled into the bladder. Prior to the recording of voiding pressures, the 8 F catheter is removed, allowing for easy voiding around the small catheter. There is no question that the catheter, especially in younger children with small-diameter urethras, will introduce some element of outflow obstruction and thereby decrease the peak flow rate. However, this appears to be negligible in most clinical settings.

Children with high voiding pressures and low flow rates may have outflow obstruction. When there is increased EMG activity during the voiding sequence, one may suspect an uncoordinated external sphincter giving rise to this degree of obstruction. On the other hand, if EMG activity is coordinated, other causes of outflow obstruction must be excluded. When voiding pressures are low and flow rates are also low, it is reasonable to conclude that detrusor contractility is lacking. This may be a result of neurologic impairment to the detrusor or myogenic detrusor decompensation. One must also take into account the possibility of poor patient cooperation during the testing sequence. In such a situation, a patient may volitionally fail to initiate a detrusor contraction and augment voiding by straining or subtle increases in intravesical pressure. This generally results in low detrusor pressures and also low flow rates.

In most instances, an experienced urodynamic technician can define the degree of patient compliance during urodynamic testing and thereby guard against misinterpretation of this type of study.

Videourodynamics

The true essence of pediatric urodynamics is achieved when the parameters of the combined study are coupled with voiding cystourethrography. The bladder is filled with contrast medium and the voiding parameters are recorded while fluoroscopic monitoring of the sequence is carried out. Limited use of the fluoroscope during bladder filling keeps the radiation exposure to a minimum (Webster and Older, 1980).

Webster et al. (1984) have defined other categories of micturitional abnormalities in neurologically normal children that may be observed with videourodynamics. In general, those conditions that fail to result in a detrusor contraction, such as detrusor areflexia and increased detrusor compliance, can be evaluated with tests that are less expensive and invasive. As before, patient cooperation is extremely important during this testing sequence, as actual voiding must occur for an adequate study to be obtained.

ENURESIS

Enuresis may be defined as the nocturnal or diurnal incontinence of urine in a child more than age 4 years. Primary enuresis is present from birth, and secondary enuresis is preceded by a dry interval of 6 to 12 months. The incidence of enuresis has been estimated at 12% of children aged 4 to 5 years (Forsythe and Redmond, 1974) and it is known to have a familial predisposition (Whiteside and Arnold, 1975). Theories regarding the cause of enuresis include such factors as delayed level of central nervous system maturation, psychogenic and behavioral components, environmental influences, deep sleep, allergies, small bladder capacity, uninhibited neurogenic bladder, and structural abnormalities of the urinary tract (Firlit et al., 1978; Kass et al., 1979; Lennert and Mowad, 1979; Marshall et al., 1973). The incidence of underlying organic problems is higher in the older patient population. This discussion focuses on those children with enuresis who have no overt neurologic or urologic disorder.

The extent of the urologic evaluation of enuretic children has recently undergone reevaluation. In the past, most children underwent intravenous urography (IVP), voiding cystourethrography (VCUG), and endoscopy. However, many investigators currently recommend a much more selective evaluation that is tailored to the individual child and family. The importance of the history, physical examination, and results of urinalysis and urine culture in this evaluation should be stressed. One should determine the pattern of incontinence—whether nocturnal, diurnal, or both; associated urinary frequency or urgency; fecal soiling or constipation; and a history of urinary tract infection and obstructive voiding symptoms. Careful examination of the spine, abdomen, genitalia, and sacral spinal cord segments is necessary and the voided stream should be observed. A urinalysis and urine culture, if indicated, are performed. A history or laboratory findings suggestive of urinary tract infection or evidence suggestive of a hyperactive external urethral sphincter, urinary tract obstruction, or a neurologic problem mandates further evaluation. Determination of the uroflow rate, possibly combined with surface perineal EMG, may be indicated (Barrett, 1980). If a screening IVP is indicated, additional information can be obtained from voiding urethral and postvoiding bladder films.

Many investigators have performed urodynamic evaluations of enuretic children in an attempt to identify any specific abnormality of vesicourethral function responsible for their incontinence. Whiteside and Arnold (1975) studied 50 patients who had normal urinary flow rates and complete bladder emptying. In 13 patients with nocturnal enuresis only, 15% had detrusor instability. In contrast, 97% of 37 patients with both diurnal and nocturnal enuresis had detrusor instability. Blaivas et al. (1977) evaluated 13 children with diurnal and nocturnal enuresis and found two with neurogenic bladder dysfunction. Seven of the remaining 11 patients had decreased bladder capacity. Firlit et al. (1978) performed pressure, flow, and EMG urodynamic studies on 34 children with diurnal and nocturnal enuresis and found 13 patients with uninhibited bladders, 17 with hyperactive external sphincters, and four with normal results. Kass et al. (1979) urodynamically evaluated 65 children with primary enuresis. Forty-two of these patients had either a history or evidence of a urinary tract infection. Among these, 30 had uninhibited detrusor contractions, 10 were normal, and 2 had mixed types of neurogenic bladder dysfunction. Of the remaining 23 patients, 5 had uninhibited detrusor contractions and 18 were normal. Smey et al. (1978) reported a subgroup of enuretic children who had hyperactive external urethral sphincters as a contributing factor to incontinence. Diurnal enuresis, urinary frequency and urgency, urinary tract infection, and fecal soiling or constipation appear to correlate with the presence of uninhibited detrusor contractions, hyperactive external urethral sphincters, or both.

The role of radiographic studies of enuretic children has also undergone reevaluation. Redman and Seibert (1979) obtained an IVP or VCUG or both in 138 enuretic children. Twenty-one children had abnormal results and each had a history of urinary tract infection, signs and symptoms of lower urinary tract obstruction, or both. No significant radiographic abnormalities were found in children with diurnal enuresis unless also accompanied by symptoms or findings suggestive of urinary tract infection or obstruction. Kass et al. (1979) similarly reported that an IVP revealed a significant abnormality only in children with a history of urinary tract infection.

Various treatment modalities have been used for the enuretic child, including reassurance, psychotherapy, behavior modification techniques, hypnotherapy, pharmacologic manipulation, and various surgical techniques. The preponderance of evidence would currently suggest that the history, physical examination, and basic laboratory findings will indicate the appropriate extent of evaluation and initial management of most enuretic children. Children with past or present urinary tract infection, evidence of lower urinary tract obstruction, or abnormalities on physical or neurologic examination should undergo thorough urologic evaluation followed by appropriate treatment. Meatotomy may be helpful in the male child with documented meatal stenosis but may be associated with a high relapse rate. The routine use of meatotomy or urethral dilations is to be condemned. Children with none of the above findings or those who have had a negative urologic evaluation may be managed in a more conservative manner.

When deciding whether or not to initiate therapy, it is important to assess the effect of the problem on the patient and the family as a whole. When some parents and children are informed that no significant organic or psychologic problem is causing enuresis, reassurance and fluid restriction before bedtime may be the only treatment required. Many are quite willing to wait for the spontaneous resolution of enuresis that occurs at a rate of 15% per year in patients between the ages of 5 and 19 years (Forsythe and Redmond, 1974). Should treatment be desired, a conditioning device such as a pad and bell bed alarm is successful in up to 60% of patients, and behavior modification therapy, aimed at making the patient responsible for changing his behavior and complemented by positive reinforcement, is helpful in up to 70% of patients (Marshall et al., 1973).

For patients who are unable to accept or who fail these approaches, pharmacologic therapy may be effective. The results of the thorough study by Kass et al. (1979) suggest that successful empiric pharmacologic treatment of these patients can be instituted on the basis of historical information, physical examination, and urinalysis. Eighty-five percent of patients with nocturnal enuresis and daytime urgency and frequency will respond well to anticholingeric medication. Seventy percent of patients with nocturnal enuresis only will be successfully treated with imipramine hydrochloride. It is the authors' experience that nortriptyline hydrochloride may also be efficacious in those patients who do not respond to imipramine hydrochloride. It has the additional benefit of a more rapid onset of action and shortened half-life should undesirable side effects be encountered. Some of those who fail imipramine hydrochloride therapy will respond to an anticholineric drug. A high relapse rate can be expected if drug therapy is withdrawn early, particularly in younger children. Pharmacologic therapy is more effective if it is suggested in a positive manner and combined with a program of behavior modification and positive reinforcement techniques. Patients with hyperactive external urethral sphincters may be successfully treated with diazepam (Smey et al., 1978) or biofeedback training (Libo et al., 1983; Sugar and Firlit, 1982). Further urologic and radiologic evaluation of these patients is frequently indicated if pharmacologic therapy fails, particularly in the older child.

MYELODYSPLASIA

Myelodysplasia (spinal dysrhaphism) is a serious congenital anomaly occurring in 1–2 per 1,000 births in the United States. Multifactorial genetic and environmental influences are thought to be responsible for the unfused neural arches and associated spinal cord defects (Emery and Lendon, 1973). Although early neurosurgical intervention has decreased the incidence of meningitis and hydrocephalus in infancy (Laurence, 1964), urologic complications resulting from neurogenic vesical dysfunction (NGVD) remain the leading cause of morbidity and mortality in the survivors (Smith, 1965). For most, urinary incontinence is a formidable social handicap and, in some, vesicoureteral reflux, hydroureteronephrosis, chronic pyelonephritis, and urolithiasis ultimately result in renal failure (Light and Van Blerk, 1977). In recent years, sophisticated urodynamic evaluation of these children has permitted more precise and rational treatment. Pharmacologic therapy—often in conjunction with intermittent catheterization—and application of new surgical techniques have rendered many of these patients continent and promoted the preservation of renal function.

The term "spinal dysrhaphism" encompasses a spectrum of anomalies from the more occult dermal sinus, lipoma of the spinal cord, aberrant roots or fibrous traction bands, and abnormal filum terminale to the more apparent and generally more serious lesions of the meningocele and myelomeningocele (Andersen, 1974). Although the occult forms may be associated with significant NGVD, this discussion will primarily be concerned with the more common form encountered by the urologist, myelomeningocele. The location of myelomeningoceles is most frequently lumbosacral (42%), thoracolumbar (27%), and sacral (21%); only 10% are in a thoracic or cervical location (Kaplan, 1978). Some investigators maintain that the level of vertebral defect largely determines the degree of neurologic damage (Barson, 1970), but most studies suggest no correlation between the level and the NGVD (Thomas et al., 1974; Bauer et al., 1977). Indeed, significant NGVD has been associated with minimal bony defects (Andersen, 1975). These disparities can be explained by the various possible neuropathologic lesions of the spinal cord, which include hydromyelia, syringomyelia, failure of upward migration or tethering of the cord, and dysplasia of the cord itself. Further, these changes may extend several segments above and below the actual site of the myelomeningocele. The importance of urodynamic evaluation to determine the precise vesicourethral dysfunction present in an individual patient is thus apparent.

Clinical Presentation

Nearly all forms of spinal dysrhaphism are associated with a cutaneous abnormality of the back such as hypertrichosis, skin pigmentation, lipoma, skin dimple, or the more obvious meningocele (Andersen, 1975). Many patients have lower extremity orthopedic deformities, paresis, or paralysis. Inability to void, urinary incontinence, and fecal incontinence unfortunately are common problems.

Urologic Evaluation

As soon as practical after repair of the myelomeningocele and shunting of the cerebrospinal fluid, if necessary, several urologic studies are done. These include IVP, VCUG, urine culture, and serum blood urea nitrogen and creatinine determinations. These are obtained both for the purpose of identifying those patients requiring immediate treatment and as a baseline in others. Approximately 20% of patients have an abnormal IVP demonstrating hydroureteronephrosis, caliectasis, or hydroureter (Gaum et al., 1982). Of particular importance, nearly two-thirds of patients with a normal IVP have an abnormal VCUG showing vesicoureteral reflux, a thickened bladder wall, diverticula, or abnormalities of the bladder shape and outlet (Gaum et al., 1982). Thus, these radiographic examinations are complementary and we think that a VCUG should be obtained even when the IVP is normal. Urodynamic evaluation of neonates has been infrequently performed, but recently Bauer et al. (1984) have obtained important data suggesting that neonates should routinely undergo urodynamic investigation.

Urodynamic evaluation of children with myelodysplasia is essential in order to render rational therapy for urinary incontinence and to preserve renal function. It is important to ascertain several urodynamic parameters, including the bladder capacity, intravesical filling pressure, intravesical pressure at the moment of urethral urinary loss, presence or absence of reflex detrusor activity, and the competence of the internal and external sphincteric mechanisms. The degree of coordination of the detrusor and sphincter mechanisms and the postvoiding residual urine volume should also be determined.

Several investigators have reported similar results of urodynamic studies in myelodysplastic children (McGuire et al., 1981; Bauer et al., 1977; Mayo et al., 1979). Reflex detrusor activity in response to bladder filling is present in 17%–40% of patients. The reported incidence of detrusor-sphincter dyssynergia depends on its definition. If it is defined as an actual increase in the EMG activity and urethral pressure at the area of the external sphincter during a reflex detrusor contraction, then the incidence is 7% (McGuire et al., 1981). If it is defined as failure of sustained sphincter relaxation during reflex detrusor contraction or voiding maneuvers such as Valsalva or Credé, then the incidence is 50% (Bauer et al., 1977). From 60%–80% of patients have detrusor areflexia. In many, this is the result of the neural injury, but in others it may represent myogenic failure resulting from chronic distention or recurrent urinary tract infection with bladder wall fibrosis. Detrusor hypertonia (decreased detrusor compliance) during bladder filling occurs in up to 85% of patients with detrusor areflexia and is manifested as a progressive increase in intravesical pressure with increasing volume, culminating in urethral urinary loss when the intravesical and intraurethral pressures are equal. A striking relationship exists between intravesical pressure at the time of urethral urinary loss and the incidence of ureteral complications. In one report, if urethral urinary loss occurred at an intravesical pressure of less than 40 cm H_2O, no patient had vesicoureteral reflux and only 10% had ureteral dilatation (McGuire et al., 1981). On the other hand, if urethral urinary loss occurred at an intravesical pressure of more than 40 cm H_2O, 68% of patients had vesicoureteral reflux and 81% had ureteral dilatation. The majority of patients had open bladder necks, determined radiographically, and these patients tend to have a lower maximum urethral closure pressure than patients with closed bladder necks. The major clinical problem in these patients tends to be urinary incontinence. In those with higher urethral closure pressures, upper urinary tract deterioration and vesicoureteral reflux tend to occur.

The results of these investigations have important prognostic and therapeutic implications for children with myelodysplasia. McGuire et al. (1983) described six patients with detrusor hypertonia on initial urodynamic evaluation, but they had no upper tract complications. Subsequently, upper urinary tract deterioration or vesicoureteral reflux developed in all patients and persisting detrusor hypertonia was demonstrated on follow-up urodynamic testing. This upper tract deterioration may occur after many years of normalcy and as late as the midteenage years. Similar urodynamic abnormalities have been demonstrated in neonates, including upper tract deterioration developing in patients who initially had detrusor-sphincter dyssynergia and normal upper tracts (Bauer et al., 1984).

Bladder wall fibrosis may cause decreased detrusor compliance in some patients. However, the fact that bilateral surgical transection of all sacral roots often results in a hypertonic, areflexic detrusor response to bladder filling suggests that this response is usually intrinsic to the vesical musculature freed from central neural regulation (McGuire and Wagner, 1977). Experimental data indicate that an increase in adrenergic innervation and α-receptor activity occurs in the bladder after parasympathetic denervation (Sundin and Dahlstrom, 1973). Histochemical fluorescent studies of excised detrusor muscle from normal and parasympathetically denervated human bladders show that the adrenergic nerve terminals of the denervated detrusors are thicker, more strongly fluorescent, and more densely distributed than in normal detrusors (Sundin et al., 1977). Interestingly, the patients with denervated bladders had filling curves typical of decreased compliance on cystometry. Although the precise mechanism responsible for increased adrenergic activity is unknown, unmasking of already existing α-receptors or an induction of α-receptors by parasympathetic denervation seems probable (Sundin et al., 1977).

Treatment is based on vesicourethral function as previously outlined and also the degree of social and functional disability.

CAUDAL REGRESSION SYNDROME

The syndrome of caudal regression was described by Duhamel (1961); in its most severe form it results in sacral agenesis, imperforate anus, fusion of the lower extremities, and absence of the genitourinary tract except for the gonads. The disordered embryogenesis appears to occur at the fourth to fifth week of fetal life when the lumbosacral spine and nephrogenic masses are forming and the cloacal septum is separating the genitourinary sinus from the rectum. Fortunately, the most severe form is rare, but imperforate anus and sacral agenesis are relatively common, both as separate and combined congenital anomalies.

Imperforate Anus

Several classifications of imperforate anus have been proposed, and that of Santulli et al. (1970) is widely used. They classified imperforate anus into four major groups based on the level of the imperforation in relation to the puborectalis muscle or the pelvic floor: low or translevator lesions, intermediate lesions (which are uncommon), high or supralevator lesions, and miscellaneous lesions. In nearly all males with supralevator lesions, a fistulous communication exists between the prostatic urethra and the blind end of the rectal pouch; in females, a rectovaginal fistula is common. Patients with translevator lesions do not have fistulas between the intestinal and urinary tracts; rather the rectal fistula opens near the posterior scrotal raphe in males and the distal vagina or posterior fourchette in females.

Patients with supralevator lesions are managed with a diverting colostomy shortly after birth, with the definitive rectal pull-through and repair of rectourethral fistula performed when the child has grown to approximately 25 pounds. Those who have infralevator lesions are treated with a primary anoplasty. All patients should have uroradiographic studies to detect associated genitourinary anomalies. Patients with supralevator lesions have a 52%–67% incidence of genitourinary anomalies, but those with infralevator lesions have a 16%–18% incidence (Belman and King, 1972; Wiener and Kiesewetter, 1973).

Imperforate anus may be associated with many urologic problems, including a broad spectrum of congenital upper tract anomalies. Additionally, complications may result from the definitive surgical correction of the lesion. Excessive surgical dissection of the fistula has resulted in urethral stricture or sphincteric damage and urinary incontinence (Persky et al., 1974; Resnick and King, 1976), and failure to adequately excise the fistula has resulted in pseudodiverticulum formation (Persky et al., 1974).

Although it is difficult to ascertain the precise cause, neurogenic vesical dysfunction is also common among patients with imperforate anus. Approximately 25% of patients have abnormalities of the lumbosacral spine and most of these are supralevator lesions, which alone could be responsible for voiding dysfunction (see Sacral Agenesis, below) (Tank, 1979). In addition, the pelvic plexuses can be injured by the surgical dissection of the rectal pull-through procedure. These plexuses lie deep in the pelvis on either side of the rectum and contain preganglionic and postganglionic parasympathetic and sympathetic neurons. Thus, abnormalities of innervation of the bladder or urethra or both may occur. These include partial or complete denervation of the bladder manifested as poor detrusor contractility or detrusor areflexia or decreased detrusor compliance with increased intravesical filling pressure. Varying degrees of urethral denervation may also occur that result in a low maximum urethral closure pressure and urinary incontinence. A similar clinical situation exists in patients who have undergone radical or Wertheim's hysterectomy or abdominoperineal resection of the rectum (Woodside and McGuire, 1982; McGuire, 1975). Because of the spectrum of potential abnormalities in patients with imperforate anus, urodynamic investigation is important in order to precisely identify the disordered vesicourethral function and thus to direct specific treatment. Most commonly encountered are patients with decreased detrusor compliance, usually detrusor areflexia, as the cause of incomplete bladder emptying and as a contributing factor to urinary continence. Some patients have also had sphincteric insufficiency, with a bladder neck that appears open radiographically, and severe urinary incontinence.

Sacral Agenesis

Sacral agenesis results from the failure of ossification of the sacral segments early in fetal development and it is manifested as a complete or partial absence of one or more sacral vertebral segments. Several authors have noted an increased incidence of sacral agenesis in the offspring of mothers with diabetes mellitus (Koff and Deridder, 1977; Mariani et al., 1979; White and Klauber, 1976). The neuropathologic abnormalities of the spinal cord, spinal roots, and spinal canal have been ascertained from postmortem anatomic dissections and from the findings encountered at neurosurgical procedures. In some patients, the sacral roots caudad to the lowest formed vertebral segment fail to develop, but in others, sacral roots are present despite the absence of the corresponding vertebral bodies (Smith, 1959). There may be dense fibrous tissue within the spinal canal as well as an intradural lipoma, a dermoid cyst, or tethering of the cord (Cumes, 1977). Sacral agenesis may also coexist with forms of spinal dysrhaphism such as myelomeningocele and diastematomyelia (White and Klauber, 1976). The resulting neurologic deficits may result from absence of spinal roots, compression or entrapment of the spinal cord or spinal roots, and traction on the spinal cord during growth of the vertebral column due to tethering.

Many patients with sacral agenesis have either no apparent or only very subtle neurologic symptoms and the condition may elude diagnosis for many years (Braren and Jones, 1979). Unfortunately, some patients with neurogenic vesical dysfunction have undergone multiple urologic surgical procedures before the underlying condition was diagnosed (Cumes, 1977; Koontz and Prout, 1968). The condition may be misdiagnosed if only anteroposterior radiographs of the lower spine are obtained, because the sacrum may be poorly visualized if an exaggerated lumbosacral angle exists. Therefore, it is important to obtain lateral sacral radiographs (Mariani et al., 1979). Patients with neurogenic vesical dysfunction may initially present with hydronephrosis, urinary tract infection, vesicoureteral reflux, difficulty in voiding, urinary incontinence, or bladder trabeculation (Cumes, 1977). Several investigators have determined that neurogenic vesical dysfunction will occur in patients with agenesis of one or two sacral segments (Mariani et al., 1979; Williams and Nixon, 1957). The findings on physical examination may include a palpable defect in the sacrum, sacral dimple, a flattened gluteal region, foot deformities, decrease in perineal sensation and resting external anal sphincter tone, and flaccid paralysis of the muscles innervated by the second through fifth sacral roots (White and Klauber, 1976; Cumes, 1977). Motor deficits are generally more pronounced than sensory deficits (Mariani et al., 1979; Sarnat et al., 1976) and in many patients these deficits do not correlate with those expected from the bony deficiency (Koff and Deridder, 1977; Smith, 1959).

Similarly, the type of neurogenic vesical dysfunction does not correlate with the bony lesion (Koff and Deridder, 1977; Williams and Nixon, 1957). Because the clinical neurologic evaluation is also not helpful in identifying the specific type of neurogenic vesical dysfunction in a given patient, urodynamic evaluation is extremely important. Koff and Deridder (1977) performed sophisticated urodynamic evaluations in 11 patients with sacral agenesis. Three patients had uninhibited detrusor dysfunction, four had detrusor areflexia, and four had a mixed type of detrusor dysfunction. Perineal EMG was performed in 12 patients and seven showed evidence of denervation, but some had normal external anal sphincter activity in the presence of detrusor dysfunction. The pattern of neurogenic vesical dysfunction may change with time, probably because of traction of the spinal cord due to tethering.

NONNEUROGENIC VOIDING DYSFUNCTION

The true challenge to the pediatric neurourologist is the definition of vesicourethral dysfunction in the child who has no outward neurologic deficits. These children present to the clinician only after voiding difficulties have led to either urinary tract infection or significant social disability. The spectrum of voiding abnormalities seen is not unlike that of patients with true neurologic disease (Allen, 1977). Thus, to label this type of vesicourethral dysfunction as nonneurogenic speaks only to the general neurologic state of the child but not to the problem of vesicourethral dysfunction. Because this group of patients has no outward indicators for the potential of underlying vesicourethral problems, it becomes important for all clinicians to assess carefully the subtle changes in voiding mentioned by the child or his parents. When in doubt as to the significance of a particular symptom, a simple noninvasive test such as uroflowmetry may better define its importance.

When voiding dysfunction is identified without outward neurologic disease or evidence of spinal dysrhaphism, confusion abounds as to its cause. Some investigators have suggested an underlying psychological defect and others emphasize an occult neuropathy (Hinman, 1974; Dorfman et al., 1969; Johnston and Farkas, 1975; Martin et al., 1971; Williams et al., 1974). Regardless of origin, many of the voiding abnormalities are thought to be related to a disorder of coordination between the detrusor contraction and external sphincter relaxation. Support for a nonneurologic acquired abnormality comes from Bauer and associates (Bauer et al., 1980), who failed to show denervation potentials on raw EMG data obtained from the external sphincter in such children. In addition, many such voiding abnormalities are associated with acquired bowel defects such as encopresis. Also supporting an acquired cause is the fact that many such voiding abnormalities can be corrected by a period of bladder retraining, which may include biofeedback methods. The full spectrum of voiding dysfunction may be seen and the diagnostic characteristics are the same as those seen with true neurologic disease (Wein, 1984). Many such patients have subtly sus-

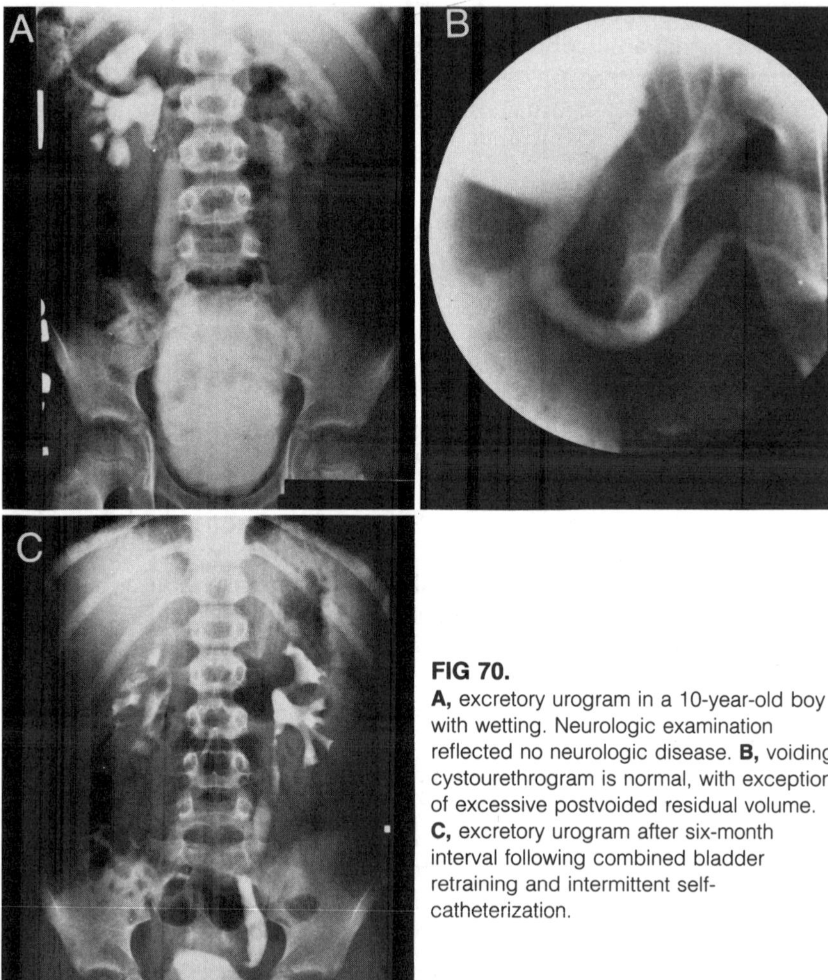

FIG 70.
A, excretory urogram in a 10-year-old boy with wetting. Neurologic examination reflected no neurologic disease. **B,** voiding cystourethrogram is normal, with exception of excessive postvoided residual volume. **C,** excretory urogram after six-month interval following combined bladder retraining and intermittent self-catheterization.

tained irreversible damage to the detrusor, resulting in myogenic decompensation (Fig 70). In others, vesicoureteral reflux may have developed and surgical repair will be necessary to ensure adequate bladder emptying (Snyder et al., 1982). In all such patients, therapy should be designed to promote adequate bladder emptying and an acceptably low voiding pressure to protect the upper urinary tracts.

Those with urgency, frequency, and wetting related to vesicourethral incoordination are ideally suited to bladder retraining with the biofeedback methods. However, those with significant failure-to-empty defects may be better managed with conventional techniques of intermittent catheterization, with or without the use of adjunctive pharmacologic agents. The length of therapy in both categories of patients will be dependent on the degree of detrusor decompensation, upper tract disease, and the likelihood of relapse into a vesicourethral incoordination state. Regular follow-up is necessary in these patients to ensure that relapse has not occurred and that the upper tracts are, in fact, being protected.

Psychogenic Voiding Dysfunction

Voiding dysfunction in the absence of organic disease has been classified as psychogenic in origin (Krane and Siroky, 1979a, 1979b). Voiding problems of all types will be associated with psychological manifestations. However, which problem arrived first, the voiding problem or the psychological problem, is not always clear. Considering all voiding problems, some are obviously organic and others psychogenic, but numerous patients with significant voiding dysfunction fall in between, resulting in diagnoses that are indeterminate. Voiding symptoms related to psychological disturbances range from frank urinary retention to marked urgency, frequency, and enuresis (Rowan, 1975).

PSYCHOGENIC RETENTION

For those patients with defects related to a "failure to empty," the symptoms may range from acute retention to those suggesting a more chronic course, such as urinary infection or overflow type incontinence (Allen, 1972; Barrett, 1976; Doran and Roberts, 1976; Larson et al., 1963; Norden and Friedman, 1961). Acute retention is often temporally related to some catastrophic psychological stress in the patient's life. These patients are often young or middle-aged women. However, select male patients may also demonstrate this phenomenon (Chapman, 1959; Fox et al., 1976; Khan, 1971; Krugman et al., 1971). Such patients may exhibit a propensity for repeated episodes of acute retention with essentially normal voiding in between.

Other patients with a more chronic pattern will continuously maintain considerable residual volumes. A propensity toward urinary infection may be seen and, depending on the degree of retention and the integrity of the ureterovesical angle, upper tract disease may develop. The patient may give a history of having been toilet-trained at an early age and exhibiting excellent urinary control. Many will be life-long infrequent voiders and notably require voiding only 1–4 times daily. Micturition in such patients may require straining, pushing, or a Credé maneuver to augment emptying. The sensation to void will become impaired and the desire to void is noticed only when large volumes occupy the bladder. Periodic "treatments" such as urethral dilation or internal urethrotomy may transiently benefit the patient; however, excessive residual urine generally returns.

The pathophysiology of psychogenic retention is open to controversy but is much easier to accept in the patient with acute retention. Theoretically, excessive stimuli, either excitatory or inhibitory, originate in centers above the brain stem and influence coordinated micturition. Speculation exists as to the point at which impairment—leading to retention—occurs in the cascade of events that take place during normal micturition. The two most plausible explanations are: (1) excessive stimulation of the centers of the pyramidal tracts that directly innervate the skeletal muscle urethral sphincter, resulting in a failure of the sphincter to relax in preparation for voiding (Lewin et al., 1967), or (2) inhibition of the autonomic motor nucleus in the brain stem that innervates the bladder body, resulting in decreased detrusor contractility (Bradley and Conway, 1966; Bradley and Teague, 1968).

Urodynamic parameters in patients with acute urinary retention generally reflect decreased detrusor contractility, normal compliance, and slightly elevated urethral closing pressure. After the acute phase resolves, the parameters—including uroflow rate—may be normal. Those with a chronic history of urinary retention will have decreased detrusor contractility, increased compliance, increased intra-abdominal pressure during voiding, and reduced average flow rate.

The diagnosis of psychogenically induced urinary retention is one of exclusion, and subtle neurologic or metabolic disease must be excluded (Barrett, 1978). Thus, consultations from appropriate specialists are indicated and often extensive neurologic testing, including scans of the brain and spinal cord, may be necessary. Since the symptoms that lead to medical scrutiny are urologic in origin, it becomes the responsibility of the urologist to coordinate this evaluation. Also, management of the voiding problem must be undertaken along the lines outlined earlier for patients with failure to empty. Psychologic consultation is required when patients have overt psychological disease or when they fail to understand the potential for a psychological disturbance as a cause for voiding abnormalities.

PSYCHOGENIC URGENCY-FREGUENCY SYNDROME

Much of the urologic practice deals with patients exhibiting symptoms of urinary urgency, frequency, and urge incontinence (Smith, 1962). Lower abdominal and perineal discomfort may also accompany this syndrome. These patients, who are predominantly female, must undergo a thorough neurologic evaluation to exclude underlying disease (Rees et al., 1976). Similar symptomatology will lead to the diagnosis of unsuspected urinary infections in many patients, and those without a psychogenic relationship will improve with antibiotic treatment (Gallagher et al., 1965). Those of psychogenic etiology again will be suspected when all tests are essentially normal. Even males with typical "prostatitis" symptoms may fall into this category (Fritjofsson et al., 1973).

Uroradiography, endoscopy, and urodynamics are normal in most of these patients. However, in a select few, micturition may be impaired by functional outflow obstruction (Farrar et al., 1976). Cystometry will reflect normal compliance but a decreased functional capacity (Rees et al., 1976). Occasionally, detrusor instability will be seen. Uroflow will reflect a small voided volume and the average rate will be decreased. Combined studies including fluoroscopy are best for detecting the functional outlet obstruction syndrome. Voiding pressure will be high and flow rate decreased. There will be little if any bladder neck funneling during the detrusor contraction. Thus, the condition suggests dyssynergia of the bladder neck and proximal urethra.

It is unclear whether this extreme version of the urgency-frequency syndrome is truly psychogenic in origin, but the lack of associated neurologic disease in most of these patients makes the diagnosis likely (Mulholland et al., 1974). Many of these patients respond, at least temporarily, to measures designed to reduce outflow resistance (Raz and Smith, 1976). Internal urethrotomy or bladder neck resection is a last resort and should be performed only in the presence of data substantiating outlet obstruction (Emmett et al., 1950). The goal of such therapy is to reduce voiding pressures and reverse the stimulus that provokes the sensation of urgency.

The psychodynamics of the psychogenic urgency-frequency abnormality are similar to the retention syndrome in that inhibitory or excitatory stimuli from the central nervous system above the brain alter the micturition sequence in such a way that either sensation or contraction is impaired.

REFERENCES

1. Abel B, Gibbon N, Jameson R, et al: The neuropathic urethra. *Lancet* 1974; 2:1229.
2. Abrams PH: Investigation of post-prostatectomy problems. *Urology* 1980; 15:209.
3. Abrams P: The practice of urodynamics, in Mundy AR, Stephenson TP, Wein AJ (eds): *Urodynamics: Principles, Practice and Application.* Edinburgh, Churchill-Livingstone, 1984a, p 76.
4. Abrams P: The urethral pressure profile measurement, in Mundy AR, Stephenson TP, Wein AJ (eds): *Urodynamics: Principles, Practice and Application.* Edinburgh, Churchill-Livingstone, 1984b, p 127.
5. Abrams P: Detrusor instability and bladder outlet obstruction. *Neurourol Urodynamics* 1985; 4:317.
6. Allen TD: Psychogenic urinary retention. *South Med J* 1972; 65:302.
7. Allen TD: The non-neurogenic neurogenic bladder. *J Urol* 1977; 117:232–238.
8. Allen TD: Commentary on dysfunctional abnormalities of the urinary tract. *Urol Clin North Am* 1980; 7:357.
9. Allen TD, Bright TC III: Urodynamic patterns in children with dysfunctional voiding problems. *J Urol* 1978; 119:247–249.
10. Althausen AF, Hagen-Cook K, Hendren WH III: Non-refluxing colon conduit: Experience with 70 cases. *J Urol* 1978; 120:35.
11. Altwein JE, Jonas U, Hohenfellner R: Long-term follow-up of children with colon conduit urinary diversion and ureterosigmoidostomy. *J Urol* 1977; 118:832.
12. Andersen JT, Nordling J: Prostatism: I. The correlation between symptomatic cystometric and urodynamic findings. *Scand J Urol Nephrol* 1979; 13:229.
13. Andersen JT, Nordling J: Prostatism: II. The correlation between cystourethroscopic, cystometric, and urodynamic findings. *Scand J Urol Nephrol* 1980; 14:23.
14. Andersen JT, Walter S, Vejesgaard R: A clinical and bacteriological trial with DMSO in the treatment of severe detrusor hyperreflexia. *Scand J Urol Nephrol* 1981; 60(suppl):63.
15. Andersen JT, Bradley WE: Abnormalities of detrusor and sphincter dysfunction in multiple scleroma. *Br J Urol* 1976; 48:193.
16. Anderson FM: Occult spinal dysrhaphism: A series of 73 cases. *Pediatrics* 1975; 55:826–835.
17. Andersen JT, Hebjorn S, Frimodt-Moller C, et al: Disturbances of micturition in Parkinson's disease. *Acta Neurol Scand* 1976; 53:161.
18. Andersen JT, Jacobson O, Worm-Petersen J, et al: Bladder function in healthy elderly males. *Scand J Urol Nephrol* 1978; 12:123.
19. Andersson K, Ek A, Hedlung H, et al: Effects of prazosin on isolated human urethra and in patients with lower neuron lesions. *Invest Urol* 1981; 19:39.

20. Ashken MH: Urinary reservoirs, in Ashken MH (ed): *Urinary Diversion.* New York, Springer-Verlag, 1982.
21. Awad SA, Bryniak SR, Downie JN, et al: Urethral pressure profile during the spinal shock stage in man: A preliminary report. *J Urol* 1977; 117:91.
22. Awad S, Downie J, Kiruluta H: Alpha adrenergic agents in urinary disorders of the proximal urethra: I. Stress incontinence. *Br J Urol* 1978; 50:332.
23. Awad S, McGinnis R, Downie J: The effectiveness of bethanechol chloride in lower motor neuron lesions: The importance of mode of administration. *Neurourol Urodynamics* 1984; 3:173.
24. Baldessarini R: Drugs and the treatment of psychiatric disorders, in Gilman AG, Goodman LS, Gilman A (eds): *The Pharmacological Basis of Therapeutics.* New York, Macmillan, 1980, pp 391–447.
25. Barrett DM: Psychogenic urinary retention in women. *Mayo Clin Proc* 1976; 51:351.
26. Barrett DM: Evaluation of psychogenic urinary retention. *J Urol* 1978; 120:191.
27. Barrett DM: Disposable (infant) surface electrocardiogram electrodes in urodynamics: A simultaneous comparative study of electrodes. *J Urol* 1980; 124:663.
28. Barrett DM: The effect of oral bethanechol chloride on voiding in female patients with excessive residual urine: A randomized double-blind study. *J Urol* 1981; 126:640.
29. Barrett DM: Urinary flow rate: Theory and methods, in Barrett DM, Wein AJ (eds): *Controversies in Neuro-urology.* New York, Churchill-Livingstone, 1984, pp 133–143.
30. Barrett DM: *AUA Update: The Artificial Sphincter,* lesson 32 Houston, AUA, 1986.
31. Barrett DM, Wein AJ: Flow evaluation and simultaneous external sphincter electromyography in clinical urodynamics. *J Urol* 1981; 125:538–541.
32. Barson AJ: Spina bifida: The significance of the level and extent of the defect to the morphogenesis. *Dev Med Child Neurol* 1970; 12:129–144.
33. Bates CP, Arnold EP, Griffiths DJ: The nature of the abnormality in bladder neck obstruction. *Br J Urol* 1975; 47:651.
34. Bauer SB: Urodynamics in children: Indications and methods, in Barrett DM, Wein AJ (eds): *Controversies in Neuro-urology.* New York, Churchill-Livingstone, 1984, pp 193–202.
35. Bauer SB, Colodny AH, Retik AB: The management of vesicoureteral reflux in children with myelodysplasia. *J Urol* 1982; 128:102–105.
36. Bauer SB, Hallett M, Khoshbin S, et al: Predictive value of urodynamic evaluation in newborns with myelodysplasia. *JAMA* 1984; 252:650–652.
37. Bauer SB, Labib KB, Dieppa RA, et al: Urodynamic evaluation of boy with myelodysplasia and incontinence. *Urology* 1977; 10:354–362.
38. Bauer SB, Retik AB, Colodny AH, et al: The unstable bladder of childhood. *Urol Clin North Am* 1980; 7:321–336.

39. Baumrucker GO: Management of the paralyzed bladder. *Arch Surg* 1948; 56:484.
40. Beisland HO, Fossberg E, Sander S: On incompetent urethral closure mechanism: Treatment with estriol and phenylpropanolamine. *Scand J Urol Nephrol* 1981; 60(suppl):67.
41. Belman AB, King LR: Urinary tract abnormalities associated with imperforate anus. *J Urol* 1972; 108:823–824.
42. Benson G, Sarshik S, Raezer D, et al: Comparative effects and mechanisms of action of atropine, propantheline, flavoxate, and imipramine on bladder muscle contractility. *Urology* 1977; 9:31.
43. Benson GS, Rogers DM, Wein AJ, et al: Effect of muscle length on adrenergic stimulation of canine detrusor. *Urology* 1975; 5:769.
44. Berg S: Polytef augmentation urethroplasty. *Arch Surg* 1973; 107:379.
45. Berry JL: A new procedure for correction of urinary incontinence: Preliminary report. *J Urol* 1961; 85:771–775.
46. Bianchine J: Drugs for Parkinson's disease: Centrally acting muscle relaxants, in Gilman AG, Goodman LS, Gilman A (eds): *The Pharmacological Basis of Therapeutics*. New York, Macmillan, 1980, pp 475–493.
47. Bigger J, Giardino E, Perel J, et al: Cardiac antiarrhythmic effect of imipramine hydrochloride. *N Engl J Med* 1977; 296:206.
48. Birkasova M, Birkas O, Flynn MJ, et al: Desmopressin in the management of nocturnal enuresis in children: A double-blind study. *Pediatrics* 1978; 62:970.
49. Blaivas JG: Management of bladder dysfunction in multiple sclerosis. *Neurology* 1980; 30:12.
50. Blaivas J: If you currently prescribe bethanechol chloride for urinary retention, please raise your hand. *Neurourol Urodynamics* 1984; 3:209.
51. Blaivas JG: Non-traumatic neurogenic voiding dysfunction in the adult: I. Physiology and approach to therapy. AUA Update Series, lesson 11, vol 4, 1985a.
52. Blaivas JG: Non-traumatic neurogenic voiding dysfunction in the adult: II. Multiple sclerosis and diabetes mellitus. AUA Update Series, lesson 12, vol 4, 1985b.
53. Blaivas JG: Electromyography and sacral evoked responses, in Mundy AR, Stephenson TP, Wein AJ (eds): *Urodynamics: Principles, Practice and Application*. Edinburgh, Churchill-Livingstone, 1984a, p 139.
54. Blaivas JG: Multichannel urodynamic studies. *Urology* 1984b; 23:421.
55. Blaivas JG, et al: Failure of bethanechol denervation supersensitivity as a diagnostic aid. *J Urol* 1980; 123:199.
56. Blaivas JG, et al: Detrusor-external sphincter dyssynergia: A detailed EMG study. *J Urol* 1981; 125:545.
57. Blaivas JG, Barbalias GA: Detrusor external sphincter dyssynergia in men with multiple sclerosis: An ominous urologic condition. *J Urol* 1984; 131:94.
58. Blaivas JG, Bhimani G, Labib KB: Vesicourethral dysfunction in multiple sclerosis. *J Urol* 1979; 122:342.

59. Blaivas J, Labib K, Michalik S, et al: Cystometric response to propantheline in detrusor hyperreflexia: Therapeutic implications. *J Urol* 1980; 124:259.
60. Blaivas JG, Labib KL, Bauer SB, et al: A new approach to electromyography of the external urethral sphincter. *J Urol* 1977; 117:773.
61. Blaivas JG, Labib KL, Bauer SB, et al: Changing concepts in the urodynamic evaluation of children. *J Urol* 1977; 117:778–781.
62. Blaivas JG, Norlen LJ: Primary bladder neck obstruction. *World J Urol* 1984; 2:195.
63. Blaivas JG, Sinha HP, Zayed AA, et al: Detrusor-external sphincter dyssynergia. *J Urol* 1981a; 125:541.
64. Blaivas JG, Zayed AAH, Labib KB: The bulbocavernosus reflex in urology: A prospective study of 299 patients. *J Urol* 1981b; 126:197.
65. Bonney V: On diurnal incontinence of urine in women. *Br J Obstet Gynecol* 1923; 30:358.
66. Bors E: Neurogenic bladder. *Urol Survey* 1957; 7:177.
67. Bors E, Comarr AE: *Neurological Urology*. Baltimore, University Park Press, 1971.
68. Bradley WE, Chou S, Markland C: Classifying neurologic dysfunction of the urinary bladder, in Boyarsky S (ed): *The Neurogenic Bladder*. Baltimore, Williams & Wilkins Co, 1967, pp 139–146.
69. Bradley WE, Conway CJ: Bladder representation in the pontine-mesencephalic reticular formation. *Exp Neurol* 1966; 16:251.
70. Bradley WE, Teague CT: Spinal cord organization of micturitional reflex afferents. *Exp Neurol* 1968; 22:504.
71. Bradley WE, Timm GW, Scott FB: Innervation of the detrusor muscle and urethra. *Urol Clin North Am* 1974; 1:3–27.
72. Bramble FJ: The treatment of adult enuresis and urge incontinence by enterocystoplasty. *Br J Urol* 1982; 54:693.
73. Braren V, Jones WB: Sacral agenesis: Diagnosis, treatment and follow up of urological complications. *J Urol* 1979; 121:543–544.
74. Brent L, Stephens FD: The response of smooth muscle cells in the rabbit urinary bladder to outflow obstruction. *Invest Urol* 1975; 12:494.
75. Bricker EM: Bladder substitution after pelvic evisceration. *Surg Clin North Am* 1950; 30:1511.
76. Briggs R, Castleden C, Asher M: The effect of flavoxate on uninhibited detrusor contractions and urinary incontinence in the elderly. *J Urol* 1980; 123:665.
77. Broecker BH, Klein FA, Hackler RH: Cancer of the bladder in spinal cord injury patients. *J Urol* 1981; 125:196.
78. Brown M, Wickham JEA: The urethral pressure profile. *Br J Urol* 1969; 51:211.
79. Bultitude M, Hills N, Shuttleworth K: Clinical and experimental studies on the action of prostaglandins and their synthesis inhibitors on detrusor muscle in vitro and in vivo. *Br J Urol* 1976; 48:631.
80. Bunce PL: Transurethral resection and Y-V plasty for neurogenic blad-

der, in Boyarsky S (ed): *The Neurogenic Bladder.* Baltimore, Williams & Wilkins Co, 1967, pp 196–199.

81. Burch JC: Urethrovaginal fixation to Cooper's ligament for correction of stress incontinence, cystocele and prolapse. *Am J Obstet Gynecol* 1961; 81:281.
82. Burgess C, Turner T: Cardiotoxicity of antidepressant drugs. *Neuropharmacology* 1980; 19:1195.
83. Caine M, Edwards D: The peripheral control of micturition: A cineradiological study. *Br J Urol* 1958; 30:34.
84. Cardozo L, Stanton S: A comparison between bromocriptine and indomethacin in the treatment of detrusor instability. *J Urol* 1980; 123:399.
85. Cardozo L, Stanton S, Robinson H, et al: Evaluation of flurbiprofen in detrusor instability. *Br Med J* 1980; 280:281.
86. Cardozo LD, Abrams PD, Stanton SL, et al: Idiopathic bladder instability treated by biofeedback. *Br J Urol* 1978; 50:521.
87. Castleden C, George C, Redwick A, et al: Imipramine—a possible alternative to current therapy for urinary incontinence in the elderly. *J Urol* 1981; 125:218.
88. Chalfin SA, Bradley WE: The etiology of detrusor hyperreflexia in patients with infravesical obstruction. *J Urol* 1982; 127:938.
89. Chan WY, Dawood MY, Fuchs F: Prostaglandins in primary dysmenorrhea. *Am J Med* 1981; 70:535.
90. Chapman AH: Psychogenic urinary retention in women. *Psychosom Med* 1959; 21:119.
91. Cole A, Fried F: Favorable experiences with imipramine in the treatment of neurogenic bladder. *J Urol* 1972; 107:44.
92. Comarr AE: The practical urologic management of the patient with spinal cord injury. *Br J Urol* 1959; 31:1.
93. Comarr AE: Diagnosis of the traumatic cord bladder, in Boyarsky S (ed): *The Neurogenic Bladder.* Baltimore, Williams & Wilkins Co, 1967, pp 147–152.
94. Constantinou CE, Faysal MH, Rother L, et al: The impact of bladder neck suspension on the mode of distribution of abdominal pressure along the female urethra, in Zinner NR, Sterling AM (eds): *Female Incontinence: Progress in Clinical and Biological Research.* New York, Alan R Liss Inc, vol 78, 1981, pp 121–132.
95. Cook WA, Firlit CF, Stephens FD, et al: Techniques and results of urodynamic evaluation of children. *J Urol* 1977; 117:346–349.
96. Council on Scientific Affairs: DMSO. *JAMA* 1982; 248:1369.
97. Cumes D: Sacral dysgenesis associated with occult spinal dysraphism causing neurogenic bladder dysfunction. *J Urol* 1977; 117:127–128.
98. Deane AM, English P, Hehn M, et al: Teflon injection in stress incontinence. *Br J Urol* 1985; 57:78.
99. Dees JE: Congenital epispadias with incontinence. *J Urol* 1949; 612:513.
100. Dees JE: Contraction of the urinary bladder produced by electric stimulation: Preliminary report. *Invest Urol* 1965; 2:539.

101. deGroat WC: Nervous control of the urinary bladder of the cat. *Brain Res* 1975; 87:201–211.
102. deGroat WC, Saum WR: Adrenergic inhibition in mammalian parasympathetic ganglia. *Nature* 1971; 231:188–189.
103. deGroat WC, Theobald RJ: Reflex activation of sympathetic pathways to vesical smooth muscle and parasympathetic ganglia by stimulation of vesical afferents. *J Physiol* 1976; 259:223–237.
104. Delaere TC, Moonen T, et al: The value of prostaglandin E_2 and $F_{2\alpha}$ in women with abnormalities of bladder emptying. *Br J Urol* 1981; 53:306.
105. Desmond A, Bultitude M, Hills N, et al: Clinical experience with intravesical prostaglandin E_2: A prospective study of 36 patients. *Br J Urol* 1980; 53:357.
106. Dhattiwala A: The effect of imipramine on isolated innervated guinea pig and rat urinary bladder preparations. *J Pharmacol* 1976; 28:453.
107. Diokno A, Koppenhoeffer R: Bethanechol chloride in neurogenic bladder dysfunction. *Urology* 1976; 8:455.
108. Diokno A, Taub M: Ephedrine in treatment of urinary incontinence. *Urology* 1975; 5:624.
109. Diokno AC, Hollander JB, Bennett CJ: Bladder neck obstruction in females: A real entity. *J Urol* 1984; 132:294.
110. Dixon JS, Hald T: Morphological studies of the bladder wall in interstitial cystitis, in George NJR, Gosling JA (eds): *Sensory Disorders of the Bladder and Urethra*. New York, Springer-Verlag, 1986, pp 63–71.
111. Donker P, Van der Sluis C: Action of beta adrenergic blocking agents on the urethral pressure profile. *Urol Int* 1976; 31:6.
112. Doran J, Roberts M: Acute urinary retention in the female. *Br J Urol* 1976; 47:793.
113. Dorfman LE, Bailey J, Smith JP: Subclinical neurogenic bladder in children. *J Urol* 1969; 101:48–54.
114. Downie J: Bethanechol chloride in urology—a discussion of issues. *Neurourol Urodynamics* 1984; 3:211.
115. Downie J, Twiddy D, Awad S: Antimuscarinic and noncompetitive antagonist properties of dicyclomine hydrochloride in isolated human and rabbit bladder muscle. *J Pharmacol Exp Ther* 1977; 201:662.
116. Drach GW, Fair WR, Meares EM, et al: Classification of benign diseases associated with prostatic pain: Prostatitis or prostatodynia? *J Urol* 1978; 120:286.
117. Duhamel B: From the mermaid to anal imperforation: The syndrome of caudal regression. *Arch Dis Child* 1961; 36:152–155.
118. Duncan G, Shahani B, Young R: An evaluation of baclofen treatment for certain symptoms in patients with spinal cord lesions. *Neurology* 1976; 26:441.
119. Dunn M, Roberts JBM, Smith PJB, et al: The long-term results of ileal conduit urinary diversion in children. *Br J Urol* 1979; 51:458.
120. Edwards L: Mechanical and other devices, in Caldwell KPS (ed): *Urinary Incontinence*. New York, Grune & Stratton, 1975, pp 115–127.
121. Ek A, Andersson KE, Gullberg B, et al: The effects of long-term treat-

ment with norephedrine on stress incontinence and urethral closure pressure profile. *Scand J Urol Nephrol* 1978; 12:105.

122. Ekman G, Andersson KE, Rud T, et al: A double blind crossover study of the effects of xerodilene in women with unstable bladder. *Acta Pharmacol Toxicol* 1980; 46(suppl):39.
123. El Badawi A, Schenk EA: A new theory of the innervation of the bladder musculature: Morphology of the intrinsic vesical innervation apparatus. *J Urol* 1968; 99:585–592.
124. El Badawi A, Schenk EA: A new theory of the innervation of bladder musculature: II. The innervation of bladder musculature: 2. The innervation apparatus of the ureterovesical junction. *J Urol* 1971; 105:368–371.
125. El Badawi A, Schenk EA: A new theory of the innervation of bladder musculature: IV. Innervation of the vesicourethral junction and external urethral sphincter. *J Urol* 1974; 111:613–615.
126. Elder DD, Moisey CU, Rees RWM: A long-term follow-up of the colonic conduit operation in children. *Br J Urol* 1979; 51:462.
127. Elder DD, Stephenson TP: An assessment of the Frewen regime in the treatment of detrusor dysfunction in females. *Br J Urol* 1980; 52:467.
128. Emmett JL: Transurethral resection in treatment of true and pseudo cord bladder. *J Urol* 1945; 53:4.
129. Emery JL, Lendon RG: The local cord lesion in neurospinal dysrhaphism (meningomyelocele). *J Pathol* 1973; 110:83–96.
130. Emmett JL, Hutchins SPR, McDonald JR: The treatment of urinary retention in women by transurethral resection. *J Urol* 1950; 63:1031.
131. Enhorning G: Simultaneous recording of intravesical and intraurethral pressure. *Acta Chir Scand* 1961; 276(suppl):1.
132. Erlandson BE, Fall M: Intravaginal electrical stimulation in urinary incontinence. *Scand J Urol Nephrol* 1977; 44(suppl):5.
133. Evans AT, Felker JR, Shank RA III, et al: Pitfalls of urodynamics. *J Urol* 1979; 122:220–222.
134. Farrar DJ: Urodynamics and the elderly, in Mundy AR, Stephenson TP, Wein AJ (eds): *Urodynamics: Principles, Practice, and Application.* New York, Churchill-Livingstone, 1984, pp 249–255.
135. Farrar DJ, Osborne JL, Stephenson TP, et al: A urodynamic view of bladder outflow obstruction in the female: Factors influencing the results of treatment. *Br J Urol* 1976; 47:815.
136. Farrar DJ, Whiteside CG, Osborne JL, et al: A urodynamic evaluation of micturition symptoms in the female. *Surg Gynecol Obstet* 1975; 141:875.
137. Feneley RCL, Shepherd AM, Powell PH, et al: Urinary incontinence: Prevalence and needs. *Br J Urol* 1979; 51:493.
138. Finkbeiner A, Welch L, Bissada N: Uropharmacology: IX. Direct acting smooth muscle stimulants and depressants. *Urology* 1978; 12:231.
139. Firlit CF, Smey P, King LD: Micturition urodynamic flow studies in children. *J Urol* 1978; 119:250–253.
140. Fischer C, Diokno A, Lapides J: The anticholinergic effects of dicyclomine hydrochloride in uninhibited neurogenic bladder dysfunction. *J Urol* 1978; 120:328.

141. Florante J, Leyson J, Martin B, et al: Baclofen in the treatment of detrusor-sphincter dyssynergy in spinal cord injury patients. *J Urol* 1980; 124:82.
142. Foley FB: An artificial sphincter: A new device and operation for control of enuresis and urinary incontinence. *J Urol* 1947; 58:250–259.
143. Forman A, Andersson K, Henriksson L, et al: Effects of nifedipine on the smooth muscle of the human urinary tract in vitro and in vivo. *Acta Pharmacol Toxicol* 1978; 43:111.
144. Forsythe WI, Redmond A: Enuresis and spontaneous cure rate: Study of 1,129 enuretics. *Arch Dis Child* 1974; 49:259–263.
145. Fossberg E, Bersland HO, Sander S: Sensory urgency in females: Treatment with phenylpropanolamine. *Eur Urol* 1981; 7:157.
146. Fowler JE Jr: Prospective study of intravesical dimethylsulfoxide in the treatment of suspected early interstitial cystitis. *Urology* 1981; 18:21.
147. Fox M, Jarvis GJ, Henry L: Idiopathic chronic urinary retention in the female. *Br J Urol* 1976; 47:797.
148. Frankel HL: Intermittent catheterization. *Urol Clin North Am* 1974; 1:115.
149. Fredericks C, Green R, Anderson G: Comparative in vitro effects of imipramine, oxybutynin and flavoxate on rabbit detrusor. *Urology* 1978; 12:487.
150. Freiha FS, Stamey TA: Cystolysis: A procedure for the selective denervation of the bladder. *J Urol* 1980; 123:360.
151. Frewen WK: An objective assessment of the unstable bladder of psychosomatic origin. *Br J Urol* 1978; 50:246.
152. Frewen WK: The management of urgency and frequency of micturition. *Br J Urol* 1980; 512:367.
153. Frimodt-Moller C: Diabetes cystopathy: I. A clinical study on the frequency of bladder dysfunction in diabetics. *Danish Med Bull* 1976; 23:267.
154. Frimodt-Moller C: Cystopathy: II. Relationship to some late diabetic manifestations. *Danish Med Bull* 1976b; 23:279.
155. Fritjofsson A, Kihl B, Danielsson G: Chronic prostato-vesiculitis: Incidence and significance of bacterial findings. *Scand J Urol Nephrol* 1973; 8:173.
156. Gallagher DJA, Montgomerie JZ, North JDK: Acute infections of the urinary tract and the urethral syndrome in general practice. *Br Med J* 1965; 1:622.
157. Gaum LD, Wese FX, Alton DJ, et al: Radiologic investigation of the urinary tract in the neonate with myelomeningocele. *J Urol* 1982; 127:510–511.
158. George NJR: Preface in George NJR, Gosling JA (eds): *Sensory Disorders of the Bladder and Urethra.* New York, Springer-Verlag, 1986a, p vii.
159. George NJR: Urethral syndrome—clinical features, in George NJR, Gosling JA (eds): *Sensory Disorders of the Bladder and Urethra.* New York, Springer-Verlag, 1986b, pp 91–102.
160. Gerstenberg TC, Andersen JT, Klarshov P, et al: High flow infravesical obstruction in the male. *J Urol* 1982; 127:943.

161. Gerstenberg TC, Lykkegaard, Nielsen M, et al: Spastic striated external sphincter syndrome initiating recurrent urinary tract infection in females. *Eur Urol* 1983; 9:87.
162. Gibaldi M, Grundhofer B: Biopharmaceutic influences on the anticholinergic effects of propantheline. *Clin Pharmacol Ther* 1975; 18:457.
163. Gibbon N: Management of the bladder in acute and chronic disorders of the nervous system. *Acta Neurol Scand* 1966; 42(suppl):133.
164. Gibbon N: Urinary incontinence in disorders of the nervous system. *Br J Urol* 1975; 37:624.
165. Gibbon NOK: Later management of the paraplegic bladder. *Paraplegia* 1974a; 12:87.
166. Gibbon NOK: Neurogenic bladder in spinal cord injury: Management of patients in Liverpool, England. *Urol Clin North Am* 1974b; 1:147.
167. Gibbon NOK: Nomenclature of neurogenic bladder. *Urology* 1976; 8:423.
168. Gibbon NOK, Ross JC, Damanski M: Bladder neck resection in the paraplegic: Report of over 100 cases. *Paraplegia* 1965; 2:264.
169. Gierup J: Micturition studies in infants and children: Intravesical pressure, urinary flow and urethral resistance in boys without infravesical obstruction. *Scand J Urol Nephrol* 1970; 4:217–230.
170. Gilpin SA, Gosling JA, Barnard RJ: Morphological and morphometric studies of the human obstructed trabeculated urinary bladder. *Br J Urol* 1985; 57:525.
171. Glahn BE: Neurogenic bladder in spinal cord injury: Management of patients. *Urol Clin North Am* 1974; 1:163.
172. Gleason D, Reilly R, Bottaccini M, et al: The urethral continence zone and its relation to stress incontinence. *J Urol* 1974; 112:81.
173. Gleason DM, Bottaccini MR, Reilly RJ: Comparison of cystometrograms and urethral profiles with gas and water media. *Urology* 1977; 9:155–160.
174. Glen E: Control of incontinence by electrical devices, in Caldwell KBS (ed): *Urinary Incontinence.* New York, Grune & Stratton, 1975, pp 89–114.
175. Godec C, Krolg B: Selection of patients with urinary incontinence for application of functional electrical stimulation. *Urol Int* 1976; 31:124.
176. Godec CJ, Fravel R, Cass AS: Optimal parameters of electrical stimulation in the treatment of urinary incontinence. *Invest Urol* 1981; 18:239.
177. Goellner MH, Ziegler EE, Fomon SJ: Urination during the first three years of life. *Nephron* 1981; 28:174–178.
178. Goldwasser B, Webster GD: Continent urinary diversion. *J Urol* 1985; 134:227.
179. Goldwasser B, Webster GD: Augmentation and substitution enterocystoplasty. *J Urol* 1986; 135:215.
180. Golz H: Complications of external condom drainage. *Paraplegia* 1981; 19:189.
181. Gordon HL, Rossen RD, Hersh EM, et al: Immunologic aspects of interstitial cystitis. *J Urol* 1983; 109:228.
182. Green T: The problem of urinary stress incontinence in the female: An appraisal of its current status. *Obstet Gynecol Surv* 1962; 23:603.

183. Green T: Urinary stress incontinence: Differential diagnosis, pathophysiology and management. *Am J Obstet Gynecol* 1975; 122:368.
184. Green T: Urinary stress incontinence: Diagnosis and classification, in Buchsbaum H, Schmidt J (eds): *Gynecologic and Obstetic Urology*. Philadelphia, WB Saunders, 1982, pp 199–223.
185. Greenhill JP: The nonsurgical therapy of stress incontinence associated with vaginal relaxation, in Cantor EB (ed): *Female Urinary Stress Incontinence*. Springfield, Ill, Charles C Thomas, 1979, pp 195–206.
186. Grimes JH, Nashold BS, Anderson EE: Clinical application of electronic bladder stimulation in paraplegics. *J Urol* 1975; 113:338.
187. Grimes JH, Nashold BS, Currie D: Chronic electrical stimulation of the paraplegic bladder. *J Urol* 1973; 109:242.
188. Grossman HB, Koff SA, Doikno AC: Cystometry in children. *J Urol* 1977; 117:646–648.
189. Hachen H: Clinical and urodynamic assessment of alpha adrenolytic therapy in patients with neurogenic bladder function. *Paraplegia* 1980; 18:229.
190. Hachen H, Krucker V: Clinical and laboratory assessment of the efficacy of baclofen on urethral sphincter spasticity in patients with traumatic paraplegia. *Eur Urol* 1977; 3:237.
191. Hachen H: Sexual impotence: A complication of external sphincterotomy. *Urol Int* 1977; 32:336.
192. Hackler R, Broecker B, Klein F, et al: A clinical experience with dantrolene sodium for external urinary sphincter hypertonicity in spinal cord injured patients. *J Urol* 1980; 124:78.
193. Hadley HR, Zimmern PE, Staskin D, et al: Transvaginal needle bladder neck suspension. *Urol Clin North Am* 1985; 12:291.
194. Hald T: *The Committee on Standardization of Terminology of Lower Urinary Tract Function*. Copenhagen, International Continence Society, 1984.
195. Hald T, Bradley WE: *The Urinary Bladder: Neurology and Dynamics*. Baltimore, Williams & Wilkins, 1982.
196. Hald T, Holm-Bentzen M: Clinical symptom complex, in George NJR, Gosling JA (eds): *Sensory Disorders of the Bladder and Urethra*. New York, Springer-Verlag, 1986, pp 49–62.
197. Halverstadt DP, Parry WL: Electronic stimulation of the human bladder: Nine years later. *J Urol* 1975; 113:341.
198. Hanna M: New concept in bladder remodeling. *Urology* 1982; 19:6.
199. Hebjorn S: Treatment of detrusor hyperreflexia in multiple sclerosis. *Urol Int* 1977; 32:209.
200. Heimburger RF, Freeman LW, Wilde NJ: Sacral nerve innervation of the human bladder. *Int J Neurosurg* 1948; 5:154.
201. Hepburn TN: Prolapse of the female urethra. *Surg Gynecol Obstet* 1920; 31:83.
202. Hilton P, Stanton SL: The use of desmopressin (DDAVP) in nocturnal urinary frequency in the female. *Br J Urol* 1982; 54:252.
203. Hindmarsh JR, Gosling PT, Deane AM: Bladder instability: Is the primary defect in the urethra? *Br J Urol* 1983; 55:648.

204. Hinman F Jr: Urinary tract damage in children who wet. *Pediatrics* 1974; 54:142–150.
205. Hinman F Jr: Syndromes of vesical incoordination. *Urol Clin North Am* 1980; 7:311.
206. Hodgkinson JC: Stress urinary incontinence. *Am J Obstet Gynecol* 1970; 108:1141.
207. Hodgson BT, Dumas S, Bolling DR, et al: Effect of estrogen on sensitivity of rabbit bladder and urethra to phenylephrine. *Invest Urol* 1978; 16:67.
208. Hollister L: Tricyclic antidepressants. *N Engl J Med* 1978; 299:1106.
209. Hunner GL: A rare type of bladder ulcer in women: Report of cases. *Boston Med Surg J* 1915; 172:660.
210. Husted S, Andersson KE, Sommer L, et al: Anticholinergic and calcium antagonistic effects of etrodilene in rabbit urinary bladder. *Acta Pharmacol Toxicol* 1980; 46:20.
211. Merillo C, Conway CJ: Clinical experience with the Mentor bladder stimulator: III. Patients with urinary vesical hypotonia. *J Urol* 1975; 113:335.
212. Ingelmann-Sundberg A: Partial denervation of the bladder: A new operation for the treatment of urge incontinence and similar conditions in women. *Acta Obstet Gynecol Scand* 1959; 38:487.
213. Ingelmann-Sundberg A: Denervation of the bladder, in Stanton SL, Tanagho EA (eds): *Surgery of Female Incontinence.* New York, Springer-Verlag, 1980, pp 93–97.
214. International Continence Society Standardization Committee: Fourth report on the standardization of terminology of lower urinary tract function. *Br J Urol* 1981; 53:333.
215. Jeffcoate N: *Principles of Gynecology.* London, Butterworths, 1975, pp 701–708.
216. Jensen D Jr: Pharmacological studies of the uninhibited neurogenic bladder. *Acta Neurol Scand* 1981a; 64:175.
217. Jensen D Jr: Altered adrenergic innervation in the uninhibited neurogenic bladder. *Scand J Urol Nephrol* 1981b; 60:61.
218. Jensen D Jr: Uninhibited neurogenic bladder treated with prazosin. *Scand J Urol Nephrol* 1981c; 15:229.
219. Johns A, Tasker J, Johnson C, et al: The mechanism of action of dicyclomine hydrochloride on rabbit detrusor muscle and vas deferens. *Arch Int Pharmacodyn Ther* 1976; 224:109.
220. Johnston JH, Farkas A: Congenital neuropathic bladder: Practicalities and possibilities of conservational management. *Urology* 1975; 5:719–727.
221. Jones KW, Schoenberg HW: Obstruction and the uninhibitable detrusor, in Hinman F Jr (ed): *Benign Prostatic Hypertrophy.* New York, Springer-Verlag, 1983, pp 706–710.
222. Jorgensen TM, Djurhuus JC, Jorgenson HS, et al: Experimental bladder hyperreflexia in pigs. *Urol Res* 1983; 11:239.
223. Jorgensen TM, Djurhuus JC, Schroder HD: Idiopathic detrusor sphincter dyssynergia in neurologically normal patients with voiding abnormalities. *Eur Urol* 1982; 8:107.

224. Kahn Z: Predictive correlation of urodynamic dysfunction after cerebrovascular accident. *J Urol* 1981; 126:88.
225. Kaplan GW: Myelomeningocele and related disorders. *J Cont Educ Urol* 1978, pp 15–28.
226. Kaplan WE, Firlit CF, Schoenberg HW: The female urethral syndrome: External sphincter spasm as etiology. *J Urol* 1980; 124:48.
227. Kass EJ, Diokno AC, Montealegre A: Enuresis: Principles of management and result of treatment. *J Urol* 1979; 121:794–796.
228. Kaufman JJ: A new operation for male incontinence. *Surg Gynecol Obstet* 1970; 131:295–299.
229. Kaufman JM, Fam B, Jacobs SC, et al: Bladder cancer and squamous metaplasia in spinal cord injury patient. *J Urol* 1977; 118:967.
230. Khan A: Psychogenic urinary retention in a boy. *J Urol* 1971; 106:432.
231. Khanna O: Disorders of micturition: Neuropharmacologic basis and results of drug therapy. *Urology* 1976; 8:316.
232. Khanna O, Barbieri E, McMichael R: The effects of adrenergic agonists and antagonists on vesicourethral smooth muscle of rabbits. *J Pharmacol Exp Ther* 1981; 216:95.
233. Khanna O, DiGregorio C, Barbieri E, et al: In vitro study of antispasmodic effects of dicyclomine hydrochloride on vesicourethral smooth muscle of guinea pig and rabbit. *Urology* 1979; 13:457.
234. Kiesswetter H, Schober W: Lioresal in the treatment of neurogenic bladder dysfunction. *Urol Int* 1975; 30:63.
235. Kinder CH, Smith RD: Hunner's ulcer. *Br J Urol* 1958; 30:338.
236. Kinn AC: The lazy bladder—appraisal of surgical reduction. *Scand J Urol Nephrol* 1985; 19:93.
237. Koelle G: Parasympathomimetic agents, in Goodman LS, Gilman A (eds): *The Pharmacologic Basis of Therapeutics.* New York, Macmillan Publishing Co, 1975, p 467.
238. Koff SA, Deridder PA: Patterns of neurogenic bladder dysfunction in sacral agenesis. *J Urol* 1977; 118:87–89.
239. Koff SA, Kass EJ: Abdominal wall electromyography: A noninvasive technique to improve pediatric urodynamic accuracy. *J Urol* 1982; 127:736–739.
240. Koff SA, Solomon MH, Lane GA, et al: Urodynamic studies in anesthetized children. *J Urol* 1980; 123:61–63.
241. Kohler R, Morales P: Cystometric evaluation of flavoxate hydrochloride in normal and neurogenic bladder. *J Urol* 1968; 100:729.
242. Koontz WW Jr, Prout GR Jr: Agenesis of the sacrum and the neurogenic bladder. *JAMA* 1968; 203:481–486.
243. Kosman ME: Evaluation of a new antidiuretic agent, desmopressin acetate (DDAVP). *JAMA* 1978; 240:1896.
244. Koyanagi T: Further observation on the denervation supersensitivity of the urethra in patients with chronic neurogenic bladders. *J Urol* 1979; 122:348.
245. Krane R, Olsson C: Phenoxybenzamine in neurogenic bladder dysfunction: I. A theory of micturition. *J Urol* 1973a; 110:650.

246. Krane R, Olsson C: Phenoxybenzamine in neurogenic bladder dysfunction: II. Clinical considerations. *J Urol* 1973b; 110:653.
247. Krane RJ, Siroky MB: Classification of neuro-urologic disorders, in Krane RJ, Siroky MB (eds): *Clinical Neuro-Urology*. Boston, Little Brown & Co, 1979a, pp 143–158.
248. Krane RJ, Siroky MB: Psychogenic voiding dysfunction, in Krane RJ, Siroky MB (eds): *Clinical Neuro-Urology*. Boston, Little Brown & Co, 1979b, chap 15.
249. Krane RJ, Siroky MB: Studies on sacral evoked potentials. *J Urol* 1980; 123:872.
250. Krane RJ, Siroky MB: Classification of voiding dysfunction: Value of classification systems, in Barrett DM, Wein AJ (eds): *Controversies in Neuro-Urology*. New York, Churchill-Livingstone, 1984, pp 223–238.
251. Krugman A, Boyarsky S, Glenn JF Jr, et al: Psychological considerations in bladder function disturbances, in Hinman F Jr (ed): *Hydrodynamics of Micturition*. Springfield, Ill, Charles C Thomas, 1971.
252. Lapides J: Urecholine regimen for rehabilitating the atonic bladder. *J Urol* 1964; 91:648.
253. Lapides J: Cystometry. *JAMA* 1967; 201:618.
254. Lapides J: Neuromuscular, vesical and ureteral dysfunction, in Campbell MF, Harrison JH (eds): *Urology*. Philadelphia, WB Saunders Co, 1970, pp 1343–1379.
255. Lapides J: Simplified operation for stress incontinence. *J Urol* 1971; 105:262.
256. Lapides J, et al: Denervation supersensitivity as a test for neurogenic bladder. *Surg Gynecol Obstet* 1962; 114:241.
257. Lapides J, Diokno AC, Gould FR, et al: Further observations on self-catheterization. *J Urol* 1976; 116:169.
258. Lapides J, Dodson A: Observations on effect of methantheline bromide in urological disturbances. *Arch Surg* 1953; 66:1.
259. Lapides J, Friend C, Ajemian E, et al: Comparison of action of oral and parenteral bethanechol chloride upon the urinary bladder. *Invest Urol* 1963; 1:94.
260. Larsen J, Mortensen S: Effect of ritodrine on the bladder capacity in unanesthetized pigs. *Acta Pharmacol Toxicol* 1978; 43:405.
261. Larsen JW, Swenson WM, Utz DC, et al: Psychogenic urinary retention in women. *JAMA* 1963; 184:111.
262. Larsen S, Thompson SA, Hald T, et al: Mast cells in interstitial cystitis. *Br J Urol* 1982; 54:283.
263. Laurence KM: The natural history of spina bifida cystica: Detailed analysis of 407 cases. *Arch Dis Child* 1964; 39:41–57.
264. Leach GE, Goldman D, Raz S: Surgical treatment of detrusor hyperreflexia, in Raz S (ed): *Female Urology*. Philadelphia, WB Saunders Co, 1983, pp 326–334.
265. Leadbetter GW Jr: Surgical correction of total urinary incontinence. *J Urol* 1964; 91:261.

266. Leadbetter GW Jr: Surgical reconstruction for complete urinary incontinence: A 10- to 22-year followup. *J Urol* 1985; 133:205.
267. Lee L: The clinical use of urocholine in dysfunctions of the bladder. *J Urol* 1949; 62:300.
268. Lennert JB, Mowad JJ: Enuresis: evaluation of perplexing symptom. *Urology* 1979; 13:27–29.
269. Levin RM, High J, Wein AJ: The effect of short term obstruction on urinary bladder function in the rabbit. *J Urol* 1984; 132:789.
270. Levin RM, Malkowicz SB, Wein AJ, et al: Recovery from short term obstruction of the rabbit urinary bladder. *J Urol* 1985; 134:388.
271. Levin R, Staskin D, Wein A: The muscarinic cholinergic binding kinetics of the human urinary bladder. *Neurourol Urodynamics* 1982; 1:221.
272. Levin RM, Jacobowitz D, Wein AJ: Autonomic innervation of rabbit urinary bladder following estrogen administration. *Urology* 1981; 17:449.
273. Levin RM, Staskin DR, Wein AJ: Analysis of the anticholinergic and musculotropic effects of desmethylimipramine on the rabbit urinary bladder. *Urol Res* 1983; 11:259.
274. Lewin RJ, Dilland GU, Porter RW: Extrapyramidal inhibition of the urinary bladder. *Brain Res* 1967; 4:301.
275. Libo LM, Arnold GE, Woodside JR, et al: EMG biofeedback for functional bladder-sphincter dyssynergia: A case study. *Biofeedback Self Regul* 1983; 8:243–253.
276. Light J, Scott F: Bethanechol chloride and the traumatic cord bladder. *J Urol* 1982; 128:85.
277. Light K, Van Blerk PJP: Causes of renal deterioration in patients with meningomyeloceles. *Br J Urol* 1977; 49:257–260.
278. Lim K, Ball AJ, Fenehey RCL: Periurethral Teflon injection: A simple treatment for urinary incontinence. *Br J Urol* 1983; 55:208.
279. Linder A, Leach GE, Raz S: Augmentation cystoplasty in the treatment of neurogenic bladder dysfunction. *J Urol* 1983; 129:491.
280. Lish P, Labbude J, Peters E, et al: Oxybutynin: A musculotropic antispasmodic drug with moderate anticholinergic action. *Arch Int Pharmacodyn* 1965; 156:467.
281. MacGregor R, Diokno A: The alpha adrenergic blocking action of prazosin hydrochloride on the canine urethra. *Invest Urol* 1981; 18:426.
282. Madersbacher H: Striated sphincter dyssynergia. *Neurourol Urodynamics* 1986; 5:307.
283. Madersbacher H, Scott FB: Twelve o'clock sphincterotomy: Technique, indications, results. *Urol Int* 1975; 30:75.
284. Mahony D, Laferte F, Majoney J: Observations on sphincter augmenting effect of imipramine in children with urinary incontinence. *Urology* 1973; 2:317.
285. Maizels M, Firlit CF: Pediatric urodynamics: A clinical comparison of surface versus needle pelvic floor/external sphincter electromyography. *J Urol* 1979; 122:518–522.

286. Maizels M, King LR, Firlit CF: Urodynamic biofeedback: A new approach to treat vesical sphincter dyssynergia. *J Urol* 1979; 122:205.
287. Malizia AA Jr, Reiman HM, Meyers RP, et al: Migration and granulomatous reaction after periurethral injection of polytef. *JAMA* 1984; 251:3277.
288. Mansson W, Sundin T, Gullberg B: Evaluation of a synthetic vasopressin analogue for treatment of nocturia in benign prostatic hypertrophy. *Scand J Urol Nephrol* 1980; 14:139.
289. Mariani AJ, Stern J, Khan AU, et al: Sacral agenesis: An analysis of 11 cases and review of the literature. *J Urol* 1979; 122:684–686.
290. Marshall S, Marshall HH, Lyon RP: Enuresis: An analysis of various therapeutic approaches. *Pediatrics* 1973; 52:813–817.
291. Marshall VF, Marchetti AA, Krantz KE: The correction of stress incontinence by simple vesicourethral suspension. *Surg Gynecol Obstet* 1949; 88:509.
292. Martin DC, Datta NS, Schweitz B: The occult neurological bladder. *J Urol* 1971; 105:733–738.
293. Mayo ME, Ansell JS: Urodynamic assessment of incontinence after prostatectomy. *J Urol* 1979; 122:60.
294. Mayo ME, Chapman WH, Shurtleff DB: Bladder function in children with meningomyelocele: Comparison of cine-fluoroscopy and urodynamics. *J Urol* 1979; 121:458–461.
295. McGuire E: Reflex urethral instability. *Br J Urol* 1978; 50:200.
296. McGuire E: Electromyographic evaluation of sphincter function and dysfunction. *Urol Clin North Am* 1979; 6:121.
297. McGuire EJ: Urodynamic evaluation after abdominal-perineal resection and lumbar intervertebral disk herniation. *Urology* 1975; 6:63–70.
298. McGuire EJ: *Urinary Incontinence.* New York, Grune & Stratton, 1981.
299. McGuire EJ: Clinical evaluation and treatment of neurogenic vesical dysfunction, in Libertino J (ed): *International Perspectives in Urology.* Baltimore, Williams & Wilkins, 1984a, vol 11.
300. McGuire EJ: Detrusor response to outlet obstruction. *World J Urol* 1984b; 2:208.
301. McGuire EJ: The neuropathic urethra, in Mundy AR, Stephenson TP, Wein AJ (eds): *Urodynamics: Principles, Practice and Application.* Edinburgh, Churchill-Livingstone, 1984c, pp 288–296.
302. McGuire EJ: Abdominal procedures for stress incontinence. *Urol Clin North Am* 1985; 12:285.
303. McGuire EJ, Lytton B: The pubovaginal sling in stress urinary incontinence. *J Urol* 1978; 119:82.
304. McGuire EJ, Savastano JA: Urodynamic findings and long term outcome management of patients with multiple sclerosis induced lower urinary tract dysfunction. *J Urol* 1984; 132:713.
305. McGuire EJ, Savastano JA: Stress incontinence and detrusor instability/urge incontinence. *Neurourol Urodynamics* 1985; 4:313.
306. McGuire EJ, Wagner FC Jr: The effects of sacral denervation on bladder and urethral function. *Surg Gynecol Obstet* 1977; 144:343–346.

307. McGuire EJ, Shi-Chun Z, Horwinski ER, et al: Treatment for motor and sensory detrusor instability by electrical stimulation. *J Urol* 1983; 129:78.
308. McGuire EJ, Woodside JR, Borden TA: Upper urinary tract deterioration in patients with myelodysplasia and detrusor hypertonia: A follow-up study. *J Urol* 1983a; 129:823–826.
309. McGuire EJ, Woodside JR, Borden TA, et al: Prognostic value urodynamic testing in myelodysplastic patients. *J Urol* 1983b; 126:205.
310. McGuire EJ, Woodside JR, Borden TA, et al: The prognostic value of urodynamic testing in myelodysplastic patients. *J Urol* 1981; 126:205–209.
311. McLellan FC: *The Neurogenic Bladder*. Springfield, Ill, Charles C Thomas, 1939, pp 57–70, 116–185.
312. Dimethylsulfoxide (DMSO). *Medical Letter* 1980; 22:94.
313. Meirowsky AM, Scheibert CD, Hinchey TR: Studies on the reflex arc in paraplegia. *Int J Neurosurg* 1950; 7:33.
314. Merrill DC: Clinical experience with the Mentor bladder stimulator: II. Meningomyelocele patients. *J Urol* 1974; 112:823.
315. Merrill DC: The treatment of detrusor incontinence by electrical stimulation. *J Urol* 1979; 122:515.
316. Merrill DC, Conway CJ: Clinical experience with the Mentor bladder stimulator: I. Patients with upper motor neuron lesions. *J Urol* 1974; 112:52.
317. Merrill D, Rotta J: A clinical evaluation of detrusor denervation supersensitivity using air cystometry. *J Urol* 1977; 111:27.
318. Merrill DC, Bradley WE, Markland C: Air cystometry: II. A clinical evaluation of normal adults. *J Urol* 1972; 108:85–88.
319. Merrill DC, Conway C, DeWolf W: Urinary incontinence treatment with electrical stimulation of the pelvic floor. *Urology* 1975; 5:67.
320. Messing EM, Stamey TA: Interstitial cystitis: Early diagnosis, pathology and treatment. *Urology* 1978; 12:381.
321. Miller NE: Applications of learning and biofeedback to psychiatry and medicine, in Freedman AM, Kaplan HI, Sadock BJ (eds): *Comprehensive Textbook of Psychiatry*. Baltimore, Williams & Wilkins, 1975, pp 349–365.
322. Miller NE, Dworkin BR: Effects of learning on visceral functions—biofeedback. *N Engl J Med* 1977; 296:1274.
323. Milner G, Hills N: A double-blind assessment of antidepressants in the treatment of 212 enuretic patients. *Med J Aust* 1968; 1:943.
324. Misak SJ, Bunts RC, Ulmer JL, et al: Nerve interruption procedures in the urologic management of paraplegic patients. *J Urol* 1962; 88:392.
325. Mobley D: Phenoxybenzamine in the management of neurogenic vesical dysfunction. *J Urol* 1976; 116:737.
326. Mogg RA, Syme RRA: The results of urinary diversion using the colonic conduit. *Br J Urol* 1969; 41:434.
327. Moisey C, Stephenson T, Brendler C: The urodynamic and subjective results of treatment of detrusor instability with oxybutynin chloride. *Br J Urol* 1980; 52:472.
328. Moisey CU, Stephensen TP, Evans C: A subjective and urodynamic as-

sessment of unilateral bladder neck incision for bladder neck obstruction. *Br J Urol* 1982; 54:114.

329. Moncada S, Flower R, Vane J: Prostaglandins, prostacyclin and thromboxane A_2, in Gilman AG, Goodman LS, Gilman A (eds): *The Pharmacological Basis of Therapeutics.* New York, Macmillan, 1980, pp 668–681.
330. Montague D, Stewart B: Urethral pressure profiles before and after Ornade administration in patients with stress incontinence. *J Urol* 1979; 122:198.
331. Mulcahy JJ, Young AB: Percutaneous radiofrequency sacral rhizotomy in treatment of hyperreflexic bladder. *J Urol* 1978; 120:557.
332. Mulholland SG, Yalla SV, Raezer DM, et al: Primary external urethral sphincter hyperkinesia in a boy. *Urology* 1974; 4:577.
333. Muller J, Schulze S: Imipramine cardiotoxicity: An electrocardiographic and hemodynamic study in rabbits. *Acta Pharmacol Toxicol* 1980; 46:191.
334. Mundy AR: Pelvic plexus injury, in Mundy AR, Stephenson TP, Wein AJ (eds): *Urodynamics: Principles, Practice, and Application.* New York, Churchill-Livingstone, 1984, pp 273–277.
335. Mundy AR: The surgical treatment of detrusor instability. *Neurourol Urodynamics* 1985a; 4:357.
336. Mundy AR: The unstable bladder. *Clin Obstet Gynecol* 1985b; 12:431.
337. Mundy AR, Blaivas JG: Non-traumatic neurological disorders, in Mundy AR, Stephenson TP, Wein AJ (eds): *Urodynamics: Principles, Practice and Application.* New York, Churchill-Livingstone, 1984, pp 278–287.
338. Mundy AR, Stephenson TP: The urge syndrome, in Mundy AR, Stephenson TP, Wein AJ (eds): *Urodynamics: Principles, Practice, and Application.* New York: Churchill-Livingstone, 1984, pp 212–228.
339. Mundy AR, Stephenson TP: Clam ileocecocystoplasty for the treatment of refractory urge incontinence. *Br J Urol* 1986; 58.
340. Mundy AR, Borzykowsky M, Saxton HM: Videourodynamic evaluation of neuropathic vesicourethral dysfunction in children. *Br J Urol* 1982; 54:645–649.
341. Murdock M, Sax D, Krane R: Use of dantrolene sodium in external sphincter spasm. *Urology* 1976; 8:133.
342. Murnaghan GF: Neurogenic disorders of the bladder in Parkinsonism. *Br J Urol* 1961; 33:403.
343. Nanninga J, Kaplan P, Lal S: Effect of phentolamine on perineal sphincter spasm. *Urology* 1976; 8:133.
344. Nemir A, Middleton RP: Stress incontinence in young nulliparous women. *Am J Obstet Gynecol* 1954; 68:1166.
345. Norden CW, Friedman EA: Psychogenic urinary retention. *N Engl J Med* 1961; 264:1096.
346. Nordling J, Meyhoff HH: Dissociation of urethral and anal sphincter activity in neurologic bladder dysfunction. *J Urol* 1979; 122:352.
347. Nordling J, Christensen B, Gosling J: Noradrenergic innervation of the human bladder in neurogenic dysfunction. *Urol Int* 1980; 35:188.
348. Nordling J, Meyhoff H, Hald T, et al: Urethral denervation supersensi-

tivity to noradrenaline after radical hysterectomy. *Scand J Urol Nephrol* 1981; 15:21.

349. Nordling J, Meyhoff HH, Christensen NJ: Effects of clonidine on urethral pressure. *Invest Urol* 1979; 16:289.
350. Norlen L, Dahlstrom A, Sundin T, et al: The adrenergic innervation and adrenergic receptor activity of the feline urinary bladder and urethra in the normal state and after hypogastric and/or parasympathetic denervation. *Scand J Urol Nephrol* 1976; 10:177.
351. Norlen L, Sundin T, Waagstein F: Beta-adrenoceptor stimulation of the human urinary bladder in vivo. *Acta Pharmacol Toxicol* 1978; 43:5.
352. Obrink A, Bunne G: The effect of alpha-adrenergic stimulation in stress incontinence. *Scand J Urol Nephrol* 1978; 12:205.
353. Olsson C, Siroky M, Krane R: The phentolamine test in neurogenic bladder dysfunction. *J Urol* 1977; 117:481.
354. Olubadewo J: The effect of imipramine on rat detrusor muscle contractility. *Arch Int Pharmacodyn Ther* 1980; 245:84.
355. Opitz JL: Treatment of voiding dysfunction in spinal cord injured patients: Bladder retraining, in Barrett DM, Wein AJ (eds): *Controversies in Neuro-urology*. London, Churchill-Livingstone, 1984, pp 437–451.
356. Oravisto KJ: Epidemiology of interstitial cystitis. *Ann Chir Gynaecol* 1975; 64:75.
357. Orr JD, Shand JEG, Watters DAK, et al: Ileal conduit urinary diversion in children: An assessment of the long-term results. *Br J Urol* 1981; 53:424.
358. Osborn DE: Prostatodynia: Clinical aspects, in George NJR, Gosling JA (eds): *Sensory Disorders of the Bladder and Urethra*. New York, Springer-Verlag, 1986, pp 139–147.
359. Ouslander IG: Urinary incontinence in the elderly. *West J Med* 1981; 135:482.
360. Palmer J, Worth P, Exton-Smith A: Flunarizine: A once daily therapy for urinary incontinence. *Lancet* 1981; 2:279.
361. Parsons CL, Schmidt JP, Pollen JJ: Successful treatment of interstitial cystitis with sodium pentosonpolysulfate. *J Urol* 1983; 130:51.
362. Parsons K, Turton M: Urethral supersensitivity and occult urethral neuropathy. *Br J Urol* 1980; 52:131.
363. Pavlakis AJ, Siroky MB, Goldstein I, et al: Neurourologic findings in Parkinson's disease. *J Urol* 1983; 129:80.
364. Pederson E, Grynderup V: Clinical pharmacology of the neurogenic bladder. *Acta Neurol Scand* 1966; 42(suppl):111.
365. Pengelly AW, Booth CM: A prospective trial of bladder training as treatment for detrusor instability. *Br J Urol* 1980; 52:463.
366. Pengelly AW, Stephenson TP, Mulroy EJG, et al: Results of prolonged bladder distention as treatment for detrusor instability. *Br J Urol* 1978; 50:243.
367. Pereyra AJ: A surgical procedure for the correction of stress incontinence in women. *West J Surg Obstet Gynecol* 1959; 67:223.
368. Perkash I: Intermittent catheterization and bladder rehabilitation in spinal cord injury patients. *J Urol* 1975; 114:230.

369. Perlberg S, Caine M: Adrenergic response of bladder muscle in prostatic obstruction. *Urology* 1982; 20:524.
370. Persky L, Tucker A, Izant RJ Jr: Urological complications of correction of imperforate anus. *J Urol* 1974; 111:415–418.
371. Petersen KE, Andersen OO, Hansen T: Mode of action and relative value of imipramine and similar drugs in the treatment of nocturnal enuresis. *Eur J Clin Pharmacol* 1974; 7:187.
372. Petti T, Law W: Abrupt cessation of high dose imipramine treatment in children. *JAMA* 1981; 246:768.
373. Philp N, Thomas D, Clarke S: Drug effects on the voiding cystometrogram: A comparison of oral bethanechol and carbachol. *Br J Urol* 1980; 52:484.
374. Pitts WR Jr, Muecke EC: A 20-year experience with ileal conduits: The fate of the kidneys. *J Urol* 1979; 122:154.
375. Plevnik S, Janež J: Maximal electrical stimulation for urinary incontinence: Report of 98 cases. *Urology* 1979; 14:638.
376. Politano VA: Periurethral polytetrafluoroethylene injection for urinary incontinence. *J Urol* 1982; 127:439.
377. Politano VA, Small MP, Harper JM, et al: Periurethral Teflon injection for urinary incontinence. *J Urol* 1974; 111:180.
378. Powell PH, Shepard AM, Lewis P, et al: The accuracy of clinical diagnosis assessed urodynamically, in Zinner NR, Sterling AM (eds): *Female Incontinence.* New York, Alan R Liss Inc, 1981, p 201.
379. Quesada EM, Scott FB, Cardus D: Functional classification of neurogenic bladder dysfunction. *Arch Phys Med Rehabil* 1968; 49:692.
380. Raezer D, Wein A, Jacobowitz D, et al: Autonomic innervation of canine urinary bladder: Cholinergic and adrenergic contributions and interaction of sympathetic and parasympathetic systems in bladder function. *Urology* 1973; 2:211.
381. Raezer DM, Benson GS, Wein AJ, et al: The functional approach to the management of the pediatric neuropathic bladder: A clinical study. *J Urol* 1977; 117:649.
382. Ramsden PD, Hindmarsh JR, Price DA, et al: DDAVP for adult enuresis—a preliminary report. *Br J Urol* 1982; 54:256.
383. Raz S, Caine M: Adrenergic receptors in the female canine urethra. *Invest Urol* 1971; 9:319.
384. Raz S, Smith R: External sphincter spasticity syndrome in female patients. *J Urol* 1976; 115:443.
385. Raz S, Caine M, Ziegler M: The vascular component in the production of urethral pressure. *J Urol* 1972; 108:93.
386. Raz S, Kaufman J, Ellison G, et al: Methyldopa in treatment of neurogenic bladder disorders. *Urology* 1977; 9:188.
387. Raz S, Ziegler M, Caine M: The role of female hormones in stress incontinence. Proceedings of 16th Congress of Societe International d'Urologie, Amsterdam. Paris, Doin, vol 2, 1973, pp 397–402.
388. Redman JF, Seibert JJ: The uroradiographic evaluation of the enuretic child. *J Urol* 1979; 122:799–801.

389. Rees D, Ransley P: Eskornade in the treatment of diurnal incontinence in children. *Br J Urol* 1980; 52:476.
390. Rees DLP, Whitfield HN, Islam AKM, et al: Urodynamic findings in adult females with frequency and dysuria. *Br J Urol* 1967; 47:853.
391. Reid GF, Fitzpatrick JM, Worth PHL: The treatment of patients with urinary incontinence post prostatectomy. *Br J Urol* 1980; 52:532.
392. Resnick MI, King LR: Use of the Leadbetter anti-incontinence procedure in children. *J Urol* 1976; 116:366–368.
393. Resnick NM, Yalla SV: Management of urinary incontinence in the elderly. *N Engl J Med* 1985; 313:800.
394. Richelson E: Antimuscarinic and other receptor blocking properties of antidepressants. *Mayo Clin Proc* 1983; 58:40.
395. Roberts JBM, Smith PJB, Dunn M, et al: Vesicoplication in the management of chronic urinary retention. *Br J Urol* 1979; 51:532.
396. Robinson AG: DDAVP in the treatment of central diabetes insipidus. *N Engl J Med* 1976; 294:507.
397. Rohner T, Hannigan J, Sanford E: Altered in vitro adrenergic responses of dog detrusor muscle after chronic bladder outlet obstruction. *Urology* 1978; 11:357.
398. Rosen M: A simple artificial implantable sphincter. *Br J Urol* 1976; 48:675–680.
399. Ross JC, Gibbon NOK, Damanski M: Division of the external urethral sphincter in the treatment of the paraplegic bladder: A preliminary report on a new procedure. *Br J Urol* 1958; 30:204.
400. Rossier A, Fam B, Lee I, et al: Role of striated and smooth muscle components in the urethral pressure profile in traumatic neurogenic bladders: A neuropharmacological and urodynamic study: A preliminary report. *J Urol* 1982; 128:529.
401. Roussan M, Abramson A, Levine S: Bladder training: Its role in evaluating the effect of an antispasticity drug on voiding in patients with neurogenic bladder. *Arch Phys Med Rehabil* 1975; 56:463.
402. Rowan EL: Psychophysiologic disorders of micturition. *Coll Health* 1975; 23:251.
403. Ruch TC, Tang PC: The higher control of the bladder, in Boyarsky S (ed): *The Neurogenic Bladder*. Baltimore, Williams & Wilkins, 1969, pp 34–45.
404. Rud T: The effects of estrogens and gestagens on the urethral pressure profile in urinary continent and stress incontinent women. *Acta Obstet Gynecol Scand* 1980a; 59:265.
405. Rud T: Urethral pressure profile in continent women from childhood to old age. *Acta Obstet Gynecol Scand* 1980b; 59:331.
406. Rud T, Andersson K, Boye N, et al: Terodiline inhibition of human bladder contraction: Effects in vitro and in women with unstable bladder. *Acta Pharmacol Toxicol* 1980; 46:31.
407. Rudy DC, Woodside JR, Crawford ED: Urodynamic evaluation of incontinence in patients undergoing modified Campbell radical prostatectomy: A prospective study. *J Urol* 1984; 132:708.
408. Salmon UJ, Walter RI, Geist SH: The use of estrogen in the treatment of

dysuria and incontinence in postmenopausal women. *Am J Obstet Gynecol* 1941; 42:845.
409. Santulli TV, Kiesewetter WB, Bill AH Jr: Anorectal anomalies: A suggested international classification. *J Pediatr Surg* 1970; 5:281–287.
410. Sarnat HB, Case ME, Graviss R: Sacral agenesis: Neurologic and neuropathologic features. *Neurology* 1976; 26:1124–1129.
411. Schmidt RA: Neural prostheses and bladder control. *Eng Med Biol* 1983; 2:31.
412. Schmidt RA: The urethral syndrome. *Clin Obstet Gynecol* 1985; 12:477.
413. Schoenberg HC, Gutrich JM: Management of vesical dysfunction in multiple sclerosis. *Urology* 1980; 16:444.
414. Schreiter F, Fuchs P, Stockamp K: Estrogenic sensitivity of alpha receptors in the urethral musculature. *Urol Int* 1976; 31:13.
415. Schulman CC, Simon J, Wesper E, et al: Endoscopic injection of Teflon for female urinary incontinence. *Eur Urol* 1983; 9:246.
416. Schwartz GE: Biofeedback and the behavioral treatment of disorders of disregulation. *Yale J Biol Med* 1979; 52:581.
417. Schwartz GR, Jeffs RD: Ileal conduit urinary diversion in children: Computer analysis of follow up from 2 to 16 years. *J Urol* 1975; 114:285.
418. Scott FB, Bradley W, Timm GW: Treatment of urinary incontinence by an implantable prosthetic urinary sphincter. *J Urol* 1974; 112:75–80.
419. Scott M, Morrow J: Phenoxybenzamine in neurogenic bladder dysfunction after spinal cord injury: I. Voiding dysfunction. *J Urol* 1978; 119:480.
420. Segura JW, Opitz JL, Greene CF: Prostatosis, prostatitis, or pelvic floor tension myalgia? *J Urol* 1979; 122:168.
421. Sehn JT: Anatomic effect of distention therapy in unstable bladder: New approach. *Urology* 1978; 11:581.
422. Sibley GNA: An experimental model of detrusor instability in the obstructed pig. *Br J Urol* 1985; 57:292.
423. *Sixth Report on the Standardization of Terminology of Lower Urinary Tract Function.* New York, The International Continence Society Committee on Standardization of Terminology, May 1985.
424. Sjogren C, Andersson K: Effects of cholinoceptor blocking drugs, adrenoceptor stimulants and calcium antagonists on the transmurally stimulated guinea pig urinary bladder in vitro and in vivo. *Acta Pharmacol Toxicol* 1979; 44:228.
425. Smey P, Firlit CF, King LR: Voiding pattern abnormalities in normal children: Results of pharmacologic manipulation. *J Urol* 1978; 120:574–577.
426. Smith DR: Psychosomatic 'cystitis.' *J Urol* 1962; 87:359.
427. Smith ED: Congenital sacral anomalies in children. *Aust NZ J Surg* 1959; 29:165–176.
428. Smith ED: *Spina Bifida and the Total Care of Spinal Myelomeningocele.* Springfield, Ill, Charles C Thomas Publisher, 1965, pp 92–123.
429. Smith JC: The place of prolonged bladder distention in the treatment of bladder instability and other disorders. *Br J Urol* 1981; 53:283.
430. Smith RB, Van Cangh P, Skinner DG, et al: Augmentation enterocystoplasty: A critical review. *J Urol* 1977; 118:35.

431. Snyder HM, Caldamone AA, Wein AJ, et al: The Hinman syndrome—alternatives for treatment. Presented at the Annual Meeting of the American Urological Association. Kansas City, May 16–20, 1982.
432. Sonda L, Gershon C, Diokno A: Further observations on the cystometric and uroflowmetric effects of bethanechol chloride on the human bladder. *J Urol* 1979; 122:775.
433. Sporer A, Leyson J, Martin B: Effects of bethanechol chloride on the external urethral sphincter in spinal cord injury patients. *J Urol* 1978; 120:62.
434. Spyraki C, Fibiger H: Functional evidence for subsensitivity of noradrenergic α_2 receptors after chronic desipramine treatment. *Life Sci* 1980; 27:1863.
435. Stamey TA: Endoscopic suspension of the vesical neck, in Starlon SL, Tanagho EA (eds): *Surgery of Female Incontinence.* New York, Springer-Verlag, 1986, pp 115–132.
436. Stanton S: Disease of the urinary system: Drugs acting on the bladder and urethra. *Br Med J* 1978; 1:1607.
437. Stanton SL: Stress incontinence: Why and how operations work. *Clin Obstet Gynecol* 1985; 12:369.
438. Stanton SL: Colposuspension, in Stanton SL, Tanagho EA (eds): *Surgery of Female Incontinence.* New York, Springer-Verlag, 1986, pp 95–103.
439. Stanton SL, Cardozo L, Williams JE, et al: Clinical and urodynamic features of failed incontinence surgery in the female. *J Obstet Gynecol* 1978; 51:515.
440. Stark G: Pudendal neurectomy in management of neurogenic bladder in myelomeningocele. *Arch Dis Child* 1969; 44:698.
441. Staskin DR, Zimmern PC, Hadley HR, et al: Pathophysiology of stress incontinence. *Clin Obstet Gynecol* 1985; 12:357.
442. Stewart B, Banowsky L, Montague D: Stress incontinence: Conservative therapy with sympathomimetic drugs. *J Urol* 1976; 115:558.
443. Stewart BH, Shirley SW: Further experience with intravesical DMSO in the treatment of interstitial cystitis. *J Urol* 1976; 116:36.
444. Stockamp K: Treatment with phenoxybenzamine of upper urinary tract complications caused by intravesical obstruction. *J Urol* 1975; 113:128.
445. Sugar EC, Firlit CF: Urodynamic biofeedback: A new therapeutic approach for childhood incontinence/infection (vesical voluntary sphincter dyssynergia). *J Urol* 1982; 128:1253–1257.
446. Sundin T, Dahlstrom A: The sympathetic innervation of the urinary bladder and urethra in the normal state and after parasympathetic denervation at the spinal root level: An experimental study in cats. *Scand J Urol Nephrol* 1973; 7:131–149.
447. Sundin T, Dahlstrom A, Norlen L, et al: The sympathetic innervation and adrenoreceptor function of the human lower urinary tract in the normal state and after parasympathetic denervation. *Invest Urol* 1977; 14:322–328.
448. Tanagho EA: Membrane and microtransducer catheters: Their effective-

ness for profilometry of the lower urinary tracts. *Urol Clin North Am* 1979; 6:110.

449. Tanagho EA: Bladder neck reconstruction for total urinary incontinence: Ten years of experience. *J Urol* 1981; 1215:321.
450. Tanagho EA: Urethral pressure profile: Membrane catheter, in Barrett DM, Wein AJ (eds): *Controversies in Neuro-urology.* New York, Churchill-Livingstone, 1984, p 55.
451. Tanagho EA: Electrostimulation, in Stanton SL, Tanagho EA (eds): *Surgery of Female Incontinence.* New York, Springer-Verlag, 1986, pp 251–257.
452. Tanagho EA, Smith DR, Meyers FH, et al: Mechanism of urinary continence: II. Technique for surgical correction of incontinence. *J Urol* 1969; 101:305.
453. Tank ES: The urologic complications of imperforate anus and cloacal dysgenesis, in Harrison JH, Gittes RF, Perlmutter AD, et al: *Campbell's Urology,* ed 4. Philadelphia, WB Saunders Co, 1979, pp 1889–1900.
454. Taylor MC, Bates CP: A double-blind crossover trial of baclofen: A new treatment for the unstable bladder syndrome. *Br J Urol* 1979; 51:505.
455. Taylor P: Cholinergic agonists, in Gilman AG, Goodman LS, Gilman A (eds): *The Pharmacological Basis of Therapeutics.* New York, Macmillan, 1980, pp 91–99.
456. Teague CT, Merrill DC: Electric pelvic floor stimulation: Mechanisms of action. *Invest Urol* 1977; 15:65.
457. Thomas DG: Spinal cord injury, in Munday AR, Stephenson TP, Wein AJ (eds): *Urodynamics: Principles, Practice and Application.* New York, Churchill-Livingstone, 1984, pp 260–272.
458. Thomas GG, Zachary RB, Lister J: Serial follow-up studies of bladder pressure in spina bifida infants. *J Pediatr Surg* 1974; 9:471–476.
459. Thomas TM, Plymat KR, Blannen J, et al: Prevalence of urinary incontinence. *Br Med J* 1980; 281:1243.
460. Thompson I, Lauvetz R: Oxybutynin in bladder spasm, neurogenic bladder and enuresis. *Urology* 1976; 8:452.
461. Thor K, Rappolo J, deGroat W: Naloxone-induced micturition in unanesthetized paraplegic cats. *J Urol* 1983; 129:202.
462. Torrens MJ: The role of denervation in the treatment of detrusor instability. *Neurourol Urodynamics* 1985; 4:353.
463. Turner-Warwick R: Bladder outflow obstruction in the male, in Mundy AR, Stephenson TP, Wein AJ (eds): *Urodynamics: Principles, Practice and Application.* Edinburgh, Churchill-Livingstone, 1984, pp 183–204.
464. Turner-Warwick RT, Ashken MH: The functional results of partial, subtotal and total cystoplasty with special reference to ureterocecocystoplasty, selective sphincterotomy and cystocystoplasty. *Br J Urol* 1967; 39:3.
465. Twiddy D, Downie J, Awad S: Response of the bladder to bethanechol after acute spinal cord transection in cats. *J Pharmacol Exp Ther* 1980; 215:500.
466. Ullery JC: *Stress Incontinence in the Female.* New York, Grune & Stratton Inc, 1953.

467. Ulmsten U, Henrickson L, Iosif S: The unstable female urethra. *Am J Obstet Gynecol* 1982; 144:93.
468. Ursillo RC: Rationale for drug therapy in bladder dysfunction, in Boyarsky S (ed): *The Neurogenic Bladder.* Baltimore, Williams & Wilkins, 1967, pp 187–190.
469. Uvelius B, Mattiasson A: Collagen content in the rat urinary bladder subjected to infravesical outflow obstruction. *J Urol* 1984; 132:587.
470. Uvelius B, Persson L, Matthiasson A: Smooth muscle cell hypertrophy and hyperplasia in the rat detrusor after short term infravesical outflow obstruction. *J Urol* 1984; 131:173.
471. Vaidyanathan S, Rao M, Bapna B, et al: Beta adrenergic activity in human proximal urethra: A study with terbutaline. *J Urol* 1980; 124:869.
472. Vaidyanathan S, Rao M, Chary K, et al: Enhancement of detrusor reflex activity by naloxone in patients with chronic neurogenic bladder dysfunction. Preliminary report. *J Urol* 1981; 126:500.
473. Vaidyanathan S, Rao M, Mapa M, et al: Study of instillation of 15(*S*)–15-methyl prostaglandin $F_{2\alpha}$ in patients with neurogenic bladder dysfunction. *J Urol* 1981; 126:81.
474. Van Gool J, Tanagho EA: External sphincter activity and recurrent urinary tract infection in girls. *Urology* 1977; 10:348.
475. Vereecken RL, Das J: Urethral instability: Related to stress incontinence? *J Urol* 1985; 134:698.
476. Veith RC, Rashkind MA, Caldwell JH, et al: Cardiovascular effects of tricyclic antidepressants in depressed patients with chronic heart disease. *N Engl J Med* 1982; 306:954.
477. Vorstman B, Lockhart J, Kaufman MR, et al: Polytetrafluoroethylene injection for urinary incontinence in children. *J Urol* 1985; 133:248.
478. Watkins RH: The bladder function in spinal injury. *Br J Surg* 1936; 23:734.
479. Wear JB Jr, Wear RB, Cleeland C: Biofeedback in urology using urodynamics: Preliminary observations. *J Urol* 1979; 121:464.
480. Webster GD: Urodynamic studies, in Resnick MI, Older RA (eds): *Diagnosis of Genitourinary Disease.* New York, Thieme-Stratton, 1982, p 173.
481. Webster GD, Koefoot RB Jr, Sihelnik S: Urodynamic abnormalities in neurologically normal children with micturition dysfunction. *J Urol* 1984; 132:74–77.
482. Webster GD, Older RA: Video urodynamics. *Urology* 1980; 16:106–114.
483. Webster GD, Sihelnik SA, Stone AR: Female urinary incontinence: The incidence, identification and characteristics of detrusor instability. *Neurourol Urodynamics* 1984; 3:235.
484. Wein A, Benson G, Jacobowitz D: Lack of evidence for adrenergic innervation of the external urethral sphincter. *J Urol* 1979; 121:324.
485. Wein A, Malloy T, Shofer F, et al: The effects of bethanechol chloride on urodynamic parameters in normal women and in women with significant residual urine volumes. *J Urol* 1980a; 124:397.

486. Wein A, Raezer D, Malloy T: Failure of the bethanechol supersensitivity test to predict improved voiding after subcutaneous bethanechol administration. *J Urol* 1980b; 123:202.
487. Wein AJ: Pharmacologic approaches to the management of neurogenic bladder dysfunction. *J Cont Educ Urol* 1979; 18:17.
488. Wein AJ: Pharmacology of the bladder and urethra, in Stanton SL, Tanagho EA (eds): *Surgery of Female Incontinence.* New York, Springer-Verlag, 1980, p 185.
489. Wein AJ: Classification of neurogenic voiding dysfunction. *J Urol* 1981; 125:605.
490. Wein AJ: Classification of voiding dysfunction: A simple approach, in Barrett DM, Wein AJ (eds): *Controversies in Neuro-urology.* New York, Churchill-Livingstone, 1984, pp 239–250.
491. Wein AJ: Specific methods of pharmacologic treatment, in Stanton SL, Tanagho EA (eds): *Surgery of Female Incontinence.* New York, Springer-Verlag, 1986, pp 229–250.
492. Wein AJ, Barrett DM: Etiologic possibilities for increased pelvic floor electromyography activity during bladder filling. *J Urol* 1982; 127:949.
493. Wein AJ, Raezer DM, Benson GS: Management of neurogenic bladder dysfunction in the adult. *Urology* 1976; 8:432.
494. Weiner N: Atropine, scopolamine and related antimuscarinic drugs, in Gilman AG, Goodman LS, Gilman A (eds): *The Pharmacological Basis of Therapeutics.* New York, Macmillan, 1980a, pp 120–137.
495. Weiner N: Drugs that inhibit adrenergic nerves and block adrenergic receptors, in Gilman AG, Goodman LS, Gilman A (eds): *The Pharmacological Basis of Therapeutics.* New York, Macmillan, 1980b, pp 176–210.
496. Weiner N: Norepinephrine, epinephrine and the sympathomimetic amines, in Gilman A, Goodman LS, Gilman A (eds): *The Pharmacological Basis of Therapeutics.* New York, Macmillan, 1980, pp 138–175.
497. White RI, Klauber GT: Sacral agenesis: Analysis of 22 cases. *Urology* 1976; 8:521–525.
498. Whiteside CG, Arnold EP: Persistent primary enuresis: A urodynamic assessment. *Br Med J* 1975; 1:364–367.
499. Whitfield H, Doyle P, Mayo M, et al: The effect of adrenergic blocking drugs on outflow resistance. *Br J Urol* 1976; 47:823.
500. Wiener ES, Kiesewetter WB: Urologic abnormalities associated with imperforate anus. *J Pediatr Surg* 1973; 8:151–157.
501. Weir J, Jaques PF: The large capacity bladder: A urodynamic study. *Urology* 1974; 5:544.
502. Williams DI, Nixon HH: Agenesis of the sacrum. *Surg Gynecol Obstet* 1957; 105:84–88.
503. Williams DI, Hirst G, Doyle D: The occult neuropathic bladder. *J Pediatr Surg* 1974; 9:35–41.
504. Williams E: Discussion on stress incontinence. *Proc R Soc Med* 1947; 40:361.
505. Williams ME, Panvill FC: Urinary incontinence in the elderly: Physiol-

ogy, pathophysiology, diagnosis and treatment. *Ann Intern Med* 1982; 97:895.
506. Wolin LH: Stress incontinence in young healthy nulliparous female subjects. *J Urol* 1969; 101:545.
507. Woodside JR, McGuire EJ: Detrusor hypertonicity as a late complication of a Wertheim hysterectomy. *J Urol* 1982; 127:1143–1145.
508. Worth PHL, Turner-Warwick R: The treatment of interstitial cystitis by cystolysis with observations on cystoplasty. *Br J Urol* 1973; 95:65.
509. Yalla S, Blunt K, Fam B, et al: Detrusor-sphincter dyssynergia. *J Urol* 1977; 118:1026.
510. Yalla SV, DiBenedello M, Blunt KJ, et al: Urethral striated sphincter responses to electro-bulbocavernosus stimulation. *J Urol* 1978; 119:406.
511. Yalla SV, Fam BA, Gagilondo FB, et al: Anteromedian external urethral sphincterotomy: Technique, rationale and results in 32 patients. *Paraplegia* 1977; 13:247.
512. Yalla SV, Kirsth L, Kearney G, et al: Postprostatectomy incontinence: Urodynamic assessment. *Neurourol Urodynamics* 1982; 1:77.
513. Yalla SV, Sharma GV, Barsamian EM: Micturitional static urethral pressure profile: A method of recording urethral pressure profile during voiding and the implications. *J Urol* 1980; 124:649.
514. Yarnell JWG, Voyle GJ, Richards CJ, et al: The prevalence and severity of urinary incontinence in women. *J Epidemiol Community Health* 1981; 35:71.
515. Yeates WK: Bladder function in normal micturition. *Clin Dev Med* 1973; 48/49:28–36.
516. Young HH: Suture of the urethral and vesical sphincters for the cure of incontinence of urine with a report of a case. *Trans South Surg Gynecol Assoc* 1907; 20:210.
517. Zinner NR, Sterling AM, Ritter RC: Role of inner urethral softness in urinary continence. *Urology* 1980; 16:115.

Index

A

C

D

E

K

L

O

P

R

S

W

Y